Clinical Orthopaedic Examination of a Child

Clinical Orthopedic Examination of a Child

Edited by
Nirmal Raj Gopinathan

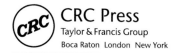

CRC Press
Taylor & Francis Group
Boca Raton London New York

CRC Press is an imprint of the
Taylor & Francis Group, an **informa** business

First edition published 2021
by CRC Press
6000 Broken Sound Parkway NW, Suite 300, Boca Raton, FL 33487-2742

and by CRC Press
2 Park Square, Milton Park, Abingdon, Oxon, OX14 4RN

© 2021 Taylor & Francis Group, LLC

CRC Press is an imprint of Taylor & Francis Group, LLC

This book contains information obtained from authentic and highly regarded sources. While all reasonable efforts have been made to publish reliable data and information, neither the author[s] nor the publisher can accept any legal responsibility or liability for any errors or omissions that may be made. The publishers wish to make clear that any views or opinions expressed in this book by individual editors, authors or contributors are personal to them and do not necessarily reflect the views/opinions of the publishers. The information or guidance contained in this book is intended for use by medical, scientific or health-care professionals and is provided strictly as a supplement to the medical or other professional's own judgement, their knowledge of the patient's medical history, relevant manufacturer's instructions and the appropriate best practice guidelines. Because of the rapid advances in medical science, any information or advice on dosages, procedures or diagnoses should be independently verified. The reader is strongly urged to consult the relevant national drug formulary and the drug companies' and device or material manufacturers' printed instructions, and their websites, before administering or utilizing any of the drugs, devices or materials mentioned in this book. This book does not indicate whether a particular treatment is appropriate or suitable for a particular individual. Ultimately it is the sole responsibility of the medical professional to make his or her own professional judgements, so as to advise and treat patients appropriately. The authors and publishers have also attempted to trace the copyright holders of all material reproduced in this publication and apologize to copyright holders if permission to publish in this form has not been obtained. If any copyright material has not been acknowledged please write and let us know so we may rectify in any future reprint.

Library of Congress Cataloging-in-Publication Data

Names: Gopinathan, Nirmal Raj, editor.
Title: Clinical orthopedic examination of a child / edited by Nirmal Raj Gopinathan.
Description: First edition. | Boca Raton, FL : CRC Press 2021. | Includes bibliographical references and index. | Summary: "As always said "Children are not young adults", and the examination of a child needs to be emphasized with special consideration to physiologic differences in a growing child. This book focuses on pediatric examination, a topic not much explored in the regular orthopedic texts. The difficulty of a child to express the symptoms needs to be kept in mind during examination, thus the examining surgeon has to be very observant in picking up even minor details that could help in diagnosis. This book serves as an essential companion to orthopedic surgeons, general practitioners and professionals as well as be helpful in pediatric orthopedic clinics"-- Provided by publisher.
Identifiers: LCCN 2020052692 (print) | LCCN 2020052693 (ebook) | ISBN 9780367001445 (paperback) | ISBN 9780367722357 (hardback) | ISBN 9780429444296 (ebook)
Subjects: MESH: Musculoskeletal Diseases--diagnosis | Physical Examination--methods | Child
Classification: LCC RJ480 (print) | LCC RJ480 (ebook) | NLM WS 275 | DDC 618.92/7075--dc23
LC record available at https://lccn.loc.gov/2020052692
LC ebook record available at https://lccn.loc.gov/2020052693

ISBN: 9780367722357 (hbk)
ISBN: 9780367001445 (pbk)
ISBN: 9780429444296 (ebk)

Typeset in Minion
by Deanta Global Publishing Services, Chennai, India

Dedication

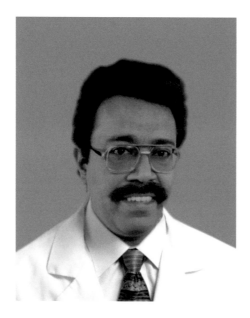

Dedicated to my father, Dr. R. Gopinathan, my family, and to the children who constantly help us learn despite their ailments.

Contents

Foreword I

The trend in orthopedics today is an evolution into multiple subspecialties, which is actually the need of the hour. The subspecialty of pediatric orthopedics is unique and new, as it involves all the issues relevant to children, in addition to the disorders of the musculoskeletal system which we know of in adults. Over the years I have seen an evolution in pediatric orthopedics in our country paralleling that in the world; from a fledgling specialty in the 1980s with a few focused surgeons looking at children with musculoskeletal problems (due to their interest alone), pediatric orthopedics has changed a lot. Initially most of these specialists' expertise needed to overlap into other spheres of orthopedics to be able to sustain a relevant medical practice, and survive; in the 21st century, however, there have been significant changes.

In 2021, we have now reached the stage where pediatric orthopedics can easily be practiced as a stand-alone specialty anywhere in the world, and even in India. Despite the fact that centers of excellence currently exist only in the larger Indian cities, it is important that the science and art focused on the musculoskeletal problems of children should be propagated all over the country. I am personally aware of the fact that many surgeons, even in the smaller cities, are taking up pediatric orthopedics as their primary practice profile; that is where we need the education and support so that these fledgling practices can flourish. This is a major reason why the current book, edited by Dr. Nirmal Raj Gopinathan, comes as a breath of fresh air, to reinforce the fact that pediatric orthopedics needs more input, more support, and more recognition.

We must understand that the problems and needs of children are extremely complex; the thinking that children can be treated as little adults needs to be changed, as not only are children's problems very different from those of adults, but often the solutions are also very different. For a pediatric surgeon, taking care of a child with an orthopedic problem involves not only interacting with the child's family, but also earning the cooperation of the child while they are undergoing an examination. Therein lies the gist of the matter, for it is only by a proper examination of a child that one can reach the correct diagnosis. Many skills are needed by the pediatric orthopedic surgeon in trying to understand what ails the child; this book, written by a diverse collection of authors, aims to provide those skills. This is a compilation which will benefit not only budding pediatric orthopedic surgeons, but even orthopedic residents as a whole, since it explains the concepts applicable to children in a clear and lucid way.

I must congratulate Dr. Nirmal Raj Gopinathan for collecting such a great list of contributors, who with their combined wisdom have made this a book worth having. In my opinion, it should be carried by all residents and even most consultants who plan to examine children.

I've known Dr. Nirmal Raj Gopinathan since his student days and from the beginning I've noted his interest in this specialty; I am so glad that I was able to encourage this interest further during his senior residency with us, and later as a consultant, as now we have a young surgeon who has evolved into an excellent pediatric orthopedic specialist with great clinical skills and an outstanding interest in academics. I'm sure this book will be the first of many subsequent editions which will go on evolving over time, as our understanding of the elements of children also evolves.

Dr. Mandeep S. Dhillon MBBS, MS (Orth), FAMS, FRCS
Professor & Head Orthopaedics; Head, Physical Medicine Dept PGIMER, Chandigarh, India

Foreword II

The speed with which medicine is progressing is enormous, and so is the speed that new medical subspecialties are emerging. When I was doing my fellowship in Pediatric Orthopedics at UCLA in 1990, it was unimaginable to envision specialists practicing pediatric orthopedics exclusively, but this is now fast becoming the reality. With more and more orthopedic residents opting for this subspecialty, I often felt the lacuna of an examination manual that would be able to precisely combine the intricacies of examination in two of the most difficult specialties of medicine, namely Orthopedics and Pediatrics: a job beautifully accomplished by Dr. Nirmal Raj Gopinathan in this volume.

Being a mentor to this growing orthopod since a very young age, I always admired him for his thorough hold on his subject and his ability to explain difficult concepts in a very free-flowing and easy way to his colleagues and juniors. It gives me great pleasure to write this Foreword for this very unique book. The most appealing part of the book is the ability of the authors to cover the most practically useful aspects of pediatric bone and joint examination while ensuring the book is not excessively long. The additional use of descriptive images helps the reader to easily understand examination methodology. This book is a real boon for future orthopedic and pediatric orthopedic residents. Lastly, I congratulate the editor on this wonderful achievement.

Shivender Singh Gill
Former Professor and Head Orthopaedics
PGIMER, Chandigarh
Former Vice Chancellor, BFUHS
Faridkot, Punjab

Preface

Physical examination has its own significance and will continue to be an important building block in a clinician's career, even in the era of cutting-edge advances in diagnostic methodologies. A clinician's skill is judged by the ability to pick up subtle abnormalities aided by keen observation and examination skills. Pediatric orthopedic examination remains a challenge due to many factors, such as an apprehensive child who has reduced comprehension in comparison to adults, parents who require patient handling, etc. Success depends on connecting with the child and noticing abnormalities which result from the pathology, aided by keen observation and correlative knowledge.

The book will focus on basic and advanced pediatric orthopedic outpatient practice. Examination of a child always poses a challenge to the orthopedic surgeon, as often the child cannot express concerns due to fear and a strange environment. Although intelligent parents and guardians can give more information during examination, it is not always the same in every case. Also, blindly following an adult orthopedic examination pattern will not yield the required information. One important thing that has to be kept in mind is that the child and body compensate in all possible ways before revealing the problem, which may not be the case compared to adults. Hence, the practicing orthopedic surgeon must be capable of thinking outside the box and be smart and trained to notice subtle clinical information that may clinch a diagnosis compared to a battery of investigations. The importance of clinical examination should never be underplayed at any point in the evolution of medical practices.

The aim of this book is to help the reader find answers to questions, such as why the clinical finding is elicitable in a given pathological condition. It is always better to understand and perform a test knowing the reason why it is positive or negative. In that way, the examiner will remember the test as well as the ability to pick up the findings even in a subtle form that might be frequently missed. The authors have covered the basics of systemic examination in the standard format of look, feel, and move along with a description of special tests and when and where they are required. Also, an attempt is made to describe the procedure in the same manner as it was described originally with reference to the published literature.

Overall, this book is an attempt to facilitate the outpatient clinic examination of a child with pediatric orthopedic complaints. Pediatric orthopedics is a vast field, and it is not possible to cover every possible diagnosis. Hence, the authors have covered examination pertaining to individual joints apart from additional chapters on short stature, deformity, and limb deficiency evaluation. A few common disorders and the salient findings are covered at the end of each chapter. In addition, a few topics are covered in the miscellaneous chapter very briefly. I must admit that it is not possible to cover everything, but an effort is made to gather routine pediatric orthopedic examination in this book.

Nirmal Raj Gopinathan

Acknowledgments

I acknowledge the understanding and constant support provided by my beloved wife, mother, and children. Without their understanding and support, compiling this book would have never been possible. Words are not enough to describe the support offered by my better half, who shouldered all the responsibilities while I had the excuse in the form of this book.

I extend my sincere thanks to my teachers who paved and crafted the path I have traveled to now. I am always thankful to Mr. Raman, whom we called Raman Sir, who gave me an interest in science, particularly biology. I remember my clinical training at Thanjavur Medical College Hospital (TMCH) under stalwarts like Prof. Perumal, who taught me general surgery and physical examination. I remember Prof. Bose and Prof. Tamilmani who are the epitome of knowledge and surprised us always with their ability to correlate findings and diagnose diseases. I am lucky to be a student of my father who made me realize medicine is fun; he surprised me with his extraordinary oratory skills. I received my orthopedic training at the Post Graduate Institute of Medical Education and Research (PGIMER), Chandigarh, and had the privilege of being trained by legends in orthopedics. I had the privilege of listening to Prof. Rai's teachings on asepsis and trauma radiograph discussion, Prof. S.S. Gill's clinics and case presentations, Prof. Raj Bahadur's bedside teachings, and Prof. Mandeep Singh Dhillon's lectures and clinical classes. I had the privilege of conducting my thesis work under Prof. Sen and being taught and guided by him. I am thankful to Prof. V. Goni who believed in my surgical and patient management skills during my residency, and the same applies to Prof. P. Sudesh in my early career as a consultant. I am especially thankful to my Head of Department,

Prof. M.S. Dhillon, who was instrumental in helping me pursue the subspecialty of my choice, i.e., pediatric orthopedics. I am also privileged to have senior colleagues and residents who always kindle the need for constant update in the subject. I believe all this training and teaching helped me compile this book as all of them constantly emphasized the importance of clinical examination. I must mention the help of my junior colleagues, Dr. Prateek Behera and Dr. Karthick Rangasamy, who were there to support my endeavor at every stage.

I acknowledge the work of artist Mr. Daramjit Singh who patiently understood our needs and penned down the artwork as we had expected. I am indebted to photographers Mr. Brij Lal, Mr. Abhijeet, Mr. Paramjeet, Mr. Pritam, and the entire photography team who helped us capture clinical examination frame by frame, which I felt was not so easy.

I acknowledge the participation of Dr. Bibek Bhandari, Dr. Nikhil Mehta, Dr. Sanjay Rawat, Dr. Karmesh, and Dr. Prashasth in the various steps undertaken while preparing the manuscripts and getting the pictures edited. I thank the publishers for entrusting me with the job of compiling this book, and I am especially thankful for their support in writing the topic I had in mind. I sincerely thank Shivangi Pramanik and Himani Dwivedi from Taylor & Francis Group for their prompt coordination and for being considerate.

Last but not least, I acknowledge all the beloved children and their parents/guardians who gave us permission and took part in the demonstrations to facilitate the dissemination of knowledge, despite their suffering and ailments.

Nirmal Raj Gopinathan

Editor

Dr. Nirmal Raj Gopinathan is currently working as additional professor in the Department of Orthopedics, PGIMER, Chandigarh, India. He has been working in the pediatric orthopedic division since 2011. He completed his undergraduate training at TMCH, Thanjavur, Tamil Nadu. He carried out his postgraduate training in orthopedics at PGIMER, Chandigarh. He did a Japanese Pediatric Orthopedic Association (JPOA) fellowship in 2012 at Minamitama Hospital, Tokyo, and AO Trauma fellowship in Muenster, Germany, in 2014, and an international observership in Scottish Rite Hospital for Children, Texas, and the Cincinnati Children's Hospital and Medical Center in 2016. He secured a diploma in SICOT in the SICOT world congress held in Sweden in 2010. He was inducted as a member of the Academy of Medical Sciences (MAMS) in 2014.

Dr. Gopinathan is actively involved in patient care and both clinical and experimental research and has secured national awards and international scholarships. He has about 50 PUBMED indexed publications that include original articles, surgical techniques, reviews, etc. He has authored four chapters in textbooks, including one in *Turek's Orthopaedics,* and is a faculty member in many national and international meetings. He is also assistant editor of the *International Journal of Paediatric Orthopaedics* and is a reviewer for many orthopedic journals.

Contributors

Anil Agarwal
Department of Pediatric Orthopedics
Chacha Nehru Bal Chikitsalaya
New Delhi, India

Prateek Behera
Department of Orthopedics
All India Institute of Medical Sciences – Bhopal
Bhopal, India

Chakshu Chaudhry
Department of Pediatrics
PGIMER
Chandigarh, India

Ashish Dagar
Spine Surgery
Medanta the Medicity Hospital
Gurugram, India

Sarvdeep Singh Dhatt
Department of Orthopedics
PGIMER
Chandigarh, India

Mandeep Singh Dhillon
Department of Orthopedics
PGIMER
Chandigarh, India

Vijay G. Goni
Department of Orthopedics
PGIMER
Chandigarh, India

Nirmal Raj Gopinathan
Department of Orthopedics
PGIMER
Chandigarh, India

Aman Hooda
Department of Orthopedics
PGIMER
Chandigarh, India

Anupriya Kaur
Medical Genetics
Advanced Pediatric Center
PGIMER
Chandigarh, India

Reet Mukopadhya
Orthopedics
RGKar Medical College and Hospital
Kolkata, India

Deepak Neradi
Department of Orthopedics
PGIMER
Chandigarh, India

Sharad Prabhakar
Department of Orthopedics
PGIMER
Chandigarh, India

Manish Pruthi
Tata Memorial Hospital
Mumbai, India

Karthick Rangasamy
Fellow AADO (Hong Kong)
Department of Orthopedics
PGIMER
Chandigarh, India

Pratik M. Rathod
Department of Orthopedics
PGIMER
Chandigarh, India

Ranjit Kumar Sahu
Department of Burns and Plastic Surgery
AIIMS
Bhubaneswar
Odisha, India

Ramesh Kumar Sen
Institute of Orthopedic Surgery
Max Super Specialty Hospital
Mohali, India

Siddhartha Sharma
Department of Orthopedics
PGIMER
Chandigarh, India

Mohsina Subair
Department of Plastic Surgery
PGIMER
Chandigarh, India

Pebam Sudesh
Department of Orthopedics
PGIMER
Chandigarh, India

Satyaswarup Tripathy
Department of Plastic Surgery
PGIMER
Chandigarh, India

1

Approach to a Child in the Outpatient Clinic

NIRMAL RAJ GOPINATHAN

1.1 INTRODUCTION

As is rightly said, clinical examination is an art that every resident/clinician needs to master to be a successful practitioner. The modern advances in diagnostic modalities can neither undermine the importance of clinical examination nor be a substitute for it. The art of examining a child should be entrusted to the trainee from the beginning of residency, as it is imperative to elicit key history and findings that can be easily masked otherwise. The examination of a child needs further training and practice as the comprehensive skills of a child may not match an adult counterpart and the clinician needs to be more talented and capable of picking up minor details. We will cover the basic aspects under four headings, as depicted below.

1.2 THE ENVIRONMENT

The examination room must be well lit and child-friendly. It will be of help to have a few puzzles, activities, or cartoon characters painted on the walls of the clinic to create a child-friendly atmosphere. A crowded clinic will not be friendly. It will add to the stranger anxiety and apprehension the child experiences in addition to their pain/suffering, and the clinician will not be able to establish a rapport or examine the child properly. A spacious, less crowded room allows the child to run and play and will provide the examiner an opportunity to observe the child's activities, motor function, coordination, gait, etc. Avoid wearing a white coat/apron while examining a child. Remember to use a hard couch for examination as a soft mattress may conceal the clinical findings like exaggerated lumbar lordosis in a child with hip flexion contracture.

1.3 COMMUNICATION WITH THE PARENTS/CARETAKERS

The clinician must learn to establish a rapport with the parent and the child, which is the basic minimum requirement of examination. The clinician must give adequate attention to every detail the parents state. Parents constantly observe the child and will be better at picking up even a minor finding or gait abnormality, and the clinician should never ignore their concerns. It is amazing to observe how well a grandparent can give a relevant history or clinical finding that helps in making a diagnosis.

Sit and talk to the parents so that they understand that you are not rushing/hurried, and you are giving adequate time for their child. Try to answer their questions and ease their concerns, which is very helpful in establishing rapport and gaining the trust of the entire family. Try not to dismiss parents' concerns immediately as it may spoil the relationship. Try to explain in simple language and assure them that few conditions like in-toeing just require observation. Sometimes parents bring recorded activities of the child at home. They can be asked to make a video on their smartphone, which can help to show the characteristic presentation that may not be elicitable in the clinic in the follow-up visit.

Remember that the parents may be stressed due to the multiple opinions given by family members and friends, and they require a warm and comforting conversation. The clinician must also develop a tolerance for the continuous interjections by parents while examining the child instead of losing patience. In cases where the clinician comes across an agitated caretaker or the parents are accusatory, argumentative, or not willing to follow instructions, it is advisable to maintain a calm demeanor and outline the recommendations in a quiet and firm manner.

1.4 COMMUNICATION WITH THE CHILD

It is obvious that the child will be anxious and frightened by attending the clinic and being examined by a stranger. It may not be of help to threaten the child, as is commonly said by parents in the clinic – "The doctor is going to give an injection," which simply increases the child's apprehension and eliminates the element of cooperation and understanding that can be established. Be friendly and talk to/engage with the child before going to the examination. Be playful and have something like a cartoon character, toy, etc. (do not offer candy as this may be a choking hazard) that can be used to distract a child. Talk to the child about his/her school, friends, teachers, and keep them engaged and distracted. This will also help in establishing a healthy rapport, and the child will start trusting the examiner. A frightened, apprehensive child will not allow a clinical examination, and the entire exercise will be futile and non-informative.

1.5 THE ART OF EXAMINING A CHILD

The examination starts by observing the child entering the clinic. The examiner should start examining the child without touching the child or engaging with them. Observe the child's activity before the examination like walking around, running, trying to climb or hop on a chair, or when a child attempts to play with a revolving chair, which can give you an idea of their coordination and upper and lower extremity function. A child with hemiplegic cerebral palsy (CP) will not sway/swing the involved upper limb in comparison with the normal side. He/she may keep it flexed from the elbow with limited exertion during running. Observe the footwear and its wear characteristics. Observe any kind of orthotics or prosthetics used.

Always examine the child in the presence of parents or guardians as this will make the child comfortable and will avoid unnecessary medicolegal issues. Respect privacy, even if it is a small child. Treat patients and parents with dignity and respect the child's privacy while undressing the child. Although adequate exposure is required to examine the child properly as a whole, try to cover the genitals and breasts (in an adolescent female). Avoid undressing the child in front of other children and attendants as this will hurt the child's dignity and self-respect.

Talk to the parents and the child and explain what you are going to do. For example, it is important to explain to the mother of a child with a clubfoot that the manipulations and maneuvers done on the foot are not painful/do not hurt the child. It is important to gain the confidence of both parents and the child to successfully manage the condition. Rub your hands to make them warm and be gentle not to aggravate any pain as the child will try to avoid examination with cold hands or if you start the examination by hurting the child. Do not examine the pathological part first if you believe it is going to hurt. Examine the normal or non-painful side/part first and then gradually drift to the affected side/part, assuring that you will try not to hurt the child. Also, it will be useful to strike up a conversation and distract the child while carrying out the examination. Do not get annoyed if the parents tell you that the other side is affected; explain why you are doing so, which will help you gain their confidence.

Try to avoid words like "pain" and "hurt" while examining the child as these words will increase the child's apprehension and will spoil an uninterrupted examination. Explain to the parents that some part of the examination may inflict pain and is necessary for diagnosing the disorder. In such circumstances, assure them that you will try to limit the discomfort, which will sound reasonable. Pouncing upon the child for examination will make the parents and the child apprehensive.

Sometimes, the child will be afraid of being examined on an examination couch or especially when you try to position the child prone. In such instances, you may examine the child in the parent's lap, or you can ask the parent to palpate to help localize the areas that hurt or do simple maneuvers such as elicit passive range of motion and give instructions for an active range of motion examination. Sometimes you may not be able to examine or elicit the findings initially as the child is not consoled and apprehensive. During those times, it is advisable to examine the child later when being fed or when the child sleeps. It is especially important not to assume findings as a result of an inadequate examination. It is also not necessary to get frustrated as not all children are the same and it takes a lot to pacify some of them.

Examine the child as a whole from head to toe. For example, a child with progressive foot deformation may have spinal dysraphism (Figure 1.1), and observing the telltale signs like a tuft of hair in the back will be of help in establishing the diagnosis (Figure 1.2). It is imperative to examine the child from head to toe to avoid missing valuable findings and the time frame in which the conditions can be managed easily. Look for dysmorphic, syndromic, and neurogenic causes and also examine whether the child is hyperlax at the time of presentation (Figures 1.3– 1.5).

Know what items are required and have all the items you require for examination.

Make it a habit to repeatedly use devices like a goniometer and measuring tape and avoid predicting angular deformation and length discrepancy by eye. Repeated use of these devices ensures that the right technique is followed all the time.

Try to go through previous medical records so as not to miss any valuable clues that may help

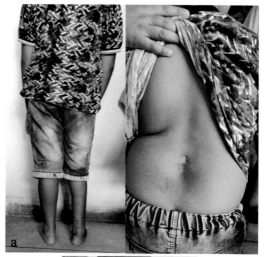

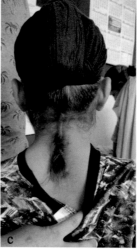

Figure 1.1 (a) Recurrent cavovarus of the foot in a child; (b) and (c) examination of the back reveals tuft of hair in the upper dorsal spine region and healed surgical scar in the lumbar spine region indicating neurogenic origin and possible spinal dysraphism.

make the diagnosis. For example, neonatal hospitalization for disseminated sepsis may help in diagnosing post-septic sequelae of the hip joint in children where initial joint suppuration might have been overlooked by the generalized morbidity induced by septicemia.

To conclude, the clinical examination of a pediatric patient is itself an art that needs patience and repeated practice. It is a worthwhile exercise to repeat and master as it is the first step in successfully managing a child with an underlying musculoskeletal disorder.

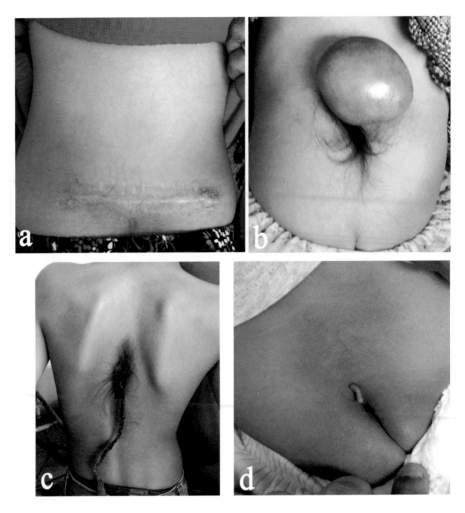

Figure 1.2 Markers of possible spinal etiology. (a) scar surgical/non-surgical, (b) swelling, (c) tuft of hair in midline back, (d) tag of skin (acrochordon).

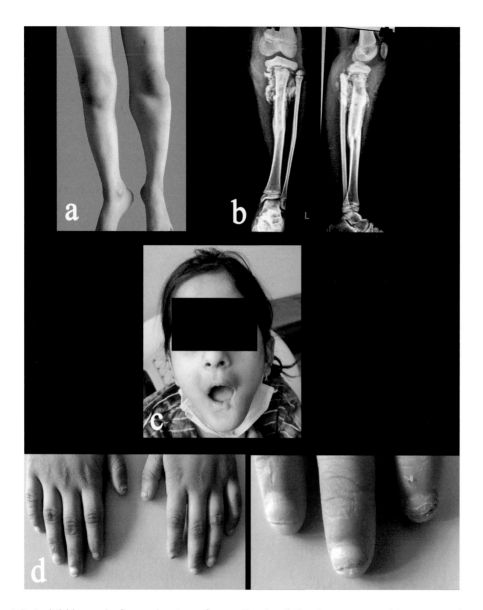

Figure 1.3 A child brought for evaluation of a swollen leg following trauma with suspected neoplastic pathology based upon radiography (a) and (b). But head-to-toe examination revealed (c) loss of teeth and unintentional self-injuries to fingertips due to repeated biting and inability to feel pain (d). History of absence of sweating. Based on the findings, the child was diagnosed with congenital insensitivity to pain with anhidrosis (CIPA)/hereditary sensory and autonomic neuropathy type IV or ectodermal dysplasia. The swelling in the leg is because of the repetitive trauma in the proximal tibial physeal region, which was missed due to the absence of pain. A healed diaphyseal fracture can also be noted.

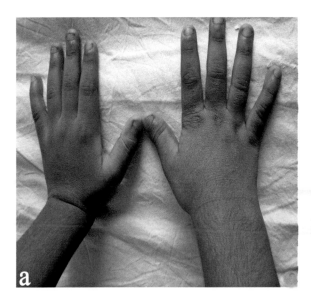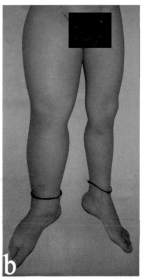

Figure 1.4 A child with hemihypertrophy must be evaluated for embryonal tumors like Wilms and hepatoblastoma and should be screened with three-monthly abdominal ultrasonogram (USG) until the child is seven years of age and a serum alpha-fetoprotein estimation three-monthly until the child is four years of age. The attending orthopedician has an opportunity to pick up these disorders at an earlier stage if he/she is aware of these associations.

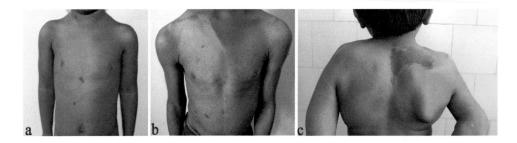

Figure 1.5 Café au lait spots. (a) and (b) neurofibromatosis (six or more spots larger than 5 mm in greatest diameter in prepubertal children, and greater than 15 mm in greatest diameter in post-pubertal children), (c) McCune–Albright syndrome, single asymmetric large spot with irregular borders (coast of Maine) not crossing the midline.

BIBLIOGRAPHY

Birch JG. The Orthopaedic Examination: Clinical application. In: Herring JA, editor. *Tachdjian's Pediatric Orthopaedics*, 5th ed. Philadelphia, PA: Elsevier Saunders; 2014. pp. 61–70.

2

Biometric Measurements and Normal Growth Parameters in a Child

PRATEEK BEHERA AND NIRMAL RAJ GOPINATHAN

2.1 INTRODUCTION

When a clinician examines a child, the basic idea behind that examination is to look for deviations from the accepted normal values. Numerous investigators have contributed to the literature on the normal values of different parameters. An orthopedic surgeon is expected to have basic knowledge of a child's development and in-depth knowledge of anatomical parameters, especially pertaining to the limbs. The ubiquitous phrase "children are not just small adults" must be remembered by clinicians, and adult values should not be automatically applied to children.

2.2 GENERAL GROWTH MEASUREMENTS

The first thing a clinician commonly looks for in any child is his/her height, weight, and body span. Examination of a child should ideally start with measurements of the head and chest circumferences, weight, height, and arm span. In a child, these parameters can either be recorded by the clinician or by the staff nurse when the child is in the waiting area. Measurement of a child's height and arm span can act as the first indicator of an underlying etiology, which might lead to a short stature. The head circumference is measured using a measuring tape. An accurate measurement can be obtained by placing the tape around the head at its greatest circumference, starting from the occipital protuberance to the midforehead. This measurement can then be plotted on specific growth charts. A child with a head circumference >95th percentile or <5th percentile for the child's age should be evaluated further.

Chest circumference is measured using a measuring tape placed across the chest at the level of the nipples. At birth, it is smaller than the head circumference, but by the age of 1 year, it should become equal to the head circumference. Further, by 2 years, the chest circumference exceeds the head circumference. It is not routinely measured after 2 years of age but is measured if there are specific indications.

Height is measured using an infantometer or a stadiometer depending on the child's age (see Chapter 16). Weight is measured using a weighing scale. The height and weight of a child when considered separately do not provide much information. When the height/length, weight, head circumference, and body mass index (BMI) are examined with respect to the child's age, then an idea about his/her physical growth can be estimated. The best way to do so is by plotting the weight, height, etc., on growth charts like the World Health Organization (WHO) growth charts (see Chapter 16). These charts primarily indicate the nutritional status, but they are indirect indicators of a child's overall growth.

In addition to the above measures, there are few indirect indicators of the nutritional status of a child. Mid-arm circumference (MAC), triceps skin fold thickness (TSF), and mid-arm muscle circumference are such indicators.[1] The MAC is the circumference (in centimeters, cm) of the non-dominant arm measured midway between the acromion and the olecranon processes using a measuring tape. The child should ideally be sitting with the arm freely hanging for an accurate measurement. This measurement indicates the bulk of muscles of the arm and has been shown to correlate well with height for weight measurements.[1] A MAC of 14 cm is considered as the minimum circumference for a normally nourished child. MAC values of less than 14 cm are indicative of undernourishment (12.5–14 cm indicates mild/acute undernourishment, and less than 12.4 cm indicates severe undernourishment). MAC measurements are usually effective up to 5 years of age.

Measurement of skin fold thickness over the triceps region is used mainly for an assessment of obesity rather than for the diagnosis of malnutrition. TSF reflects the status of subcutaneous fat stores. This value is measured in millimeters using a Harpenden caliper midway between the acromion and olecranon processes with the arm hanging freely. Mid-arm muscle circumference is a derived value using MAC and TSF and equals MAC (cm) − TSF (mm) × 0.314. It is believed to be a better indicator of the actual muscle mass in the arm.

BMI is now increasingly being used in clinical pediatrics. It is calculated as weight (kg)/height (meter)^2. The pattern of change of BMI in children has been defined using the median BMI values. At birth, the median BMI is 13 kg/m^2, which increases to 17 kg/m^2 by one year. This then decreases to a median value of 15 kg/m^2 by age 6 and thereafter, increases to a value of 21 kg/m^2 in adulthood.[1] In adolescents, BMI values of <15 are considered an indicator of under-nutrition. Values of 22 and 25 are the lower limits defining overweight and obesity, respectively.[1] A BMI value of 15–18 is considered underweight, 18–22 is normal, 22–25 is overweight, and >25 is obese.

An assessment of the child's sexual maturity during evaluation is an essential component of the clinical examination pertaining to certain disorders. While it is essential for a detailed examination of patients who are admitted for evaluation of their condition, it might be omitted when examining in the outpatient department. The universally accepted method is the one described by Tanner and Marshall, which is also called the sexual maturity rating (SMR). Tanner staging is based on the gradual and often sequential changes in the external genitalia in males, breasts in females, and pubic hair in both males and females. In females, the development of breasts (thelarche) occurs around 8–12 years of age and is the first pubertal change. This is followed by the appearance of pubic hairs (pubarche). In males, puberty starts when the testicular volume becomes more than 4 ml (estimated with an orchidometer), and pubic hairs start to appear usually between 9 and 14 years of age. In both males and females, five SMR ratings have been defined from 1 to 5 (Figure 2.1). While SMR provides some idea about a child's chronological age, many decisions in adolescent pediatric orthopedics are based on the child's bone age, which is estimated using radiographs. Tanner staging has been used by investigators in decision-making for the management (of various pathologies),[2,3] but there is criticism too. Assigning a Tanner stage to a child has large interobserver and intraobserver variability,[4] and it should hence be used judiciously for this purpose.

In addition to the growth of a child, the evaluation of his/her developmental parameters is equally essential. This can easily be done using the revised Denver Developmental Screening Test (DDST), which assesses the gross motor, language, fine motor (adaptive), and personal-social development.[5]

2.3 UPPER LIMB

At the time of birth, the upper limbs are in a state of universal flexion like the lower limbs. This flexed posture is seen primarily at the elbows. Gradually, this posture corrects as the child becomes older.

The growth of the upper limb is primarily longitudinal along its length. The proximal end of the humerus is its principal growing end, contributing

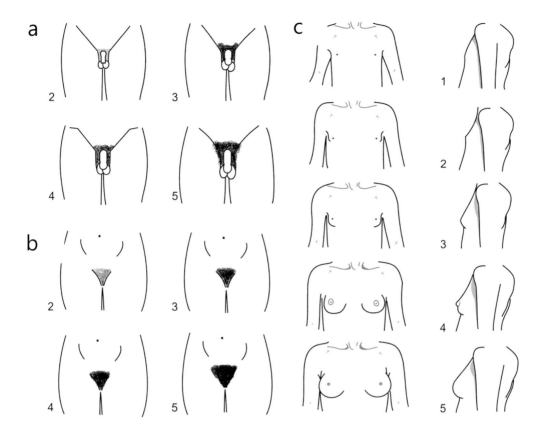

Figure 2.1 Tanner and Marshall sexual maturity rating. (a) External genitalia development in boys, (b) external genitalia development in girls, (c) breast development in girls.

about 80% of its length. For radius, the principal growing end is the distal end, which contributes 75% to its length. The proximal end of the ulna is the primary growing end, contributing 80% to its growth.[6,7] The angle between the arm and the forearm (carrying angle) gradually develops over the years in children. It has been reported that the mean carrying angle in newborns is 15° and increases to 17.8° in adults (Figure 2.2). This increase in the carrying angle follows the development and growth of the bones of the pelvis.

An evaluation to assess if the child is ambidextrous is an essential component of the examination. Most children are ambidextrous until 18 months to 3 years of age. Definite dexterity before 18 months is an indicator of probable pathology like cerebral palsy, brachial plexus injury, etc. of the opposite upper limb.[8]

There is usually more range of movement of the joints of the upper limb in children than in adults, which is a result of the laxity seen in them.

2.4 LOWER LIMB

In cephalic presentation, the intra-uterine fetal position is of universal flexion, which is carried by the child to the immediate post-partum period. The hips and knees are flexed. The lower legs are internally rotated. The feet are further internally rotated with respect to the lower legs. At times there is an external rotational contracture of the hip that tends to mask the true femoral rotational profile. The anatomy of the lower limbs changes significantly as the child grows. This is primarily in response to the development of motor abilities and the ability of the child to crawl, cruise, stand, walk, and finally run. These changes are seen right from the hip joints, the femoral neck, knees, and tibia to the feet.

The neck-shaft angle changes as a child continues to grow. The upper femoral and the greater trochanteric epiphysis grow synchronously such that the neck-shaft angle, which averages about

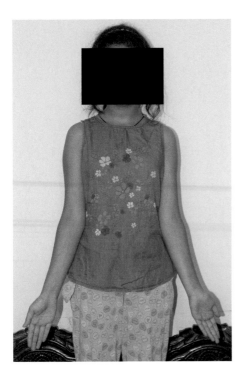

Figure 2.2 Normal carrying angle.

child is sitting in a "W" posture (Figure 2.5). Children have the maximum amount of anteversion at birth, and it gradually decreases as the child approaches adulthood. The mean anteversion at birth is about 40°, and it comes down to a value of around 15° in adulthood.[10,11] Failure of this gradual decrease results in an in-toeing gait. Clinically, the increased femoral anteversion can be estimated by Craig's test.

Another method of estimating whether the anteversion is appropriate for the age of the child is by measuring the internal rotation and external rotation of the hip (Figure 2.6). This is performed with the patient prone. Staheli and colleagues[10] have reported that infants have an average of 40° of internal rotation (range 10–60°) and 70° of external rotation (range 45–90°) at the hip joint. There is a gradual change in these values, and by the age of 10 years, internal hip rotation averages 50° (range 25–65°) and external rotation 45° (range 25–65°). Thus, if a child has an internal rotation measuring more than 70° at 10 years of age, then it is an indicator of increased femoral torsion, and further clinical and radiological evaluation must be done. Confirmation of the same is best estimated by CT scan or MRI studies. Based on the studies by Fabry et al.,[11] Shands and Steele,[12] and Crane,[13] femoral anteversion values can be summarized as in Table 2.1.

It has been suggested that children with a normal gait and children who in-toe have a gradual reduction in femoral anteversion between 7 and 14 years of age.[14] While most children with in-toeing gait can be managed non-operatively, there are a few who can be offered a femoral osteotomy.

150° at birth, gradually decreases to the adult average value of 135°.[9] This significant information is essential for guiding treatment in patients of coxa vara and valga (Figure 2.3).

The proximal femoral torsional profile, i.e., the femoral anteversion, changes in growing children. Excessive femoral anteversion has been believed to be a cause of in-toed gait in children, which is a common complaint with which they are brought to the outpatient clinic by their parents (Figure 2.4). Additionally, the parents may complain that their

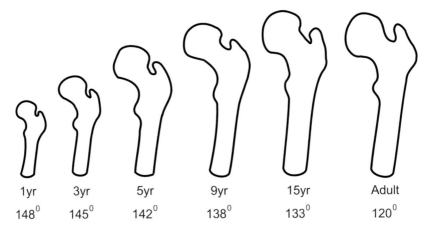

| 1yr | 3yr | 5yr | 9yr | 15yr | Adult |
| 148° | 145° | 142° | 138° | 133° | 120° |

Figure 2.3 Pattern of the evolution of the femoral neck-shaft angle with age.

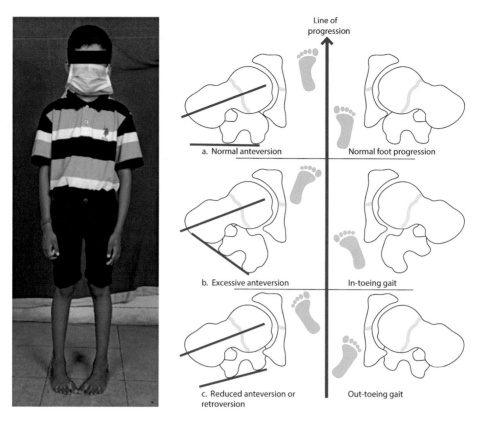

a. Normal anteversion

Normal foot progression

b. Excessive anteversion

In-toeing gait

c. Reduced anteversion or retroversion

Out-toeing gait

Line of progression

Figure 2.4 In-toeing and associated exaggerated femoral anteversion. Reproduced with permission from Torde I (2020). Femoral anteversion. In: Joseph B, Nayagam S, Loder R, Torde I, editors. *Paediatric Orthopaedics: A System of Decision-Making* (2nd ed., 133), Taylor & Francis.

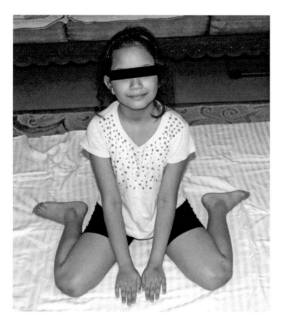

Figure 2.5 "W"-sitting in a child.

Table 2.1 Summary of the Femoral Anteversion Values in Children at Different Ages

Age	Femoral Anteversion
3–12 months	40° (mean)
At 2 years	31° (mean)
3–10 years	Mean decrease of around 1–2° per year
10–14 years	Around 20° (mean)
At 16 years	Around 16° (mean)

Staheli[15] has concluded that surgery can be offered if the child has age >8 years; deformity resulting in a significant cosmetic and functional disability; anteversion >50°; internal rotation of hip >85° and external rotation <10°; and if the family consents after being made aware of the risks of the procedure.

Bowed legs and knock knees are the most common deformities of the lower limbs for which consultations are sought by parents. It is not

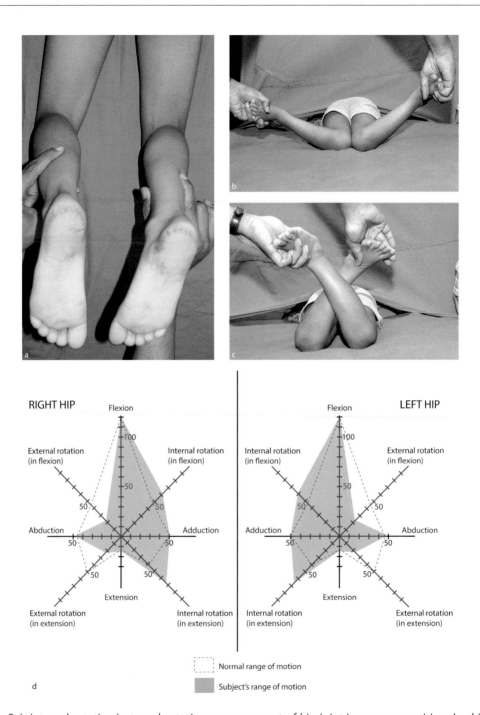

Figure 2.6 Internal rotation/external rotation measurement of hip joint in a prone position. In children with exaggerated anteversion, internal rotation is more than the external rotation. Reproduced with permission from Torde I (2020). Femoral anteversion. In: Joseph B, Nayagam S, Loder R, Torde I, editors. *Paediatric Orthopaedics: A System of Decision-Making* (2nd ed., 133), Taylor & Francis.

uncommon for a pediatric orthopedic surgeon to see apprehensive parents complaining about the apparent deformity of the knees of their children. As previously discussed, a child with a cephalic presentation has his/her legs internally rotated and the knees have some inherent varus. Parents, especially those of the first child, are apprehensive about this condition. Thus, it is essential that the clinician be aware of the normal developmental pattern of the tibiofemoral angle and can allay the apprehension of such parents appropriately.

Salenius and Vankka[16] were the first investigators to document the pattern of tibiofemoral angle evolution from childhood to adulthood. They noted that children had a varus angulation of about 15° at birth, which gradually improved to 0° at around 18–20 months, further developing into a valgus angle of around 10° by 3 years of age and finally stabilizing at around 6–7° of valgus by 8–10 years (Figure 2.7). Numerous subsequent studies[17,18] have reported a similar pattern of evolution of the tibiofemoral angle though the absolute values are different. Varus in children in their early years is labeled as physiological genu varum, especially if it is symmetrically present on both sides. At times it is important to differentiate physiological bowing of the tibia from pathological genu varum (e.g., Blount's disease) in a walking child. A cover-up test[19] is a good outpatient screening tool for differentiating the physiological from the pathological (Figure 2.8). This test is performed with the child supine and the legs exposed from groin to toes. A note is made of the apparent genu varum, and then the lower half of the leg and foot are covered. The axes of the femur and the visible tibia are drawn (imagined). A valgus angulation between the axes indicates that the apparent bow leg is diaphyseal and hence physiological. The absence of valgus alignment in a walking child is considered pathological and needs to be evaluated further. Variations in the absolute values of the time of evolution of the tibiofemoral angle vary with race and ethnicity.[17,18] Mathew et al.[17] noted that in south Indian children, the reversal of physiologic genu varum started before 2 years of age and reached a peak valgus around 5–6 years of age. Saini et al.[18] reported in their study of north Indian children that the peak valgus of 8° was achieved at around 6 years of age. Both these studies have thus found that the peak valgus angulation occurs at a later age when compared to Caucasian children.

Intermalleolar and intercondylar distance measurements are useful outpatient tools for quick evaluation of genu valgum and genu varum, respectively. Usually, an intermalleolar distance of <8 cm and intercondylar distance of <6 cm is considered normal. These measurements are obtained in a standing position (Figure 2.9). The child stands such that the patellae are facing forwards, and either the femoral condyles (in genu valgum) or the malleoli (in genu varum) are touching each other. In a child with physiological alignment, the two femoral condyles should just be in contact with an intermalleolar distance of <8 cm. One must be cautious in using intermalleolar distance in obese children with bulky thighs; their thighs touch each other, preventing any contact between the condyles and can provide a false reading for the intermalleolar distance. The alignment is better evaluated by the tibiofemoral angle and confirmed with full-length radiographs.

The tibial torsional profile is an important contributor to the overall appearance of the lower limbs of a child, especially when the child ambulates. At

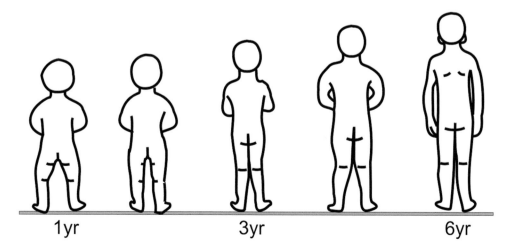

Figure 2.7 Knee alignment progression from varus to valgus in a child.

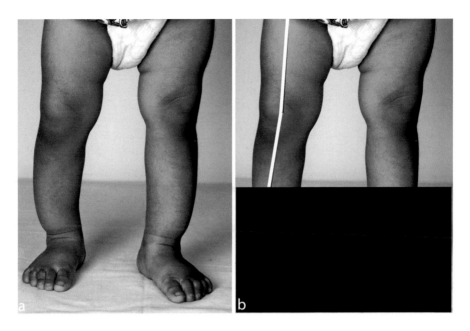

Figure 2.8 Cover-up test (a) with the entire leg exposed, (b) the lower part is covered up. Long axes are estimated (imagined) for the femur and the proximal part of the tibia. The presence of a valgus alignment indicates the absence of any pathologic varus deformity at the knee.

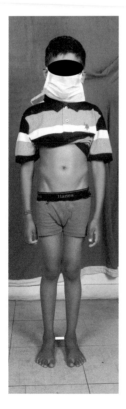

Figure 2.9 Normal alignment of the lower limb and intermalleolar distance.

birth, children usually have an internal torsion of the tibia. The best method to evaluate this torsional profile is with the child prone, and the knees flexed at 90° with the examiner looking down the foot. A measurement of the thigh-foot angle (angle between the axis of the thigh and the axis of the foot) gives the torsional profile of the tibia. In infants, the average thigh-foot angle measures 5° internal (range −30° internal to +20° external).[10,20] Commonly, the tibial rotational profile changes from internal torsion to external torsion, and most of the change takes place by 4–5 years of age.[21] By the age of 8 years, the thigh-foot angle averages 10° external (range, −5 to +30°) (Table 2.2). The transmalleolar axis is also used as a parameter for measuring the rotational profile of the tibia. Its values mimic the pattern of the thigh-foot angle and then change from internal rotation to external rotation from childhood to adult life. The mean measurement of this angle is 25°, with the range being from 0 to 45°.[10]

The foot progression angle (FPA) is an indicator of the way a child walks. It is measured by measuring the angle between the axis of the foot and a line along which the child walks. A measurement of FPA must be done whenever a child is being evaluated for gait abnormalities. The normal foot progression is outward with a mean angle of 6°

Table 2.2 Summary of the Pattern of Thigh-Foot Angle Change[a]

Age	Thigh-Foot Angle
Infants	Average −5° (−30 to +20°)
1–8 years	Internal torsion changes to external torsion with maximum change occurring between 1 and 5 years
8–10 years	+10° (−5 to +30°)

[a] Minus values indicate internal torsion and plus values indicate external torsion.

(range −5 to +15°) in children aged 1–3 years and 4° (range −2 to +12°) for children aged more than 4 years (Figure 2.10).[10]

2.5 LIGAMENTOUS LAXITY

Children are born with inherent ligamentous laxity. This laxity is necessary for the satisfactory completion of parturition when the child must come out through a relatively narrow vaginal opening. Most of the children lose this laxity with age. Consequently, the range of motion of different joints in children tends to change over time before reaching adult values. Lack of knowledge on the accepted range in children can result in overdiagnosis or underdiagnosis.

The persistence of ligamentous laxity can be indicative of underlying disorders like Ehlers–Danlos syndrome or Marfan syndrome.

Wynne–Davies criteria[22] and the Beighton score[23] are commonly used methods for detecting laxity (Figure 2.11).

2.5.1 Wynne–Davies' Criteria

The following criteria are evaluated:

- The ability of the thumb to touch the forearm on flexion of the wrist.
- Extension of the fingers parallel to the forearm on extension of wrist and metacarpo phalangeal (MCP) joints.
- Extension of the elbows beyond 180°.
- Extension of the knees beyond 180°.
- Dorsiflexion of the foot to 45°.

If three pairs of the five joints showed this much laxity, it is considered indicative of hyperlaxity.

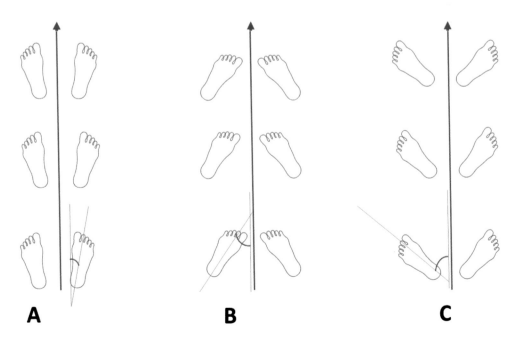

A **B** **C**

Figure 2.10 Foot progression angles. (a) Normal foot progression angle, (b) in-toeing, (c) out-toeing.

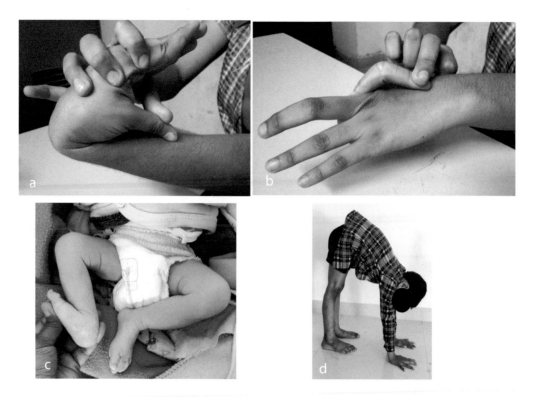

Figure 2.11 Ligamentous laxity.

2.5.2 Beighton's Score

Beighton's scoring method uses the following criteria:

- Passive dorsiflexion of the little finger beyond 90°.
- Passive apposition of the thumb to the flexor aspect of the forearm.
- Hyperextension of the elbow beyond 10°.
- Hyperextension of the knee beyond 10°.
- Forward flexion of the trunk with fully extended knees with the ability to place the palms of the hands flat on the floor.

The first four criteria are given one point each, and since they can be done on both right and left, it amounts to a total of eight points, and the forward trunk flexion is given a point amounting to a total score of nine points. In general, a score of four or more indicates a diagnosis of hyperlaxity. In an infant or toddler who has not started walking/not capable of obeying a command to bend forward with extended knees, the Wynne–Davies criteria is used.

REFERENCES

1. Sharma M. Nutritional assessment of children. In: *Pediatric nutrition in health and disease*, 1st ed. New Delhi: Jaypee Brothers; 2013. pp. 26–29.
2. Kocher MS, Garg S, Micheli LJ. Physeal sparing reconstruction of the anterior cruciate ligament in skeletally immature prepubescent children and adolescents. Surgical technique. *J Bone Joint Surg Am.* 2006;88(Suppl 1 Pt 2):283–293. doi:10.2106/JBJS.F.00441
3. Madelaine A, Fournier G, Sappey-Marinier E, et al. Conservative management of anterior cruciate ligament injury in paediatric population: About 53 patients. *Orthop Traumatol Surg Res.* 2018;104(8S): S169–S173. doi:10.1016/j.otsr.2018.09.001
4. Slough JM, Hennrikus W, Chang Y. Reliability of Tanner staging performed by orthopedic sports medicine surgeons. *Med Sci Sports Exerc.* 2013;45(7):1229–1234. doi:10.1249/MSS.0b013e318285c2f7
5. Frankenburg WK, Fandal AW, Sciarillo W, et al. The newly abbreviated and revised Denver developmental screening test. *J Pediatr.* 1981;99:995.
6. Herring JA. Growth and development. In: Herring JA, editor. *Tachdjian's Pediatric Orthopaedics*, 5th ed. Philadelphia, PA: Elsevier Saunders; 2014. pp. 3–22.

7. Hensinger RN. *Standards in pediatric orthopedics*, 1st ed. New York: Raven Press, 1986.
8. Ho C. Disorders of the upper extremity. In: Herring JA, editor. *Tachdjian's pediatric orthopaedics*, 5th ed. Philadelphia, PA: Elsevier Saunders; 2014. pp. 356–362.
9. Herring JA. Congenital coxa vara. In: Herring JA, editor. *Tachdjian's pediatric orthopaedics*, 5th ed. Philadelphia, PA: Elsevier Saunders; 2014. pp. 666–669.
10. Staheli LT, Corbett M, Wyss C, et al. Lower-extremity rotational problems in children. Normal values to guide management. *J Bone Joint Surg Am* 1985;67(1):39–47.
11. Fabry G, MacEwen GD, Shands AR Jr. Torsion of the femur. A follow-up study in normal and abnormal conditions. *J Bone Joint Surg Am* 1973;55:1726.
12. Shands AR Jr, Steele MK. Torsion of the femur; a follow-up report on the use of the Dunlap method for its determination. *J Bone Joint Surg Am* 1958;40:803.
13. Crane L. Femoral torsion and its relation to toeing-in and toeing-out. *J Bone Joint Surg Am* 1959;41:423.
14. Matovinović D, Nemec B, Gulan G, et al. Comparison in regression of femoral neck anteversion in children with normal, intoeing and outtoeing gait prospective study. *Coll Antropol* 1998;22:525.
15. Staheli LT. Torsion—treatment indications. *Clin Orthop Relat Res* 1989;247:61.
16. Salenius P, Vankka E. The development of the tibiofemoral angle in children. *J Bone Joint Surg Am* 1975;57(2):259–261.
17. Mathew SE, Madhuri V. Clinical tibiofemoral angle in south Indian children. *Bone Joint Res.* 2013;2(8):155–161. doi:10.1302/2046-3758.28.2000157.
18. Saini UC, Bali K, Sheth B, Gahlot N, Gahlot A. Normal development of the knee angle in healthy Indian children: A clinical study of 215 children. *J Child Orthop.* 2010;4(6):579–586. doi:10.1007/s11832-010-0297-z.
19. Gugenheim JJ. Clinical evaluation including imaging. In: Sabharwal S editor. *Pediatric lower limb deformities.* Switzerland: Springer; 2016. pp. 18–19.
20. Lincoln TL, Suen PW. Common rotational variations in children. *J Am Acad Orthop Surg.* 2003;11(5):312–320. doi:10.5435/00124635-200309000-00004
21. Mooney JF III. Lower extremity rotational and angular issues in children. *Pediatr Clin North Am.* 2014;61(6):1175–1183. doi:10.1016/j.pcl.2014.08.006
22. Wynne-Davies R. Acetabular dysplasia and familial joint laxity: Two etiological factors in congenital dislocation of the hip. A review of 589 patients and their families. *J Bone Joint Surg Br.* 1970;52:704–716.
23. Beighton P, Solomon L, Soskolne CL. Articular mobility in an African population. *Ann Rheum Dis.* 1973;32:413–438.

Examination of Gait in a Child

PRATEEK BEHERA AND NIRMAL RAJ GOPINATHAN

3.1 INTRODUCTION

Gait examination is an important and integral part of clinical evaluation that gives enormous information about the dynamic and functional implications of the underlying pathology. As is always taught in clinics, an attentive clinician begins examination by observing the child walking into the clinic to assess the gait. The statement "A child's footwear is itself a gait lab" by Dr. Alvin H. Crawford holds good in most walking children as the simple footwear can provide a lot of information about the way a child walks. It is especially important to understand that visual/observational gait analysis holds its importance even in the era of instrumented gait analysis labs.

"Doctor, my child is not walking normally – Please help!" is not an uncommon complaint an orthopedist encounters in outpatient clinics. The examiner must evaluate the underlying reason for the gait abnormality. To satisfactorily answer the questions and alleviate the parents' anxiety, one must be well-versed in normal and abnormal gait patterns. The learning objectives of this chapter are to learn about the basics of gait and identify different gait patterns and the possible associated conditions.

3.2 DEVELOPMENT OF GAIT

In children, the ability to walk is achieved concurrently with the gradual and craniocaudal stepwise development of the neurological system. The old aphorism, "a child walks at one and talks at two," holds good in most cases. However, walking can be delayed in many children, and it is not uncommon to find a child to start walking by 18 months. If a child has not walked by 18 months, then a detailed examination is warranted.

While learning to walk, an infant walks short, fast steps about a wide base of support (placing the feet wide apart helps the child to balance). There is increased flexion of the hips and knees, the arms are carried in high guard position, and the swing of the upper limbs is absent.[1,2] The heel-to-toe pattern of foot positioning is not established, and children have a flatfooted gait. The long axis of the feet is often directed toward the midline (inwards directed). At around 2 years, the heel-to-toe pattern sets in, the walking base reduces in width, and the arms tend to get lowered. By around 3 years, the arm swing pattern is established, the walking base becomes narrow, and step length and walking velocity increase.[1] Between the ages of 4 and 7, the walking pattern gradually matures toward the adult pattern, and by 7 years, the adult gait pattern is usually attained.[1]

3.3 GAIT CYCLE

Gait can be defined as a cyclical pattern of musculoskeletal motion that carries the body forwards. Simply stated, gait can be considered as the way an individual walks. Normal gait is smooth, symmetrical, and ergonomically economical, with each leg out of phase with the other.[3–5] To walk

properly, the efficient and complete coordination of the brain, spinal cord, peripheral nerves, muscles, bones, and joints is necessary. Any abnormality anywhere in these locations leads to an abnormal gait.

3.3.1 Phases of Gait

Each lower limb alternates between two phases – stance and swing during the gait cycle.[1] In stance phase, the limb is in contact with the ground, and while in swing phase, there is no contact of the foot with the ground, and the limb advances forward off the ground. Stance phase occupies 60%, and swing phase occupies 40% of the time of a gait cycle, which is the time interval between two consecutive initial contacts with the ground of the same foot.

Stance phase consists of five substages[3,5]: initial contact (heel strike), loading response (foot flat), mid-stance (single leg stance), terminal stance (heel-off), and pre-swing (toe-off). The swing phase consists of three substages: initial swing (acceleration), mid-swing, and terminal swing (deceleration) (Figure 3.1). Each normal gait cycle has two periods of double limb support that occurs when one foot is in the heel strike state and the other in the toe-off state, i.e., when stance phase is starting for one and is ending for the other. The duration of double limb support varies with the speed of walking. When one walks slow, the duration of double limb stance increases; it disappears and is replaced by double limb float (both the limbs are in air) while running.

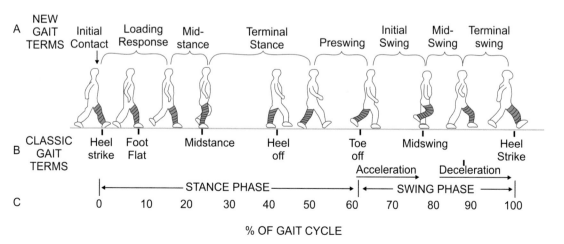

Figure 3.1 Phases of gait.

3.3.2 Commonly Used Terminologies for Describing Gait

Step length (distance between the feet when the heel of one foot strikes the ground and the toes of the other are about to come off the ground), stride length (distance traveled from heel strike of a limb to the next heel strike of the same limb) (Figure 3.2), cadence (the number of steps taken per minute), walking speed (the distance traveled per minute usually mentioned as meter/second), and foot progression angle (the angle that the foot makes with the line of progression on the path the subject is walking) are a few parameters that should be understood by the examiner.

3.4 HOW TO EXAMINE A CHILD'S GAIT

Examination of a child's gait is often difficult, especially in a busy outpatient setting. Children are frequently afraid of the examiner. They do not readily follow commands and have a very low level of patience and hence, will not normally walk back

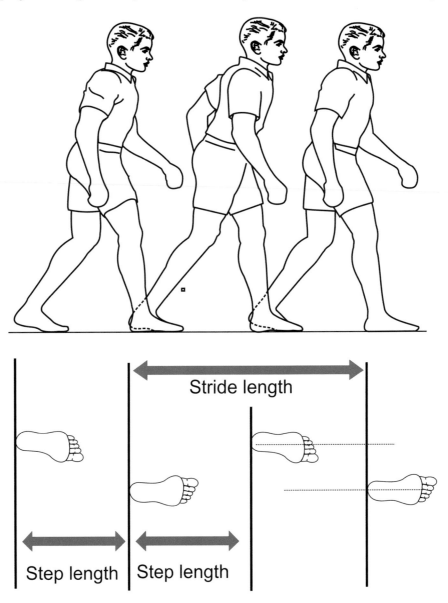

Figure 3.2 Step length/stride length.

and forth if asked to do so. Also, some children tend to voluntarily check on their walking pattern, fearful of any intervention by the examiner. Videos recorded by parents in a relaxed environment (home/playground) often come in handy, and with the ready availability of smartphone technology, parents can be requested to record and bring videos during their next hospital visit.

In cooperative children, gait is best examined in a well-illuminated hall/walkway with adequate space to allow the free movement of the child. The child should be undressed to a comfortable level (genitals covered) so that the lower limbs from the iliac crests and below are adequately visualized. The examiner either sits in a chair or kneels so that the level of his/her eyes are at the level of the child's iliac crests. The child is instructed to walk back and forth in the hall as much as naturally possible. The examiner takes a note of the child's head, shoulders, trunk, and the position of the three major joints of the lower limb – hips, knees, and ankles – by inspecting from the sides and from the front and back while the child continues to walk. Wherever possible, the child should also be asked to run. In case the child uses a walking aid, his/her gait should be evaluated both with and without the aid. This type of evaluation of a child's gait is called observational gait analysis. Further detailed evaluation of gait can be done in specialized gait laboratories. These analyses are beyond the scope of this book. Table 3.1 presents a summary of the position of hip, knee, and ankle during a normal gait cycle (Figure 3.3).

3.5 COMMON PROBLEMS IN GAIT NOTICED BY PARENTS

There are a few notable complaints that bother parents and are a reason for a hospital visit, but they often need no more than a calm listening of complaints and patient reassurance.

3.5.1 Toe-Walking

Tiptoe walking or toe-walking is often a common complaint. In fact, many children, while learning to walk, tend to walk on their toes. Painless toe-walking, especially if it is on both sides, is benign and often labeled as idiopathic. However, every child examined must be carefully evaluated to rule out conditions like mild spastic diplegic cerebral palsy and hereditary spastic paraparesis, tendoachilles contracture, etc. If toe-walking is present on one side, then shortening of the lower limb might be a possibility (Figure 3.4).

3.5.2 In-Toeing Gait

Parents often bring their child saying, "He/she walks abnormally with feet falling in reverse direction or the feet cross each other while he/she walks." When a child walks with the foot progression angle values in negative, i.e., when the feet are directed toward each other instead of being directed away from each other, the gait pattern is said to be in-toe. In most children, it is harmless and tends to improve with age, especially if it is bilateral, symmetrical, and painless due to increased femoral anteversion. The child should also be examined to rule out other causes of torsional anomalies of the lower limb, like intorsion of the tibia, torsional malunion (unilateral), and metatarsus adductus deformity, among other possible causes.[6]

3.5.3 Out-Toeing Gait

This is an uncommon cause of hospital visit compared to in-toeing, and the usual gait pattern is of out-toeing. The usual amount of out-toeing recorded is between 0° and 30°, and this tends to improve with age. The persistence of out-toeing is suggestive of torsional anomalies of the tibia.

3.5.4 Flat Feet

A common complaint that brings children to hospital is that of flat feet. Almost all children have flat feet at birth, and the arch tends to develop over the years, with the adult shape achieved by 10 years of age. It should also be noted that not all adult flat-feet are pathological and that flat feet represent a variant of normal feet if they are flexible, painless, symmetrical, and not associated with any underlying condition. Parents need to be reassured and the child examined for pain, symmetry, tendoachilles tightness, and flexibility of the feet. Pathological conditions leading to flat feet are numerous including congenital vertical talus, tarsal coalition, joint hypermobility syndrome, fibular hemimelia, peroneal contracture, muscular dystrophy, and others.

Table 3.1 Summary of the Position of the Hip, Knee, and Ankle at Different Phases of a Normal Gait Cycle

Phases of the Gait Cycle	Position of Hip	Status of Pelvis	Position of Knee	Status of Leg (Tibia)	Position of Ankle	Status of the Foot
Stance Phase						
Heel strike	Flexed to about 20–40°; medially rotated	Pelvis is level and medially rotated	Knee is slightly flexed or extended	Tibia is laterally rotated	Ankle is at 90° (Neutral)	Forefoot is supinated with hindfoot everted
Foot flat	Flexed hip starts to move to extension; medially rotated	Pelvis drops slightly on the swing leg side	Knee is flexed from 15° to 25°	Tibia is medially rotated and starts to move over the foot	Ankle is plantar flexed	Forefoot moves into pronation from supination and hindfoot is inverted
Mid-stance	Hip gradually moves through neutral to extension. Greatest force is on the hip in this phase	Pelvis starts to rotate posteriorly with a slight drop to the swing leg side	Knee is slightly flexed	Tibia is in neutral position	Ankle has 5–8° of dorsiflexion	Forefoot is pronated and hindfoot is inverted
Heel-off	Hip moves to an extension of about 10–15° with lateral rotation	Pelvis is posteriorly rotated and dips slightly to the swing leg side, remaining posteriorly rotated	Knee is extended	Tibia is laterally rotated	Ankle moves from dorsiflexion to plantar flexion	Forefoot is in supination; hindfoot moves from inversion to eversion
Toe-off	Hip is extended to about 10° and has lateral rotation	Pelvis remains posteriorly rotated	Knee flexes to about 30–40°	Tibia is laterally rotated	Ankle has about 20° of plantar flexion	Forefoot gradually pronates and hindfoot continues to evert
Swing Phase						
Initial swing	Hip moves from slight flexion to 30° of flexion and from lateral rotation to neutral rotation	Pelvis medially rotates and dips to the swing leg side	Knee has about 30–60° flexion	Tibia moves from lateral rotation to neutral	Ankle moves from 20° plantar flexion position to about 10° plantar flexion	Forefoot starts supinating and hindfoot continues to evert
Mid-swing	Hip further flexes and medially rotates	Pelvis has the same position as the previous phase	Knee continues to flex further	Tibia is in neutral position	Ankle moves from 10° plantar flexion to a neutral position	Forefoot is supinated and hindfoot is everted
Terminal swing	Hip continues to flex and medially rotate	Pelvis has the same position as above	Knee has maximal extension	Tibia starts to rotate laterally from neutral	Ankle moves to a position of about 10° dorsiflexion	Forefoot is supinated and hindfoot is everted

Source: Modified and adapted from Karol LA[1] and Magee DJ[3].

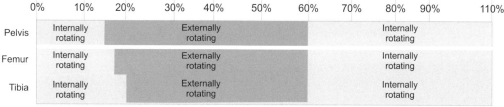

	0%	10%	20%	30%	40%	50%	60%	70%	80%	90%		110%

Pelvis	Internally rotating		Externally rotating				Internally rotating
Femur	Internally rotating		Externally rotating				Internally rotating
Tibia	Internally rotating		Externally rotating				Internally rotating

Gait cycle

Figure 3.3 Position of pelvis, hip, knee, and ankle during different phases of gait.

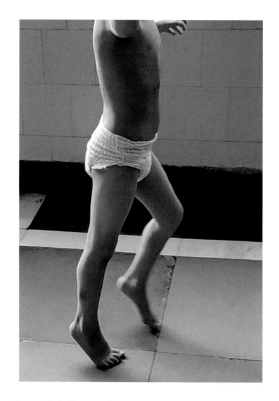

Figure 3.4 Toe walker.

3.6 ABNORMAL GAIT PATTERNS INDICATIVE OF PATHOLOGY

3.6.1 Antalgic Gait

Antalgic gait literally means "relieving or reducing pain." Antalgic gait is the most common gait disturbance in a limping child.[7] It results from the child's subconscious efforts to reduce pain by putting limited weight on the affected side. It might be secondary to pathology in the hip, knee, ankle, or back. It is a protective gait and aims to prevent any further damage by removing weight from the affected leg as quickly as possible. This leads to a short stance phase on the affected limb and, consequently, a relatively long stance phase on the contralateral limb. In case the pathology is in the hip, the patient shifts the body weight over the painful hip to decrease the abductor pull and the effective joint reaction force on the affected hip. This leads to a sway toward the affected side. Common etiology includes infective and inflammatory arthritis, avascular necrosis, proximal femoral osteomyelitis, chondrolysis, acute slipped capital femoral epiphysis, and fracture of femoral neck. The examiner should look at the child's sway and the time spent by each limb in stance phase to identify this gait pattern.

3.6.2 Trendelenburg Gait

Trendelenburg gait, also called "abductor lurch," essentially results from insufficiency of the abductor mechanism of the hip. In this gait pattern, the patient lurches on the affected side to avoid dropping the pelvis toward the opposite side. It may result from an abnormality in the hip joint or in the femoral neck or the abductor musculature. The child tends to lean over to the affected side and by doing so, brings his or her center of gravity closer to the femoral head. Consequently, the leverage of the patient's upper body weight is reduced, and thus the counterbalancing force exerted by the hip abductors also decreases. To be labeled as Trendelenburg gait, the gait should be pain-free. However, it is not uncommon for both antalgic and Trendelenburg gait to be present together. Causes of unilateral Trendelenburg gait include Perthes' disease, unilateral developmental dysplasia of hip (DDH), slipped capital femoral epiphysis (SCFE),

non-union of femoral neck fractures, mal-united neck or intertrochanteric fractures neglected by longstanding dislocation of hip, poliomyelitis, and paralysis of hip abductors, etc.

If there is an abnormality of the abductor mechanism on both sides, the gait shows accentuated side-to-side movements resulting in a waddling gait. A waddling gait may be seen in cases of bilateral DDH and myopathies affecting the abductors of the hip. The identification of a painless sway of the child to the affected side helps in making the diagnosis[3,5,7] (Figure 3.5).

3.6.3 Short Limb Gait

Short limb gait is seen when one of the limbs of the patient is shorter than the other. It is present when there is a true limb length discrepancy with the affected limb being shorter in length. The pelvis and the shoulder drop down vertically on the affected side. The patient thus has a sway to the affected side. The joints of the unaffected side may demonstrate exaggerated flexion, or hip hiking may occur during the swing phase to allow the foot to clear the ground. The stance phase duration on

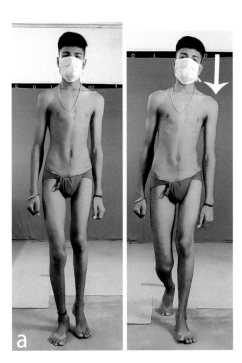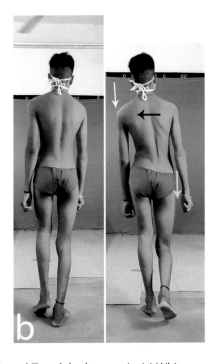

Figure 3.5 Patient with components of both short limb and Trendelenburg gait. (a) White arrow shows a vertical dip in the shoulder, (b) white arrow shows shoulder dip, black arrow shows the sway of the trunk to the affected side, and the yellow arrow denotes the drop in pelvis.

both sides is equal, as is the differentiating point between the antalgic and short limb gait. The sway noted in short limb gait is not as pronounced as in Trendelenburg gait and is more of a vertical drop of one half of the body rather than a classical sway.

If the patient is asked to walk with a shoe raise equal to the amount of shortness of the limb, then the pelvic drop and the shift to the opposite side gets reduced/disappears, and this may be used for differentiating a short limb gait from a Trendelenburg gait. Any congenital, infective, or traumatic condition that leads to shortening of one of the limbs would lead to a short limb gait (Figure 3.5).

3.6.4 High Stepping Gait

High stepping gait is also called a foot-drop gait or dragging gait and results primarily from weakness or paralysis of the ankle dorsiflexors. The child is unable to dorsiflex the foot during the initial swing, and to avoid dragging the toes against the ground, he/she lifts the knee higher than usual, thus generating the high stepping. The initial heel strike is absent as the patient is unable to maintain the foot in neutral, and thus the toes instead of the heel meet the ground. Common causes include post-injection sciatic nerve palsy, post-traumatic peroneal palsy, myelodysplasia, Charcot–Marie–Tooth disease, etc.

3.6.5 Gluteus Maximus Gait

A gluteus maximus gait occurs in children with a weak gluteus maximus. The gluteus maximus normally locks the hip in extension as the contralateral limb is advanced for the next step. A patient with a weak gluteus maximus may thrust the pelvis forward and trunk backward, shifting the center of gravity posterior to the hip and thereby reducing the force that the gluteus maximus needs to generate to lock the hip in extension. This gait is seen in cases of polio affecting the gluteus maximus[1,3,7] (Figure 3.6).

3.6.6 Quadriceps Avoidance Gait or Hand-to-Knee Gait

In a normal gait cycle, the knee is fully extended and locked in extension by the quadriceps during mid-stance. In children with weakness of the

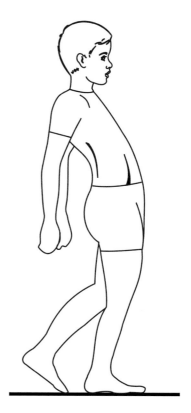

Figure 3.6 Gluteus maximus gait.

quadriceps, like those with poliomyelitis, femoral nerve injuries, and trauma, the quadriceps fail to extend and lock the knee. The patient develops a compensatory mechanism in which the patient leans over the affected limb and uses his/her ipsilateral hand/fingers to produce the extension of the knee. A child may use his/her hand through the pant pockets and thus avoid pressing the distal femur from outside.

3.6.7 Role of Using a Cane

A cane is an assistive device used for improving the gait. From a biomechanical viewpoint, it is especially helpful in patients with hip pathologies. Previously, it has been discussed that most of the hip pathologies produce a lurch (sway) of the trunk to the affected side. This lurch tends to shift the center of gravity toward the affected hip and in this process, decreases the amount of force being exerted on the diseased hip. However, the unsightly appearance due to sway is unacceptable to most. Additionally, the repetitive sway tends to put strain on the lumbar spine and the paraspinal muscles and is responsible for backache in many patients.

Another method of reducing the force on the diseased hip is by using a cane in the unaffected hand. When an individual walks with a cane in the opposite hand, then the moderate amount of push applied to the cane during the swing phase of the unaffected limb helps decrease the total amount of force that the abductors of the affected side must generate to keep the pelvis stable.[8] A decrease in this force leads to a decrease in the overall force acting on the diseased hip, thereby decreasing the sway and the pain (if any).

3.7 GAIT IN CEREBRAL PALSY

Children with cerebral palsy (CP) present with a spectrum of gait-related problems. On the one hand, there are children who cannot walk, and on the other hand, there are those who walk near normally. Issues with walking ability are one of the most common reasons for which medical care is sought. Children with CP have issues related to balance (stability), forward propulsion, shock absorption, muscle function, and energy consumption. Stability is disturbed in CP because of impaired balance, increased muscle tone, and muscle weakness.[9] There are numerous patterns of gait disturbances noted in patients of CP and detailed examination and record of gait is needed not only to determine the intervention needed but also to keep track of progress made due to such interventions. Computerized gait analysis has maximum utility for CP patients. Video recording of gait with the option to play back the video at slow speeds helps to gain information in the absence of a gait lab.[8]

The gait patterns/postural patterns in CP will depend on the topographical involvement, say hemiplegia/diplegia, the amount of spasticity/contracture, and the associated lever arm (bone and joint) alterations. It is imperative to understand that in spastic hemiplegia there is more distal involvement and hence true equinus is the basis for the described gait patterns; in diplegia and quadriplegia, proximal involvement is more pronounced, leading to apparent equinus and crouch gait patterns. It is important to keep in mind that these postural patterns are better recognized in the middle- and end-of-stance phase and on the sagittal plane observation of the gait. The coronal and transverse plane observations are more important in diplegia/quadriplegia and type 4 hemiplegia. The commonly seen gait patterns are mentioned below.

3.7.1 Gait Patterns in Spastic Hemiplegia

The description of gait in spastic hemiplegia by Winters et al.[10] is the most widely accepted classification and is based mainly on the sagittal plane kinematics (Figure 3.7, Table 3.2).

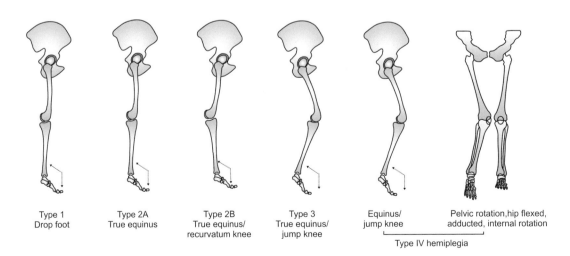

Type 1	Type 2A	Type 2B	Type 3	Equinus/	Pelvic rotation, hip flexed,
Drop foot	True equinus	True equinus/	True equinus/	jump knee	adducted, internal rotation
		recurvatum knee	jump knee		

Type IV hemiplegia

Figure 3.7 Gait patterns in spastic hemiplegia.

Table 3.2 Summary of the Classification of Gait Observed in Children with Spastic Hemiplegia

Type 1 hemiplegia	"Drop foot" in swing phase	Inability to selectively control the ankle dorsiflexors. No calf contracture
Type 2a hemiplegia	Equinus in stance phase and neutral knee and extended hip	Spasticity/contracture of the gastrocsoleus
Type 2b hemiplegia	Equinus in stance phase and recurvatum knee and extended hip	Spasticity/contracture of the gastrocsoleus Overactive plantarflexion–knee extension couple
Type 3 hemiplegia	Equinus and impaired dorsiflexion in swing Flexed "stiff knee gait"	Spasticity/contracture of the gastrocsoleus Hamstring/quadriceps co-contraction
Type 4 hemiplegia	Pelvic retraction Sagittal plane – equinus, flexed stiff knee, flexed hip, and an anterior pelvic tilt Coronal plane – hip adduction Transverse plane – hip internal rotation	High incidence of hip subluxation

3.7.2 Gait Patterns in Spastic Diplegia/Quadriplegia

The description of gait in spastic hemiplegics and quadriplegics is based on the work by Sutherland and Davids[11] and its interpretation by Rodda and Graham[12] (Figure 3.8). It is important to make a note of the "lever arm disease" described by Gage[13] that is frequently present in children with spastic diplegia/quadriplegia (Table 3.3).

In a scissoring gait pattern, with each step, one leg crosses directly over the other due to the tight adductors of the hip and the medial hamstrings and weak abductor muscles. Excessive femoral anteversion is a frequently associated finding. The following abnormalities are to be kept in mind, namely adduction contracture with or without subluxation in the coronal plane. In the transverse plane, look for pelvic rotation, medial femoral torsion, lateral tibial torsion, and foot deformities.

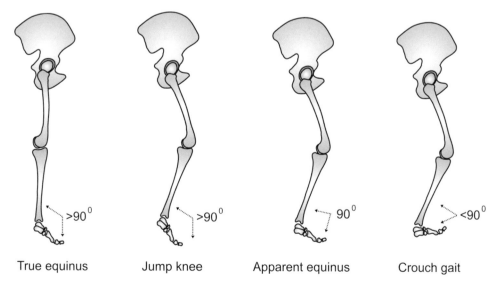

True equinus   Jump knee   Apparent equinus   Crouch gait

Figure 3.8 Gait patterns in spastic diplegia.

Table 3.3 Common Gait Patterns in Children with Spastic Diplegia/Quadriplegia

True equinus	Ankle in plantar flexion throughout stance and the hips and knees extended
	Equinus may be masked by recurvatum at knee
Jump gait (with or without stiff knee)	Ankle in equinus, knee and hip in flexion, anterior pelvic tilt, and increased lumbar lordosis
	There is often stiff knee because of rectus femoris activity in the swing phase of gait
Apparent equinus (with or without stiff knee)	Child walks on toes but has normal range of dorsiflexion at the ankle
	Plantigrade ankle/foot, flexed hip, and knee. Weakening of gastrocnemius by lengthening/botulinum toxin type A injection will result in crouch gait
Crouch gait (with or without stiff knee gait)	Excessive dorsiflexion or calcaneus at the ankle along with excessive flexion at the hip and the knee

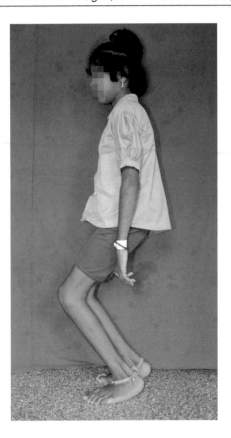

Figure 3.9 Crouch gait pattern. Reproduced with permission from Joseph B (2020). Spastic knee. In: Joseph B, Nayagam S, Loder R, Torde I, editors. *Paediatric Orthopaedics: A System of Decision-Making* (2nd ed., 475), Taylor & Francis.

3.7.3 Lever Arm Disease

See description in Chapter 13, "Examination of a Child with Cerebral Palsy."

3.7.4 Plantarflexion–Knee Extension Couple

The plantarflexion–knee extension couple is an important biomechanical concept in understanding the foot-ankle and knee level relationship. When a competent gastrocnemius acts on a stable foot in the line of progression, it controls the anterior progression of the tibia over the planted foot during the stance phase. The ground reaction vector is directed anterior to the knee, thereby providing the extensor moment at the knee and reducing the demands on the quadriceps. However, a weak or overlengthened gastrocnemius and a misdirected breached foot may result in crouch gait (Figure 3.9).

REFERENCES

1. Karol LA. Gait analysis. In: Herring JA, editor. *Tachdjian's pediatric orthopedics*, 5th ed. Philadelphia: Saunders; 2014. pp. 71–78.
2. Evans A. Gait development. *In: Pocket podiatry paediatrics*, 1st ed. Edinburgh: Churchill Livingstone, 2010.
3. Magee DJ. Assessment of gait. In: *Orthopaedic physical assessment*, 6th ed. St. Louis: Saunders; 2014. pp. 981–1016.
4. Martell JM. Pelvis, hip, and thigh. In: Reider B, editor. *The orthopaedic physical examination*, 2nd ed. Philadelphia: Saunders; 2005. pp. 177–180.
5. Gopinathan NR, Behera P. Gait. In: Dhatt S, Prabhakar S, editors. *Handbook of clinical examination in orthopedics*. Singapore: Springer; 2019. pp. 291–299.
6. Evans AM. Mitigating clinician and community concerns about children's flatfeet, intoeing gait, knock knees or bowlegs. *J Paediatr Child Health*. 2017;53(11):1050–1053. doi:10.1111/jpc.13761.

7. Herring JA, Birch JG. The limping child. In: Herring JA, editor. *Tachdjian's pediatric orthopedics*, 5th ed. Philadelphia: Saunders; 2014. pp. 79–89.

8. Blount WP. Don't throw away the cane. *J Bone Joint Surg Am.* 1956;38(3):695–708.

9. Berker N, Yalcin S. HELP guide to cerebral palsy. https://global-help.org/products/help_guide_to_cerebral_palsy/. Last accessed 15 May 2020.

10. Winters TF, Gage JR, Hicks R. Gait patterns in spastic hemiplegia in children and young adults. *J Bone Joint Surg (Am)* 1987;69:437–441.

11. Sutherland DH, Davids JR. Common gait abnormalities of the knee in cerebral palsy. *Clin Orthopaedics Related Res* 1993;288:139–147.

12. Rodda JM, Graham HK. Classification of gait patterns in spastic hemiplegia and spastic diplegia: A basis for a management algorithm. *Eur J Neurol* 2001;8(Suppl. 5):98–108.

13. Gage JR. *Gait analysis in cerebral palsy.* London: MacKeith Press, 1991. pp. 61–100.

Evaluation of Congenital Limb Deficiencies

NIRMAL RAJ GOPINATHAN AND PRATIK M. RATHOD

4.1 INTRODUCTION

Congenital limb deficiency disorders encompass a wide group of dysplastic/hypoplastic/aplastic disorders. They range anywhere from the constriction ring of a digit to aplasia of the complete limb.[1–5] Often, these disorders are associated with the underlying syndromic entity/systemic abnormalities but can also occur spontaneously. It is vital to identify these disorders as early as possible to look for systemic disorders (cardiovascular, central nervous system)/syndrome associated pathologies. Also, the evaluation of such a child to manage the deficiency with appropriate rehabilitation and the best possible outcome would be the goal. As is the rule, the evaluation demands an interdisciplinary approach with the involvement of a pediatrician, geneticist, cardiologist, etc.

4.2 CLASSIFICATION

The classification of limb deficiency disorders has evolved with time. The difficulty in classifying these disorders is due to the variety of presentations. There are two groups of diseases: skeletal dysostosis, which is fixed at birth, and the other being skeletal dysplasia, which is an ongoing abnormality of the skeletal system. But some disorders are such that they share common features of both spectrums of the disorder.[6] Numerous classification systems exist for congenital limb deficiencies. But the most commonly used classification system was created by Frantz et al., which is given in Table 4.1.[7]

Broadly, these diseases are classified into either terminal or intercalary deficiency (Figure 4.1). An intercalary deficiency is the one where the deficiency occurs within the extremity and does not extend to its end. On the contrary, in terminal deficiency, the missing segment extends to the end of the extremity. These are further classified into:[8]

- Transverse – the deficiency mimics an amputation/disarticulation across the long axis of the limb. Limb development is normal to a particular level beyond which skeletal elements are absent. At times there may be the presence of distal digital buds
- Paraxial/longitudinal – a defect parallel to the long axis of the limb

Table 4.1   Frantz et al. Classification of Congenital Limb Deficiency[7]

Terminal Deficiency

Transverse	Longitudinal
• Amelia (total absence of a limb)	• Complete paraxial[a] hemimelia (failure of formation of
• Hemimelia (failure of formation of the forearm with hand or leg with foot)	one of the two bony parts of forearm/leg and the corresponding portion of hand or foot)
• Partial hemimelia (presence of part of forearm or leg)	• Incomplete paraxial hemimelia (similar to above but existence of part of the defective elements)
• Acheiria (absent hand)/apodia (absent foot)	• Partial adactylia (deficiency of 1 to 4 digits with their metacarpals/metatarsals)
• Complete adactylia (failure of formation of all five digits with metacarpals/metatarsals)	• Partial aphalangia (deficiency of one or more phalanges from 1 to 4 digits)
• Complete aphalangia (failure of formation of one or more phalanges from all digits)	

Intercalary Deficiency

Transverse	Longitudinal
• Complete phocomelia (hand or foot attached directly to the trunk)	• Complete paraxial hemimelia (it differs from the corresponding terminal defect by the existence of more or less complete hand/foot)
• Proximal phocomelia (forearm with hand or leg with foot attached directly to the trunk)	• Incomplete paraxial hemimelia (it differs from the corresponding terminal defect by the existence of a more or less complete hand/foot)
• Distal phocomelia (hand/foot attached with arm/thigh)	• Partial adactylia (failure of formation of all or part of a metatarsal/metacarpal; first digit ray or fifth digit ray)
	• Partial aphalangia (deficiency of proximal and/or middle phalanx from one or more digits)

[a] Paraxial – formerly longitudinal – preaxial pertains to the ulnar/fibular side and postaxial pertains to the radial/tibial side of the limb.

4.3 DIAGNOSTIC EVALUATION

Once a congenital limb deficiency is identified, the child should be thoroughly evaluated both clinically and radiologically.

4.3.1 History Taking

Clinical evaluation includes taking a detailed history of the demography, birth history including antenatal history, previous miscarriages, placental pathologies, or congenital anomalies in previous pregnancies. Any history of drug intake in the first trimester is important as the period between 18 and 55 days of gestation is the time of organogenesis, and limb formation occurs from the end of the fourth week to the sixth week of fertilization (thalidomide intake is associated with phocomelia). Antenatal history should include diagnostic interventions like chronic villus sampling or soft signs (fever, rashes, etc.), especially in the initial trimester, antenatal infections, diabetes, etc.

Transverse deficiencies (Figure 4.2) are most commonly found to be associated with placental pathologies like amniotic band syndrome/Streeter's dysplasia. This condition results from the formation of aberrant amniotic bands/strands resulting from an early rupture of the amniotic membrane. These bands can affect a fetus from head to toe, including the limbs (chorionic villus sampling can be associated with this deformation). The constriction impedes venous circulation resulting in deep clefts or complete amputation distal to the band (Figure 4.3).

Also, family history (last three generations' history with pedigree charts)[6] and the marital history of the parents must be obtained. Consanguinity of the marriage plays a direct role in extrapolating the existing genetic deformity in the family. The

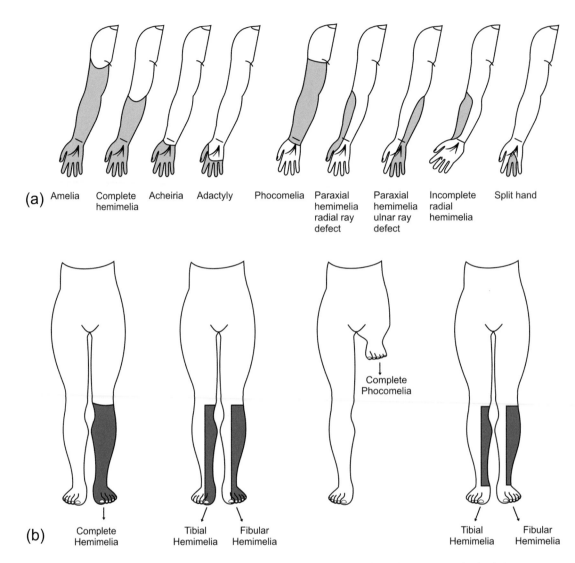

Figure 4.1 Schematic diagram of terminal, intercalary, longitudinal, and transverse limb deficiencies. (a) arms (b) legs.

degree of consanguineous marriage is crucial as the rate of diseases and congenital defects of recessive origin increases many a fold.

4.3.2 General Physical Examination

Once the clinical history is elicited, we may proceed to a detailed physical examination. A complete general physical examination is a must. The child must be evaluated as a whole and not just the affected part. At times we may be able to pick up other soft signs indicating the presence of a syndromic association. A head-to-toe examination is a must in these cases. Subtle signs such as peculiar

facies, low set ears, small mouth, webbed neck, syndactyly, a tuft of hair in the midline, hypoplastic thumb, isolated short metacarpal and metatarsal are just some traits to look for, to name a few. The examiner must be aware of heritable limb deficiencies and other associated systemic anomalies. For example, a child with Fanconi pancytopenia syndrome is small at birth and has patchy brown discoloration of the skin. It should be kept in mind that upper extremity deficiencies are more prone to having associated abnormalities. A child presenting to an orthopedic surgeon with a deformed upper limb (radial club hand/paraxial deficiency) may have associated hematologic abnormalities

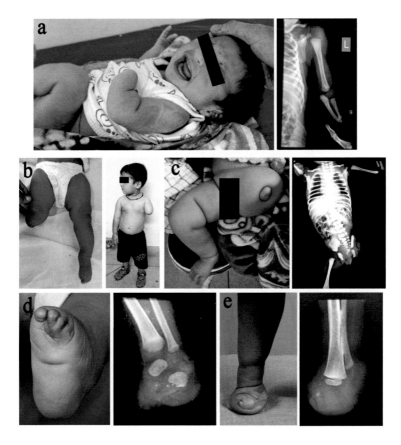

Figure 4.2 Transverse limb deficiencies. (a) acheiria (absence of hand), (b) partial hemimelia right lower limb and hemimelia left upper limb, (c) amelia (complete absence of left lower limb), (d) absence of midfoot and forefoot, (e) apodia (deficiency of foot).

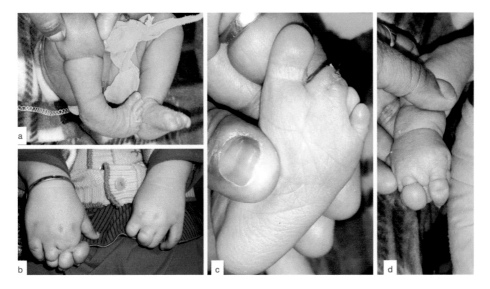

Figure 4.3 Amniotic band syndrome (Streeter's dysplasia); (a) constriction band of leg and talipes equinovarus deformation, (b) amputation of digits, (c) amputation of toes, (d) constriction bands and amputation in fingers.

Table 4.2 Concerns to Be Addressed[9,10,11]

Special Concerns in Young Children	Special Concerns in Adolescents
• Counsel parents regarding the guilt of "producing deformed baby" • Clear misconceptions regarding the prognosis from other social acquaintances • Amputation as an option in grossly deformed/difficult to reconstruct anomalies • Special schooling problem for an orthopedically handicapped child should be addressed • Address prosthetic requirements	• Separate counseling session for the adolescent and their parents • Address the challenges faced in peer relationships to the child • Manage "acting out" of the adolescent with adequate complacency • It is difficult to change the parents' understanding of the disease if seeing them for the first time (neglected cases) • Address prosthetic requirements

Table 4.3 Common Associated Features with Limb Deficiencies[11–15]

Limb Deficiency	Associated Anomaly/Syndromic Disorder
Humeral deficiency	May be associated with: • Poland syndrome • SAMS – short stature, auditory anomalies, mandibular anomalies, skeletal anomalies
Radial deficiency (Figure 4.4)	Associated with aplasia or hypoplasia of the thumb. May be associated with: • TAR (thrombocytopenia absent radius) • Fanconi's anemia • Holt–Oram syndrome • VACTERL (vertebral anomalies, anal atresia, cardiac defects, tracheal anomalies including tracheoesophageal fistula, renal and limb anomalies)
Ulnar deficiency (Figure 4.5)	Associated with hypoplasia to aplasia of the ulna and at times radiohumeral synostosis along with the absence of fourth and fifth digits. May be associated with: 1. Crouzon syndrome 2. Holt–Oram syndrome
Femoral deficiency – congenital femoral deficiency (CFD) (Figure 4.6)	May be associated with: • Fibular deficiency • Absent hip • Femoral neck pseudoarthrosis • ACL (anterior cruciate ligament) deficiency • Coxa vara • Contractures around the knee
Tibial deficiency (Figure 4.7)	May be associated with: • Foot and ankle deformity, commonly equinovarus • Polydactyly
Fibular deficiency (Figure 4.8)	May be associated with: • Femoral and tibial shortening • Valgus knee • ACL deficiency with absent tibial spine • Limb length discrepancy (LLD) • Fibular hemimelia syndrome with a normal-appearing fibula (missing lateral rays of the foot, ball, and socket ankle with a tarsal coalition, clubfoot deformity, shortening of the tibia) • Anterolateral bowing of tibia with equinovalgus deformity of the foot, and tarsal coalition
Split hand/foot (Figure 4.9)	Loss of the central rays of the fingers and the foot

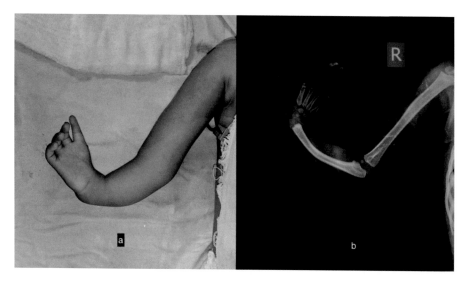

Figure 4.4 (a) Radial deficiency with absent thumb; (b) radiography.

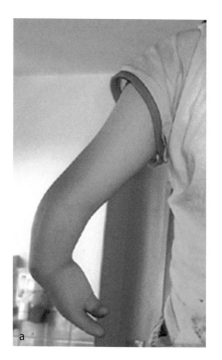

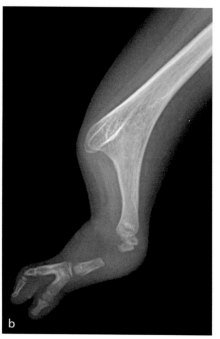

Figure 4.5 (a) Ulnar deficiency, (b) radiography. Source: Reproduced with permission from Joseph B (2020). Ulnar club hand. In: Joseph B, Nayagam S, Loder R, Torde I, editors. *Paediatric Orthopaedics: A System of Decision-Making* (2nd edn., 316), Taylor & Francis.

like thrombocytopenia. The importance of picking up these conditions lies in the identification and prevention of a potentially fatal/morbid event like an intraventricular hemorrhage. Longitudinal deficiencies are commonly associated with syndromes but can also be found in isolation.

4.3.3 Systemic and Local Examination

This general physical examination should be followed by a detailed systemic examination including the cardiovascular, abdominal, and nervous

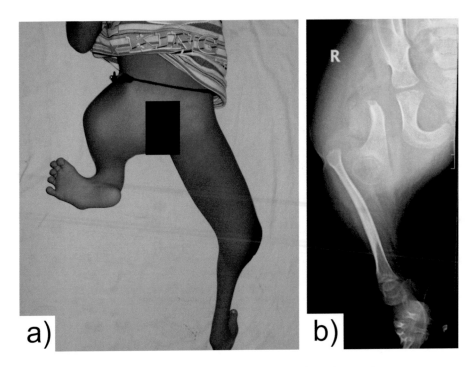

Figure 4.6 (a) Femoral deficiency along with fibular deficiency; (b) radiography.

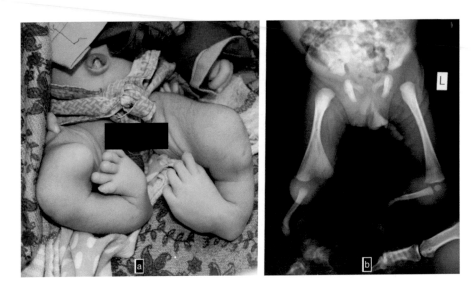

Figure 4.7 (a) Tibial deficiency with the appearance of clubfoot; (b) radiography.

system along with a musculoskeletal examination. Often, such examination may require multide-partmental teamwork to come to a final diagnosis, management, and rehabilitation. After the examination of the child is completed, it is worthwhile examining his/her sibling(s) and his/her parents, which may provide a clue to the diagnosis (e.g., parents with a hypoplastic thumb may have a child with a hypoplastic thumb and radius or both).[6] The examiner then examines the extremity and should classify the limb deficiency and identify the status of the joints in proximity.

Once all the detailed examination is done, keeping in mind a working diagnosis/set of working differentials, we proceed to the next part. This includes radiography/skeletal survey/advanced

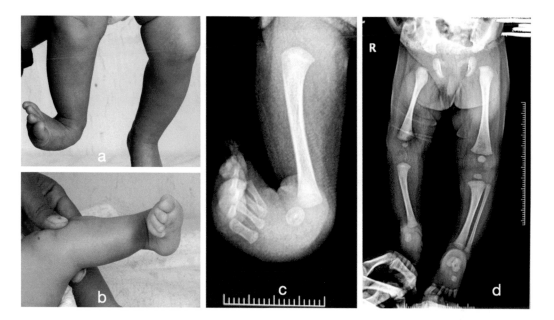

Figure 4.8 (a), (b) Fibular deficiency with valgus foot and absent lateral ray. (c), (d) X-ray of fibular deficiency with congenital femoral deficiency.

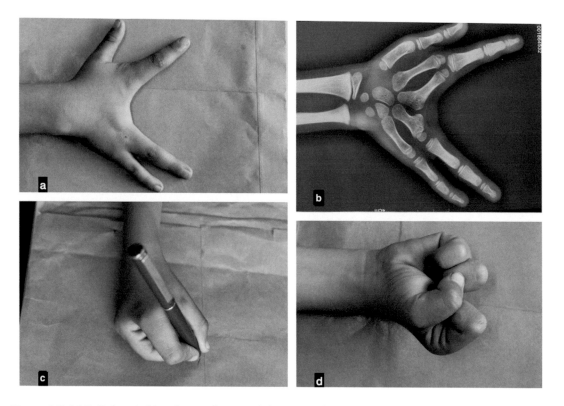

Figure 4.9 (a) Split hand; (b) radiography; (c), (d) function of hand and fist making.

Algorithm of working up of a patient with congenital limb deficiency.[6,7,9,10,15]

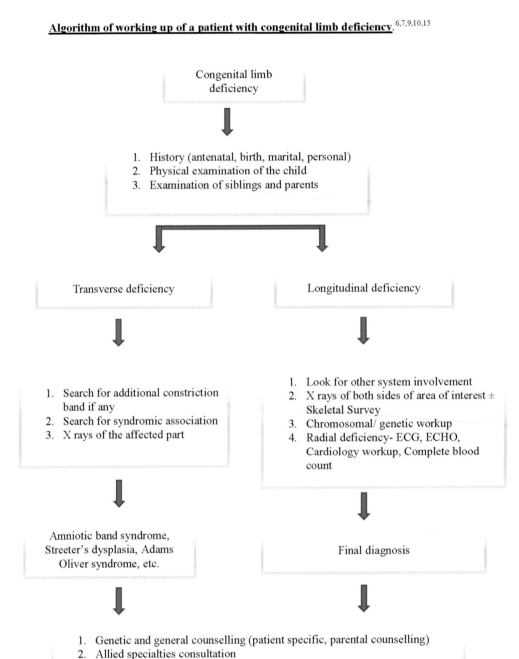

Congenital limb
deficiency

1. History (antenatal, birth, marital, personal)
2. Physical examination of the child
3. Examination of siblings and parents

Transverse deficiency

Longitudinal deficiency

1. Search for additional constriction
   band if any
2. Search for syndromic association
3. X rays of the affected part

1. Look for other system involvement
2. X rays of both sides of area of interest ±
   Skeletal Survey
3. Chromosomal/ genetic workup
4. Radial deficiency- ECG, ECHO,
   Cardiology workup, Complete blood
   count

Amniotic band syndrome,
Streeter's dysplasia, Adams
Oliver syndrome, etc.

Final diagnosis

1. Genetic and general counselling (patient specific, parental counselling)
2. Allied specialties consultation
3. Rehabilitation with prosthesis/ orthosis as appropriate/ surgical intervention
   if required

Figure 4.10 Algorithm for outpatient clinic approach toward a child with limb deficiency.

imaging studies if required.[6] If multiple deformities are seen, it is worthwhile getting the opinion of a medical geneticist, who may advise chromosomal studies to arrive at a diagnosis. Table 4.2 identifies multiple issues that are to be kept in mind while addressing these children.

4.3.4 Specific Congenital Limb Deficiencies

Longitudinal deficiencies are grouped according to the bones involved and are namely: radius, ulna, humerus, femur, tibia, fibula, and a separate group for split hand/foot. It is beyond the scope of this book to discuss all congenital limb deficiencies individually. But the attending clinician must be aware of the associated anomalies that are seen in some of these disorders; a few of them are listed in Table 4.3.

Management of such a deficiency needs a multidisciplinary team effort, which includes physicians, obstetricians, orthopedicians, neurologists, cardiologists, physiotherapists, medical geneticists, clinical psychologists, etc. (Figure 4.10). The management of each child has to be tailored accordingly to provide an accurate diagnosis, treat the deficiency, offer adequate surgical procedures after counseling of both the patients and child/adolescent, give adequate prosthetic/orthotic rehabilitation, and frequent follow-ups to monitor the acceptability of the treatment.

REFERENCES

1. Gold NB, Westgate M-N, Holmes LB. Anatomic and etiological classification of congenital limb deficiencies. *Am J Med Genet Part A.* 2011;155(6):1225–1235.
2. Hershkovich O, Tenenbaum S, Gordon B, Bruck N, Thein R, Derazne E, et al. A large-scale study on epidemiology and risk factors for chronic ankle instability in young adults. *J Foot Ankle Surg.* 2015;54(2):183–187.
3. Evans JA, Vitez M, Czeizel A. Congenital abnormalities associated with limb deficiency defects: A population study based on cases from the Hungarian Congenital Malformation Registry (1975–1984). *Am J Med Genet.* 1994;49(1):52–66.
4. Froster UG, Baird PA. Congenital defects of lower limbs and associated malformations: A population based study. *Am J Med Genet.* 1993;45(1):60–64.
5. Froster UG, Baird PA. Upper limb deficiencies and associated malformations: A population-based study. *Am J Med Genet.* 1992;44(6):767–781.
6. Wilcox WR, Coulter CP, Schmitz ML. Congenital limb deficiency disorders. *Clin Perinatol.* 2015;42(2):281–300.
7. Frantz CH, O'Rahilly R. Congenital skeletal limb deficiencies. *JBJS.* 1961;43(8):1202–1224.
8. Day HJB. The ISO/ISPO classification of congenital limb deficiency. *Prosthet Orthot Int.* 1991;15(2):67–69.
9. Hamamy H. Consanguineous marriages: Preconception consultation in primary health care settings. *J Community Genet.* 2012;3(3):185–192.
10. Bennett RL, Motulsky AG, Bittles A, Hudgins L, Uhrich S, Doyle DL, et al. Genetic counseling and screening of consanguineous couples and their offspring: Recommendations of the National Society of Genetic Counselors. *J Genet Counseling.* 2002;11(2):97–119.
11. Kalamchi A. *Congenital lower limb deficiencies.* New York: Springer, 1989.
12. Koskimies E, Lindfors N, Gissler M, Peltonen J, Nietosvaara Y. Congenital upper limb deficiencies and associated malformations in Finland: A population-based study. *J Hand Surg.* 2011;36(6):1058–1065.
13. Epps CH. Proximal femoral focal deficiency: Evaluation and management. *Orthopedics.* 1991;14(7):775–784.
14. Herring JA. *Tachdjian's pediatric orthopaedics e-book: From the Texas Scottish Rite hospital for children.* Philadelphia: Elsevier Health Sciences, 2013.
15. Rogala EJ, Wynne-Davies R, Littlejohn A, Gormley J. Congenital limb anomalies: Frequency and aetiological factors: Data from the Edinburgh Register of the Newborn (1964–68). *J Med Genet.* 1974;11(3):221–233.

5

Examination of Pediatric Shoulder

SHARAD PRABHAKAR AND AMAN HOODA

5.1 INTRODUCTION

Shoulder injuries are common and account for up to 10% of all sports injuries in high school athletes.[1] Shoulder injuries in the pediatric age group differ from adults. In children and adolescents, open growth plates predispose them to unique injuries requiring special techniques to diagnose and treat them.[2]

Physical examination of the shoulder requires the evaluation of the glenohumeral, acromioclavicular, and sternoclavicular joints and the scapulothoracic articulation. Physical examination tests of the shoulder have high sensitivity but low specificity.[3] A good medical history, combined with a detailed physical examination, usually provides the necessary information to obtain an accurate diagnosis.[3]

5.2 CLINICAL ANATOMY

The glenohumeral joint is a ball and socket joint that depends on the muscles and ligaments rather than its bony architecture for its support, stability, and integrity. It resembles a golf ball on its tee. The circumferential fibrocartilaginous labrum deepens the glenoid cavity of the scapula by about 50%. The glenoid has a 5° superior inclination and is retroverted by 5–7°. The humeral neck-shaft angle is about 130°, and the humeral head is retroverted 30–40°. The soft tissue structures around the shoulder are the glenohumeral ligaments, coracohumeral ligaments, glenoid labrum, and the rotator cuff muscles. While the superior, middle, and inferior glenohumeral ligaments are static stabilizers, the rotator cuff muscles, pectoralis major, latissimus dorsi, scapular muscles, and the deltoid are dynamic stabilizers.

5.3 HISTORY

A good clinical history, coupled with a systematic shoulder examination, helps to pinpoint the diagnosis. Most commonly, patients complain of pain, especially on movement, restricted motion, and/or shoulder instability. The patients' age is important as various pathologies have predominant age groups; for instance, instability issues are more common in younger patients, while rotator cuff pathologies are not common in children.[4]

In the young athlete, a detailed history of athletic complaints should include age, the onset of symptoms, mechanism of injury, site of pain, its nature and onset, along with activities that exacerbate the pain and those that relieve it. The athlete's sport, position as a player, and the level of competition are important. A review of general health and other joint involvement is necessary to document during history-taking.

If there was a traumatic incident, the details regarding the injury, whether the patient was able to move his/her arm immediately after the injury, and the treatment received should be noted. For instance, in throwing athletes, the possibility of superior labral tear from anterior to posterior (SLAP) lesion should be suspected. A note should also be made of any injections to the shoulder, if any.

The cervical spine should be evaluated as part of the overall shoulder problem because cervical pathologies and thoracic outlet syndrome can have radiating pain in the shoulder. Remember that subdiaphragmatic collection can present as shoulder pain due to irritation of the phrenic nerve. In cases of instability, the attitude of the limb that reproduces the instability, the number of episodes, and the ease of dislocation/reduction should be noted. Beware of the habitual dislocator, who can dislocate and reduce his shoulder himself. Such patients require muscle training rather than any surgical intervention! The patient's hand dominance, occupation, functional demand, and functional disability should be carefully noted.

5.4 EXAMINATION

Before starting a local examination, a general examination is imperative. The Beighton scoring system[5] should be used to determine generalized laxity. Patients with scores of four or more have generalized laxity, and such patients may have multidirectional shoulder instability as well.

5.4.1 Inspection

The patient should be adequately exposed. Always respect the patient's right to privacy. If the patient is under 18 years of age, there should be a parent or guardian in the room. Female patients can be advised to wear a tank top, or an examination gown should be available. The shoulder is seen with the patient standing, sitting, or even lying in a supine position.

5.4.2 Attitude

A patient with an anterior dislocation supports his/her arm away from the body with corresponding flattening of the deltoid contour, more common in children. A patient with an inferior dislocation usually keeps the arm abducted, often touching the side of his ear. A posterior dislocation is often missed as the arm is in an adducted, internally rotated position while external rotation is severely limited. In infants, Erb's palsy presents with the arm lying by the side of the body and internally rotated with the elbow extended, forearm pronated, and the wrist and fingers partially palmar flexed (policeman's tip hand).[6]

5.4.3 From the Front

Observe the relationship of the head and neck to the shoulders. Asymmetry may be found in case of congenital torticollis, scoliosis, etc. Asymmetry in the bony contour of the clavicle may suggest a malunion or non-union of a clavicle fracture. An anterior fullness in the axillary fold with loss of deltoid contour suggests an anterior shoulder dislocation. Wasting of the deltoid will be seen in deltoid paralysis, axillary nerve injury, tuberculosis, or other chronic inflammatory cuff pathologies.

5.4.4 From the Side

Assess the deltoid contour. In instability patients, look for the presence of any sulcus below the acromion process when traction is applied to the arm. This is known as the sulcus sign. Causative factors include multidirectional instability or nerve injury, allowing inferior subluxation of the glenohumeral joint. Always remember to assess the sensations for the axillary nerve (regimental badge sign), especially in patients with traumatic shoulder dislocations so as not to miss an axillary nerve injury.

5.4.5 From the Back

The examiner again should note bony and soft tissue contours and body alignment. Attention should be directed to the muscles around the shoulder. A Sprengel's deformity is associated with a high riding scapula, whereas a short neck with a low hairline would suggest Klippel–Feil syndrome.

Winging of the scapula is a condition in which the scapula's medial border moves away from the posterior chest wall. Dynamic winging is seen in injury to the long thoracic nerve with serratus anterior weakness and spinal accessory nerve palsy causing trapezius weakness. Less commonly, involvement of the rhomboids, multidirectional instability, voluntary action, or a protective reflex in shoulder pain results in reversal of scapulohumeral rhythm. Spinal accessory nerve palsy and trapezius muscle deficiency cause the scapula to move laterally, with the inferior angle rotated laterally (occurs before 90° abduction, and there is little winging on forward flexion). Long thoracic nerve palsy causes the scapula to elevate and move medially, with the inferior angle rotating medially on abduction and forward flexion. Dynamic winging is also seen with painful shoulder pathologies leading to reverse origin-insertion of the rotator cuff muscles so that instead of the humerus, the scapula starts to move. Static winging is usually caused by a structural deformity of the scapula, clavicle, spine, or ribs.

5.4.6 Palpation

Use a systematic approach and always follow the same sequence during examination. We usually start the palpation from the midline, i.e., the sternoclavicular joint. An increase in temperature, tenderness, or step deformities can be identified. This is followed by palpation of the suprasternal notch, sternocleidomastoid muscle, and the first rib. Palpate the costochondral junctions if suspecting costochondritis or Teitze syndrome. Next, both clavicles are palpated. At the concavity of the clavicle, palpate the coracoid a finger's breadth below the clavicle. Be gentle in doing this because even the normal coracoid may be a bit tender on palpation. Always compare with the opposite side.

Continue along the clavicle to the acromioclavicular joint. Identification of this joint can be by feeling a small dip just beyond the lateral edge of the clavicle. Next, palpate the lateral tip of the acromion and move inferiorly to the greater tuberosity of the humerus.

External–internal rotation of the humerus allows sequential palpation of the long head of the biceps in the bicipital groove, followed by the lesser tuberosity and the subscapularis tendon (*De Anquin test*).

Now palpate the anterior humeral head with the fingers while the thumb is over the posterior humeral head. The humeral head can also be grasped and translated anteriorly and posteriorly to assess joint laxity. The joint line can be determined by rotating the humerus while palpating. Often a line is drawn on the sagittal plane over the acromioclavicular joint as surface-marking for the shoulder joint (Figure 5.1).

Palpate the spine and medial border of the scapula. Also, palpate the trapezius muscle and the rhomboids and at the inferior scapular angle, the latissimus dorsi. Palpate the serratus anterior along the lateral scapular border. Also, palpate the supraspinatus and infraspinatus fossae and the cervical and thoracic spinous processes.

The axilla should also be examined. The shoulder is abducted slightly to 15–20°, and the axilla is felt for any lymph nodes, the pectoralis major tendon in the anterior fold, and the latissimus dorsi muscle in the posterior fold.

5.4.7 Movements

Movements of any joint are assessed and documented as active and passive movement. Often,

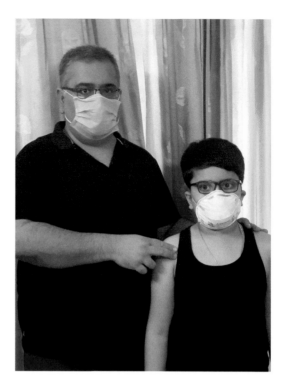

Figure 5.1 Demonstrating tenderness over the shoulder region.

patients with reduced active range of motion due to pain or cuff tears have normal passive range of motion. However, secondary frozen shoulder sets in quickly, limiting both active and passive motion. Passive movement allows the character of the restriction of motion to be assessed. The shoulder may feel soft and supple or "creaky" and "grinding" especially with chronic tears and impingement. Always compare with the other side.

5.4.7.1 FORWARD ELEVATION (RANGE 160–180°)

The primary elevators are the anterior deltoid and coracobrachialis, with the secondary flexors being the pectoralis major and the biceps. Stand in front of the patient and ask them to raise both arms to the ceiling. If there is a difference between the two sides, passively test elevation by standing behind the patient and stabilizing the scapula with the palm over the acromion and elevating the arm with the other hand. Limitation of forward elevation may be seen in cuff tears (passive elevation is full) or shoulder stiffness secondary to adhesive capsulitis (both active and passive are restricted).

5.4.7.2 EXTERNAL ROTATION (RANGE 80–90°)

The primary external rotators are the infraspinatus and the teres minor, with the posterior portion of the deltoid as a secondary rotator. Ask the patient to flex both elbows with the patient's arms by the side of the chest with the elbows tucked in to prevent the patient from substituting with adduction. The patient is now asked to rotate the arms outwards. Again, if there is a difference between the two sides, passively test by continuing the stabilization of the elbow into the waist and holding the forearm with the other hand and moving it outwards (Figure 5.2). In massive cuff tears, active external rotation is less than the other side. Furthermore, the patient is unable to maintain maximum external rotation even if the forearm is passively externally rotated (*lag sign*). Limitation of both active and passive external rotation is characteristic of a frozen shoulder.

5.4.7.3 INTERNAL ROTATION (NORMAL RANGE 60–100°)

The subscapularis, pectoralis major, latissimus dorsi, and the teres major are the principal internal rotators, with the anterior deltoid as the secondary internal rotator. The patient is asked to touch the midline of his/her back and to take the hand up as high as possible. Internal rotation is recorded as to hip pocket/beltline/D12/D7 (Figure 5.3). Painful internal rotation with stiffness is classically seen in cuff tears and advanced frozen shoulder.

5.4.7.4 ABDUCTION (NORMAL RANGE 170–180°)

The principle abductors are the middle deltoid and the supraspinatus.

Normally, the abduction at the shoulder happens via the scapulohumeral rhythm, which comprises movement of the humerus, scapula, and clavicle. This is divided into three phases as follows:

Phase 1: Humerus 30° abduction (initiation by the supraspinatus)
Scapula minimal movement (setting phase)
Clavicle 0–5° elevation

Phase 2: Humerus further 40° abduction (deltoid takes over)
20° of scapular rotation, with minimal protraction or elevation, making a total of 60° of abduction in this phase (2:1 ratio)

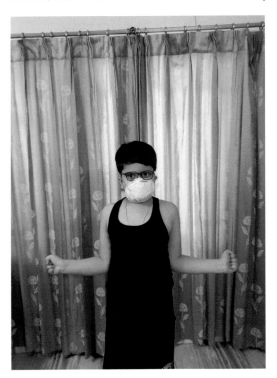

Figure 5.2 External rotation movement at shoulder joint.

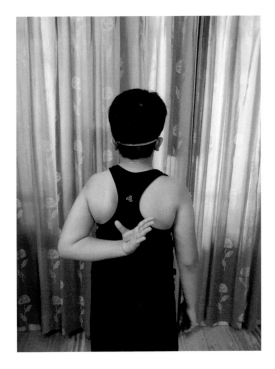

Figure 5.3 Internal rotation movement at shoulder joint.

Clavicle 15° elevation

Phase 3: Humerus further 60° abduction and 90° external rotation to clear the greater tuberosity from the acromion process

Scapula 30° rotation making total abduction 90° in this phase at 2:1 ratio

Clavicle 30–50° posterior rotation and up to 15° elevation

5.4.7.4.1 The Painful Arc Sign

As the patient abducts the shoulder, the impingement of the inflamed structures under the acromion between 60° and 120° of abduction presents as the painful arc sign. There is no pain in abduction up to 60°, followed by a painful arc, and if full abduction is possible, the pain diminishes after 120° as the tuberosity rotates out from under the acromion. If the patient has pain in terminal abduction, it is often caused by pathology in the acromioclavicular joint.

5.4.7.5 ADDUCTION (NORMAL RANGE 50–75°)

The pectoralis major and the latissimus dorsi are the primary adductors, whereas the teres major and the anterior deltoid are the secondary muscles. To accomplish this movement, the patient is asked to touch the opposite shoulder. This is known as the cross body adduction test and elicits tenderness over the acromioclavicular joint if symptomatic (Figure 5.4).

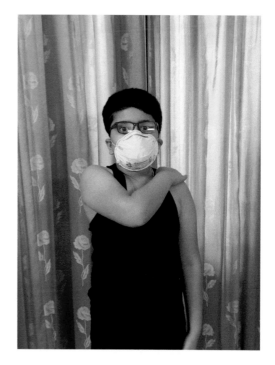

Figure 5.4 Adduction movement at shoulder joint demonstrated by touching the opposite shoulder.

5.4.7.6 SCAPULAR ELEVATION

The primary elevators are the trapezius and the levator scapulae, with the rhomboids being secondary elevators. Observe shoulder shrugs from the back while looking for any abnormal winging (Figure 5.5).

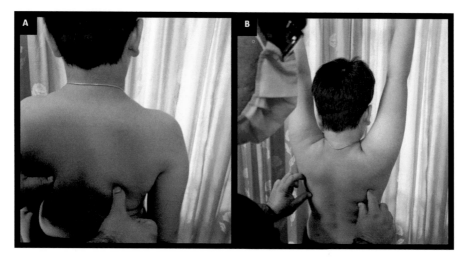

Figure 5.5 Scapular elevation. (a) Thumbs pointing to the lower pole of the scapula, (b) demonstration of the scapular elevation.

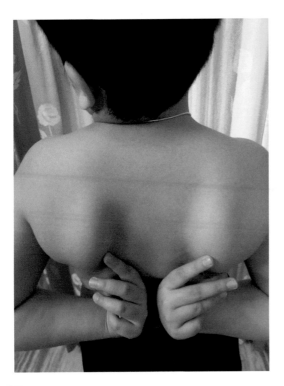

Figure 5.6 Scapular retraction.

5.4.7.7 SCAPULAR RETRACTION AND PROTRACTION

The rhomboids are the primary retractors, and the trapezius muscle is the secondary muscle. Observe from the back while instructing the patient to stand at attention.

Protraction of the scapula is enabled by the serratus anterior. Ask the patient to touch the opposite shoulder while observing from the back. Place one hand over the patient's spine to prevent substitution by trunk rotation and instruct the patient to reach further behind the opposite shoulder and look at the protraction of the scapula. Feel for any crepitus over the scapular body, which may suggest a snapping scapula (Figure 5.6).

5.4.7.7.1 Apley's Scratch Test

A quick method to test all the movements of the shoulder is to perform the *Apley's scratch test*, which involves reaching behind the head and touching the superior medial angle of the opposite scapula to assess abduction and external rotation. This is followed by reaching in front of the head and touching the opposite acromion to assess internal rotation and adduction. Touching the inferior

angle of the scapula by reaching behind the back also allows the assessment of internal rotation.

5.4.7.8 MEASUREMENTS

The length of the arm is measured from the angle of the acromion to the lateral epicondyle of the humerus. Using a fixed bony point like the lateral epicondyle, circumferential measurement of the mid-arm should also be done to document muscle wasting at the same distance on both sides.

5.4.8 Anterior Instability Tests

5.4.8.1 APPREHENSION TEST

With the patient in a standing or supine position, the examiner abducts the arm to 90° and slowly externally rotates the shoulder. A positive test is indicated by a look or feeling of apprehension and resistance to further motion. The abduction is initially started with as little as 10°, and the shoulder externally rotated. The angle of abduction is gradually increased, from 10° to 90°. Those with a bony deformity have apprehension at a lesser degree of abduction (Figure 5.7).

5.4.8.2 FULCRUM TEST

The apprehension test can be converted into the fulcrum test with the patient in a supine position and a fist under the glenohumeral joint to act as a fulcrum (Figure 5.8).

5.4.8.3 LOAD AND SHIFT TEST

Ask the patient to rest the forearm on the thigh in a seated position. The examiner sits behind the patient and stabilizes the scapula with one hand over the shoulder while the other hand grasps the head of the humerus, carefully moving it anteriorly and posteriorly in the glenoid if necessary, to seat it properly in the glenoid fossa. This is the load portion of the test. The examiner then tries to translate the humeral head anteriorly or posteriorly, and the amount of translation and end feel are noted. This is the shift portion of the test (Figure 5.9).

The anterior glenohumeral translation is graded as follows:

Normal laxity	Mild translation (0–25%)
Grade I	Humeral head riding up to the rim (25–50%)

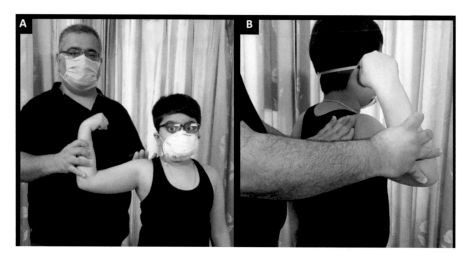

Figure 5.7 Apprehension test. (a) Anterior view, (b) lateral view.

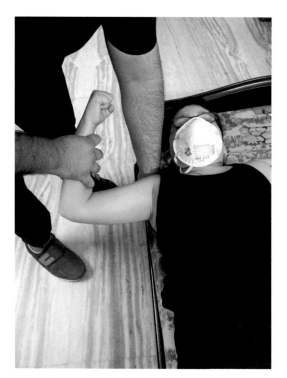

Figure 5.8 Fulcrum test.

| Grade II | Head riding over the rim but reduces spontaneously (>50%) |
| Grade III | Head riding over the rim and remains dislocated |

For posterior translation, usually 50% of translation of the humeral head may be considered normal but should be compared with the other side.

Reproduction of the patient's symptoms in addition to translation is considered confirmatory.

5.4.9 Posterior Instability Tests

The load and shift test is conducted, as described in Section 5.4.9.3.

5.4.9.1 POSTERIOR APPREHENSION TEST

The test can be performed with the patient in the supine or sitting position. The examiner stabilizes the scapula with one hand (when done in a sitting position) and elevates the patient's shoulder in the plane of the scapula to 90° with the other. The examiner then applies a posterior force on the patient's elbow and horizontally adducts and internally rotates the shoulder. This essentially recreates the provocative position for a posterior dislocation. A positive result is indicated by the appearance of apprehension, and the patient resisting any further motion.

5.4.9.2 POSTERIOR DRAWER TEST

The patient is placed in the supine position. The forearm is held with one hand while the elbow is flexed to 120° and the shoulder to between 80° and 120° of abduction and between 20° and 30° of forward elevation. The scapula is stabilized by placing the index and middle fingers on the spine of the scapula and the thumb on the coracoid process. The arm is internally rotated and flexed to between 60° and 80°, and at the same time, the

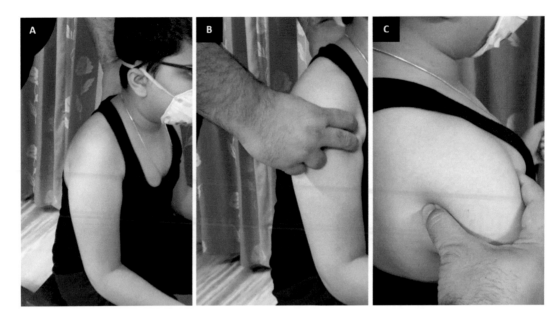

Figure 5.9 Load shift test. (a) Sitting position of patient, (b) hold the proximal humerus of the patient and shift anteriorly, (c) closer view of load shift test.

thumb is taken off the coracoid process, and the head of the humerus is pushed posteriorly. The head of the humerus is felt by the index finger of the same hand. A translation greater than 50% of the humeral diameter is considered as positive.

5.4.9.3 JERK TEST

The patient is seated with the arm internally rotated and forward flexed to 90°. The examiner axially loads the humerus in a proximal direction by grasping at the elbow. While maintaining the axial loading, the arm is horizontally adducted across the body. The production of a sudden jerk or clunk as the humeral head slides off the back of the glenoid is regarded as a positive test. When the arm is returned to the original 90° abducted position, a second jerk of reduction of the head may be felt.

5.4.10 Tests for Inferior and Multidirectional Instability

5.4.10.1 SULCUS SIGN

With the patient standing, the arm by the side, the patient's forearm is held firmly, and the arm is pulled distally. The presence of a sulcus below the acromion process indicates inferior instability. The sulcus sign with a sensation of subluxation is more clinically significant.[7]

The sulcus sign is graded by measuring from the inferior margin of the acromion to the humeral head:

+1 sulcus   distance of less than 1 cm
+2 sulcus   distance of 1 cm to 2 cm
+3 sulcus   distance of more than 2 cm

5.4.10.2 FEAGIN TEST

The Feagin test is a modification of the sulcus sign test with the arm abducted to 90° and is supported on the examiner's shoulders. This test can be done either in a sitting or standing position. The examiner's hands are clasped together over the patient's humerus, between the upper and middle thirds. The examiner pushes the humerus down and forward. A sulcus may be seen as described before. If both the sulcus sign and Feagin test are positive, it is a greater indication of multidirectional instability.

5.4.11 Tests for the Anteriorly Dislocated Shoulder

5.4.11.1 HAMILTON RULER TEST

Normally, a straight ruler cannot be made to touch both the acromion process and the lateral epicondyle of the humerus simultaneously as the greater tuberosity pushes the ruler away. In the case of an

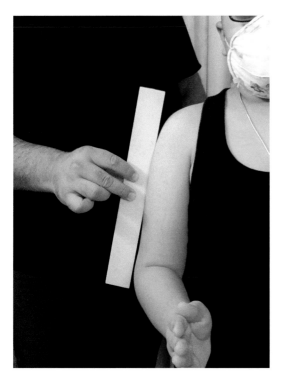

Figure 5.10 Hamilton ruler test.

anterior dislocation, this would become possible (Figure 5.10).

5.4.11.2 DUGAS TEST

In the event of dislocation, the patient will not be able to touch the contralateral shoulder while the arm is kept in contact by the side of the chest.

5.4.12 Tests for Scapular Instability

The scapula must be stabilized by its muscles to act as a firm base for the glenohumeral muscles in order for the muscles of the glenohumeral joint to work in a normal coordinated fashion.

5.4.12.1 LATERAL SCAPULAR SLIDE TEST/ SCAPULAR LOAD TEST

The patient sits or stands with the arm at the side. The examiner measures the distance from the D2 spinous process to the superior angle of the scapula, from the base of the spine of the scapula to the spinous process of D3, or from the inferior angle of the scapula to the spinous process of D7–D9. The patient is then asked to hold the arm at 45° abduction, 90° abduction with internal rotation, 120° abduction, and 150° abduction. In each of these positions, the distance measured should not

vary more than 1 cm to 1.5 cm from the original measurement. However, there may be increased distances above 90° as the scapula rotates during scapulohumeral rhythm.

The test may also be performed by providing resistance at 45° and greater abduction. This is known as the scapular load test to see how the scapula stabilizes under dynamic load.

5.4.12.2 WALL PUSHUP TEST

Ask the patient to do wall pushups 15–20 times, standing at an arm's length from a wall.

Any weakness of the scapular muscles or winging will usually show up with 5–10 pushups.

5.4.13 Impingement Tests

5.4.13.1 NEERS IMPINGEMENT SIGN AND TEST

The test is designed to detect the involvement of the supraspinatus tendon. With the patient in a sitting position, the examiner stands behind the patient. One hand of the examiner stabilizes the scapula while the patient's arm is passively fully elevated in an internally rotated position in the scapular plane resulting in compression of the greater tuberosity against the anteroinferior border of the acromion. Pain produced by this maneuver reflects a positive test result (Neers impingement sign).[8] Patients with other shoulder conditions like instability may also have pain during this test. However, pain due to these other causes is not relieved by the injection of 10 ml of 1.0% xylocaine beneath the anterior acromion. This is known as a positive impingement test (Figure 5.11).

5.4.13.2 HAWKINS–KENNEDY IMPINGEMENT TEST

With the patient standing, the examiner forward flexes the arm to 90° and then internally rotates the shoulder. This compresses the supraspinatus tendon against the coracoacromial ligament and coracoid process. Pain indicates a positive test for supraspinatus tendinosis.

5.4.14 Tests for Muscles Around the Shoulder

5.4.14.1 BICEPS TENDON

5.4.14.1.1 Yergason's Test

This test assesses the ability of the transverse humeral ligament to hold the biceps tendon in the

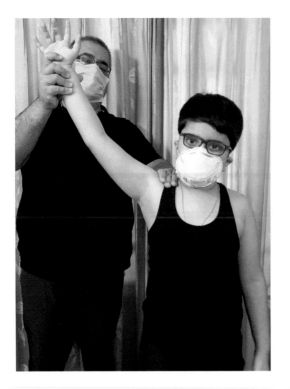

Figure 5.11 Neer's impingement test.

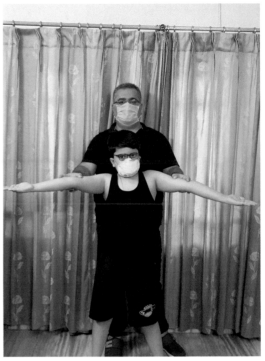

Figure 5.12 Speed test.

bicipital groove. The examiner flexes the patient's elbow to 90°, stabilizes it against the waist, and pronates the forearm. Now the patient is asked to supinate the forearm against resistance. Tenderness in the bicipital groove with or without a pop-out sensation indicates bicipital tendinosis.

5.4.14.1.2 Speed's Test (Biceps or Straight-Arm Test)

Resisted shoulder forward flexion with fully extended elbow is done initially in supinated position (thumbs up position) and next with the forearm in pronation (thumbs down position). The test is said to be positive when the patient complains of pain in the bicipital groove, especially with the arm supinated. This test may give a false-positive result in SLAP lesions (Figure 5.12).

5.4.14.2 SUPRASPINATUS AND ROTATOR CUFF COMPLEX

5.4.14.2.1 Supraspinatus ("Empty Can"/ Jobe) Test

The patient is asked to forward elevate and internally rotate the shoulders in the plane of the scapula with the thumbs pointing toward the floor. This is known as "empty can" position. If the patient has pain or weakness on resistance to abduction, it is a positive test result. This would be indicative of a tear of the supraspinatus tendon or neuropathy of the suprascapular nerve.

5.4.14.2.2 Drop-Arm (Codman's) Test

The patient's shoulder is passively abducted to 90°, and then the patient is asked to slowly lower the arm to the side. The inability to do so in a controlled manner is a positive test and suggestive of a large cuff tear.

5.4.14.3 SUBSCAPULARIS MUSCLE

5.4.14.3.1 Lift-Off Test

In the standing position, the patient is asked to take his/her hand to the back. The patient is then asked to use their hand to push the examiner's hand away from the back. The inability to do so is indicative of a subscapularis lesion.

5.4.14.3.2 Belly Press Test

This test is utilized when the patient cannot internally rotate the shoulder adequately to take it behind the back. The patient is asked to place their hand on their belly while keeping the wrist and elbow in a straight line. The examiner attempts to pull the forearm away from the abdomen. The inability to sustain the positioning hand on the belly against the examiner's force indicates a sub-scapularis tear (Figure 5.13).

5.4.14.4 INFRASPINATUS AND TERES MINOR MUSCLES

5.4.14.4.1 Infraspinatus Test

The patient stands with the arm at the side with the elbow at 90°, and the humerus internally rotated to 45°. The examiner then applies an internal rotating force that the patient is asked to resist. Alternatively, the patient may be asked to externally rotate against resistance. Pain or weakness is indicative of a positive test for an infraspinatus tear (Figure 5.14).

15.4.14.4.2 Teres Minor Test

The patient is asked to lie in a prone position and place their hand on the opposite posterior iliac crest. The patient is then instructed to extend and adduct the arm against resistance. Pain and/or weakness indicates a positive test for teres minor strain.

5.4.14.5 TRAPEZIUS

The patient is seated and is asked to place the hands together over the head. The examiner stands behind the patient and attempts to push the elbows forward while looking for the contraction of the trapezius. To separately test the upper trapezius, elevate the shoulder with the arm slightly abducted or simultaneously resist shoulder abduction and head side flexion. If the shoulder is elevated with the arm by the side, levator scapulae and rhomboids are more likely to be involved.

The middle trapezius is tested with the patient in a prone position with the arm abducted to 90° and externally rotated. Then resistance is applied to the horizontal extension of the arm while watching for scapular retraction. If protraction of the scapula occurs, the middle fibers of the trapezius are weak.

To test the lower trapezius, the patient is again placed in a prone lying position with the arm abducted to 120° and the shoulder externally rotated. The examiner applies resistance to diagonal extension, watches for scapular retraction, and feels for the contraction of the muscle fibers. If scapular protraction occurs, the lower trapezius is weak.

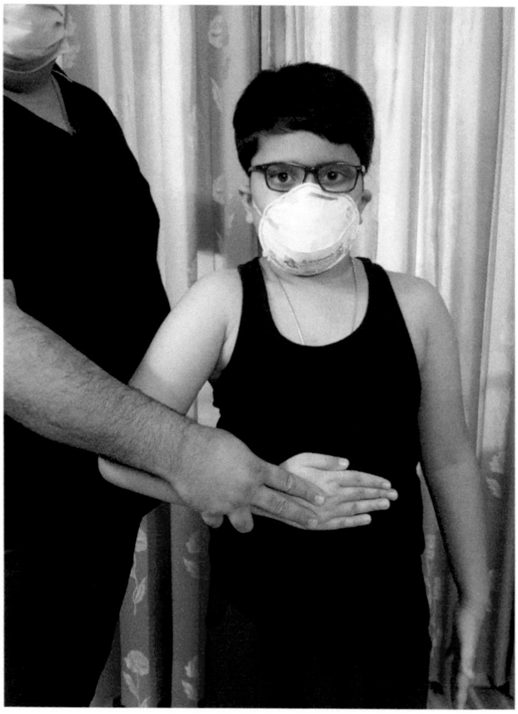

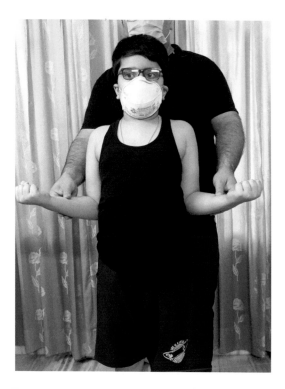

Figure 5.13 Belly press test.

Figure 5.14 External rotation against resistance.

5.4.14.6 SERRATUS ANTERIOR

With the patient standing, forward flex the arm to 90° and apply a backward force to the arm, instructing the patient to maintain the position. If the serratus anterior is weak or paralyzed, the medial border of the scapula will wing. A similar finding can be elicited by doing a wall or floor pushup.

5.4.14.7 RHOMBOIDS

The patient is asked to lie in a prone or sitting position, with the test arm behind the body so the hand is on the opposite side (opposite back pocket). The examiner places the index finger along and under the medial border of the scapula by asking the patient to push the shoulder forward slightly against resistance to relax the trapezius. The patient is then asked to raise the forearm and hand away from the body. If the rhomboids are normal, the finger is pushed away from under the scapula.

5.4.14.8 LATISSIMUS DORSI

The patient is in a standing position with the arms elevated in the plane of the scapula to 160°. Against the resistance of the examiner, the patient is asked to internally rotate and extend the arm downward as if climbing a ladder; feel for the contracting muscle.

5.4.15 Tests for the Labrum

Snyder classified the SLAP lesions into four types:

Type I: Superior labrum markedly frayed but attachments intact.
Type II: Superior labrum has a small tear, and there is instability of the labral-biceps complex (most common).
Type III: Bucket-handle tear of the labrum that may displace into joint; labral-biceps attachment intact.
Type IV: Bucket-handle tears of the labrum that extends to the biceps tendon, allowing the tendon to subluxate into the joint.

5.4.15.1 CLUNK TEST

The patient lies in the supine position, and the examiner places one hand on the back of the shoulder over the humeral head, and the other hand holds the humerus above the elbow. The examiner fully abducts the arm over the patient's head. The examiner then pushes anteriorly with the hand over the humeral while the other hand rotates the humerus into external rotation. A clunk or grinding sound indicates a positive test and is indicative of a tear of the labrum.

5.4.15.2 O'BRIEN'S ACTIVE COMPRESSION TEST

The patient is in the standing position with the arm forward flexed to 90°, elbow fully extended, and the arm is then horizontally adducted 10–15° and internally rotated with the thumb facing downward. The examiner stands behind the patient and applies a downward eccentric force to the arm while the patient is instructed to hold the position. Now the forearm is supinated, and the downward eccentric force is repeated.[9] If pain or painful clicking is produced inside the shoulder (not over the acromioclavicular joint) in the first part of the test and eliminated or decreased in the second part, the test is considered positive for labral abnormalities (Figure 5.15).

5.4.16 Tests for the Acromioclavicular Joint

5.4.16.1 ACROMIOCLAVICULAR SHEAR TEST

With the patient in a sitting position, the examiner cups his or her hands over the deltoid muscle,

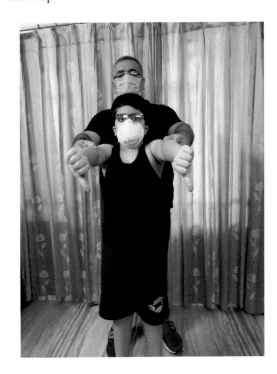

Figure 5.15 O'Brien test.

with one hand on the clavicle and one hand on the spine of the scapula. The examiner then squeezes the heels of the hands together. Pain or abnormal movement at the acromioclavicular (AC) joint indicates a positive test and is suggestive of AC joint pathology.

5.4.16.2 ACROMIOCLAVICULAR CROSSOVER/CROSS BODY OR HORIZONTAL ADDUCTION TEST

The patient stands/sits and reaches the hand across to the opposite shoulder. The test may also be performed passively by the examiner. If localized pain is felt over the acromioclavicular joint, the test is positive.

5.4.17 Miscellaneous Tests

5.4.17.1 TESTS FOR THORACIC OUTLET SYNDROME

5.4.17.1.1 Roos Test/Hands Up Test/ Abduction and External Rotation Test/Elevated Arm Stress Test

The patient stands and abducts the arms to 90°, externally rotates the shoulder, and flexes the elbows to 90°. The patient then alternatively opens and closes the hands slowly for 3 minutes. If the patient is unable to keep the arms in the starting position for 3 minutes or suffers ischemic pain, heaviness or profound weakness of the arm, or numbness and tingling of the hand during the 3 minutes, the test is considered positive for thoracic outlet syndrome on the affected side.[10]

5.4.17.1.2 Wright Maneuver

Here the arms are hyper abducted so that the hand is brought over the head with the shoulder externally rotated. The pulse is palpated for differences. The pulse disappearance indicates a positive test result for thoracic outlet syndrome.

5.4.17.1.3 Allen Maneuver

This is a modification of the Wright test. The examiner flexes the patient's elbow to 90° while the shoulder is extended horizontally and rotated externally. The patient is asked to rotate the head away from the test side. The examiner palpates the radial pulse, which becomes absent (disappears) when the head is rotated away from the test side.

The neurological examination of the various muscle groups and examination of the cervical spine will be dealt with Chapters 12 and 14.

REFERENCES

1. Bonza JE, Fields SK, Yard EE, Dawn Comstock R. Shoulder injuries among United States high school athletes during the 2005–2006 and 2006–2007 school years. *J Athl Train.* 2009;44(1):76–83.
2. Maffulli N, Caine D. The younger athlete. In: Brukner P, Khan K, editors. *Clinical sports medicine*, 4th ed. Sydney: McGraw-Hill; 2012, pp. 888–909.
3. Dhatt SS, Prabhakar S, editors. *Handbook of examination in orthopaedics: An illustrated guide.* Singapore: Springer publications, 2019.
4. Chen FS, Diaz VA, Loebenberg M, Rosen JE. Shoulder and elbow injuries in the skeletally immature athlete. *J Am Acad Orthop Surg.* 2005;13(3):172–185.
5. Singh H, McKay M, Baldwin J, Nicholson L, Chan C, Burns J, Hiller CE. Beighton scores and cut-offs across the lifespan: Cross-sectional study of an Australian population. *Rheumatology.* 2017; 56(11):1857–1864.
6. Chater M, Camfield P, Camfield C. Erb's palsy – who is to blame and what will happen? *Paediatr Child Health.* 2004;9(8):556–560.
7. Emery R, Mullaji A. Glenohumeral joint instability in normal adolescents. Incidence and significance. *J Bone Joint Surg Br.* 1991;73B(3):406–408.
8. Patel DR, Breisach S. Evaluation and management of shoulder pain in skeletally immature athletes. *Transl Pediatr.* 2017;6(3):181–189.
9. Edmonds EW, Roocroft JH, Parikh SN. Spectrum of operative childhood intra-articular shoulder pathology. *J Child Orthop.* 2014;8(4):337–340.
10. Rehemutula A, Zhang L, Chen L, Chen D, Gu Y. Managing pediatric thoracic outlet syndrome. *Ital J Pediatr [Internet].* 2015 Mar 27. [cited 2020 Jul 30];41.

Examination of Pediatric Elbow

KARTHICK RANGASAMY, NIRMAL RAJ GOPINATHAN, AND PEBAM SUDESH

6.1 INTRODUCTION

The elbow joint is a complex hinge (trochogingly-moid) joint that permits flexion, extension, and an axial rotation of the forearm. It consists of three articulations, namely humeroulnar, radiocapitel-lar, and proximal radioulnar joint. Flexion and extension movement takes place at the ulnohu-meral joint. Movement of pronation and supina-tion occur at the radiocapitellar joint and proximal radioulnar joint.

Although pediatric elbow fractures are the second most common injuries next only to fractures of the forearm and wrist,[1,2] they are particularly important as they need careful attention to ensure a correct diagnosis. Due to its unique anatomy and mostly cartilaginous nature, pediatric elbow stands as a challenging diagnostic environment for clinicians. A thorough understanding of anatomy, systematic clinical examination, and correct radiology allows the clinician to manage these injuries better.

6.2 ANATOMY OF THE ELBOW JOINT

On extension, the elbow joint line is tilted laterally as the trochlear medial flange is 6 mm longer than the lateral flange and results in the carrying angle of the elbow.

6.2.1 Stability of the Elbow Joint

Elbow joint stability is assisted by static or passive elbow stabilizers and dynamic or active elbow stabilizers. Static stabilizers include osteoarticular surfaces at the elbow joint, medial collateral ligament, lateral collateral ligament, and the joint capsule. Articular surfaces of the olecranon and trochlea of the humerus provide bony stability. Muscles crossing the elbow joint provide dynamic stability.[3]

6.2.2 Ligaments of the Elbow Joint

- *The medial collateral ligament* (Figure 6.1) gives protection during valgus stress of the elbow. It consists of three parts[4]:
  - *The anterior oblique ligament* provides stability on the medial side of the elbow joint and protects from excessive valgus stress. It is the strongest ligament extending from the humeral medial epicondyle to the sublime tubercle on the coronoid process of the ulna.
  - *The posterior oblique ligament* extends from the medial epicondyle to the olecranon process of the ulna by running posteriorly.
  - *The transverse ligament*, which is also called Cooper's ligament, runs from the olecranon to the coronoid process of the ulna between the anterior and posterior oblique ligament.
- *The lateral collateral ligament* (Figure 6.2) includes three parts, namely the annular ligament, lateral ulnar collateral ligament, and radial collateral ligament. It provides posterolateral rotational stability and protects against varus stress on the elbow.[5]

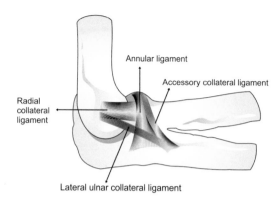

Figure 6.2 Anatomy of lateral collateral ligament.

- *The lateral ulnar collateral ligament* is the major stabilizer extending from the humeral lateral epicondyle to the supinator crest on the ulna.
- *The radial collateral ligament* originates from the lateral humeral epicondyle and inserts on the annular ligament.
- *The annular ligament* has its origin and insertion at the sigmoid notch of the ulna and it wraps around the radial neck. It stabilizes the proximal radioulnar joint.
- *The accessory lateral collateral ligament* begins at the annular ligament and inserts at the supinator crest on the ulna. It reinforces the annular ligament.

6.2.3 Joint Capsule

The elbow joint is enclosed by a fibrous capsule that is lined with synovial membrane. The anterior capsule gets taut during extension, and the posterior capsule gets taut during flexion. The capacity of the elbow joint is around 20 cc.[6]

Anteriorly, the capsule extends from the margins of the capitellum and trochlea of the humerus to the coronoid process of the ulna and annular ligament. Posteriorly, it extends from above the olecranon fossa to the annular ligament and olecranon tip. Most of the remaining part of the olecranon remains extracapsular. Three fibrous bands reinforce the capsule both anteriorly and posteriorly. The fibrous capsule is thickened to form collateral ligaments medially and laterally, which strengthen the elbow joint. The anterior capsule provides valgus stability during extension.[7] The

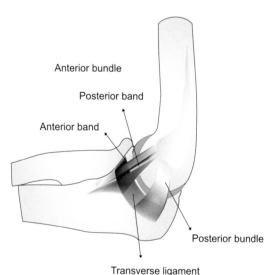

Figure 6.1 Anatomy of medial collateral ligament.

posterior capsule counters flexion and forces that are directed posteriorly.[8]

6.2.4 Muscles of the Elbow Joint

Muscles that cross over and attach around the elbow joint are responsible for providing secondary stabilization of the joint by protecting it against varus and valgus forces. The anconeus provides dynamic restraint to the varus and posterolateral rotatory instability.

Muscles that protect against valgus forces are the flexor carpi radialis, flexor carpi ulnaris, flexor digitorum superficialis, and also pronator teres.[4] Muscles that provide varus stability are the extensor digitorum communis, extensor carpi radialis longus, extensor carpi radialis brevis, anconeus, and extensor carpi ulnaris.[4]

6.3 HISTORY

- *Age.* The age of the child is very important. A pulled elbow or "nursemaid's elbow" occurs mostly due to longitudinal traction of the forearm. It is common between the age of 1–4 years[9] and rarely occurs after 5 years due to the development of the orbicular ligament. Supracondylar humerus fractures are common in the age group of 5–8 years. Distal humerus physeal separation is commonly seen in an age of less than 2 years and may be mistaken for elbow dislocation due to the cartilaginous nature of the distal humerus and not being visualized in radiographs.
- *Mechanism of injury.* The nature of the injury and the mechanism/attitude of the limb at the time of injury determines the injury sustained. For example, a fall on an outstretched hand (FOOSH) with the elbow in extension can result in an extension type of supracondylar humerus fracture. A FOOSH injury with hyperpronation most commonly causes Monteggia fractures. The fracture pattern is also influenced by the patient's age and the level of skeletal maturity.

For chronic injuries, overuse, or sports participation should be asked. Pain in the medial elbow is common in overhead athletes and little league baseball pitchers. The pain usually occurs due to repeated trauma to the ossification center and also medial condyle apophysis.

- *Pain.* If the child complains of pain, inquire about the location, onset, duration, characteristic/quality, radiation, association with fever, or trauma. Referred pain to the elbow from other sites such as the cervical spine, shoulder, and wrist must be ruled out by asking for any restriction of movements, pain at those sites, muscle weakness, or numbness at extremities.
- *Swelling.* Inquire about the onset, duration, location, progression, single or multiple sites, and any associated constitutional symptoms like fever or weight loss. Any history of massage or manipulation that may be overlooked is important and may suggest myositis.
- *Deformity.* Find out whether it is congenital or acquired. Few disorders may not be appreciable at birth but may present later with deformities/restricted range of motion (Figures 6.3 and 6.4). Also, it is important to document its association with fever, trauma, or swelling. It is important to inquire whether the deformity is progressive or static.
- *Restriction of movements.* Ask about any limitation in flexion/extension and/or axial rotation of the forearm. Inquire whether there is any difficulty in performing activities of daily living or difficulty in sports participation.

6.4 INSPECTION

Prerequisite. With adequate exposure of both upper limbs up to shoulder level, examine the elbow on both sides together in an identical position. The normal elbow and the affected elbow must be compared and assessed from all the sides (anterior, posterior, lateral, and medial aspect).

Attitude. A careful inspection of the child when he/she enters the clinic gives, to a certain extent, a clue to the diagnosis. A young child with a swollen flexed elbow supported by his/her other hand is suggestive of acute injury to the elbow, probably a case of supracondylar fracture of the humerus.

In the case of a pulled elbow, the child will often hold the arm in slight flexion with the forearm pronated (known as the "nursemaid's position").

6.4.1 Look from the Front

- *Position of the joint.* Whether flexed or extended, pronated, or supinated. In most

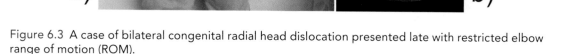

Figure 6.3 A case of bilateral congenital radial head dislocation presented late with restricted elbow range of motion (ROM).

cases of injury to the elbow, the joint is held in a flexed position.

- *Carrying angle*. For children who can fully extend their elbow, the carrying angle is measured and compared with the opposite side. The carrying angle is the angle formed between the long axes of the arm and the supinated forearm in a fully extended elbow. Measurement is done with arms by the side, elbow in full extension, and forearm in supination. The normal carrying angle varies but is generally between 5° and 15° (more in females than in males). The angle disappears on pronation and cannot be documented on elbow flexion. In cubitus valgus, the carrying angle is abnormally increased compared to the normal opposite side. Causes are non-union lateral condyle of the humerus or any injury resulting in premature closure of the lateral portion of the distal humeral physis. In cubitus varus or gunstock deformity, the carrying angle is abnormally decreased compared to the contralateral side, and most results are a malunited supracondylar (SC) humerus fracture. (Figure 6.5).

6.4.2 From Behind

Look for olecranon prominence. In children, unduly prominence of the olecranon most commonly results from the extension type of supracondylar humerus fracture. It can also be seen in a posterior elbow dislocation. Tenting of triceps can be seen in old neglected posterior elbow dislocation.

6.4.3 From the Side

Look for elbow hyperextension or flexion deformity. Any visible swelling in the lateral soft spot is

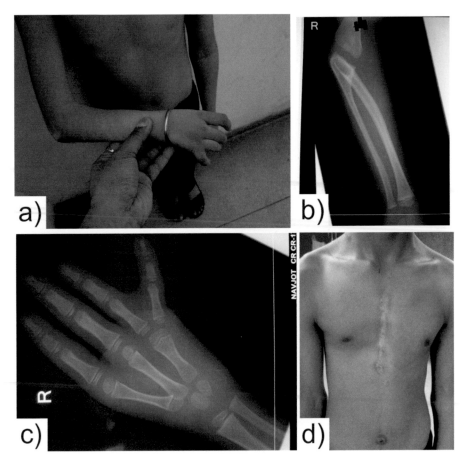

Figure 6.4 A case of proximal radioulnar synostosis along with cardiac anomaly and with an absent thumb.

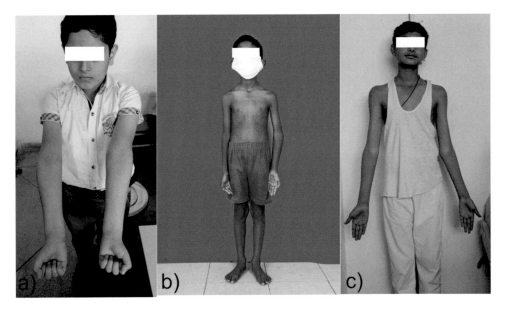

Figure 6.5 (a) Cubitus rectus, (b) cubitus varus of left elbow, (c) cubitus valgus of left elbow.

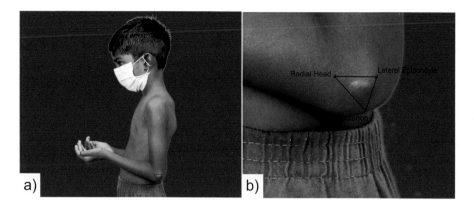

Figure 6.6 Lateral soft spot.

suggestive of joint effusion. It is a triangle connecting the lateral epicondyle, the tip of the olecranon, and the head of the radius (Figure 6.6).

Anteroposterior widening of the elbow can be seen in posterior dislocation and can also be seen in an SC humerus fracture with distal fragment in gross hyperextension. From all sides, look for any swelling, ecchymosis, abrasions in case of acute injury, surgical scar in case of previous surgery, or any discharging sinus/puckered scar in case of chronic infection. In chronic cases, look for atrophy of muscles and joint contracture.

Muscles around the elbow joint mostly cross the wrist joint and small joints of the hand as well. So, look for any muscle wasting and contracture in the forearm and hand. Brachial artery injury in SC humerus fracture or missed compartment syndrome may lead to Volkmann's contracture.

6.5 PALPATION

Always compare with the contralateral side.

Feel for local warmth with the back of the hand and exert gentle pressure to elicit superficial tenderness. Feel for any swelling and examine scars and sinuses if present. Palpate the soft tissues across the elbow gently and check for abnormality like any bony mass (myositis mass) within the soft tissue, especially brachialis muscle. The lateral soft spot is a triangular area formed between the lateral epicondyle, head of the radius, and olecranon tip. Palpate the *lateral soft spot* area for any fullness that may suggest joint effusion. When it comes to palpating bony landmarks, begin from the normal area, then progress toward the affected area.

Bony landmarks around the elbow are systematically palpated for any tenderness, bony irregularity, displacement, abnormal mobility, and crepitus, etc. Palpate the supracondylar ridges, medial and lateral epicondyles, assess the three bony point relationship, olecranon process, proximal ulna, and head of the radius.

6.5.1 Lateral and Medial Epicondyle

The lateral epicondyle is the most prominent bony point on the lateral aspect of the distal humerus, and it is palpated by flexing the elbow to 90°. The lateral supracondylar ridge will be traced downwards, and the most prominent bony landmark beneath, which is the bone, starts receding and will be marked as the lateral epicondyle. Tenderness over this area may be due to lateral epicondylitis/apophysitis, depending on the age of the child or fracture of the lateral condyle or supracondylar humerus.

The medial epicondyle is the most prominent subcutaneous landmark on the medial aspect and is marked by tracing downwards from the medial supracondylar ridge. Tenderness is present in case of medial epicondylitis/apophysitis or ulna collateral injury, depending on the child's age. Ulnar collateral incompetence or avulsion injury is more common in older children. The ulnar nerve can be palpated or rolled under the finger for any thickening on the back of the medial epicondyle.

6.5.2 Palpation of Supracondylar Ridges

Keep the elbow in a semi-flexed position and the forearm in supination. Hold the forearm with one

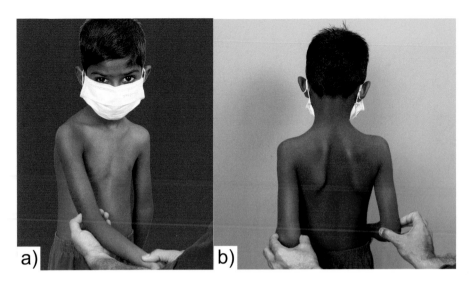

Figure 6.7 Palpation of supracondylar ridges.

hand. Use the thumb along with the index finger from the other hand to palpate the medial epicondyle and lateral epicondyles, respectively. Then palpate upwards to feel for the supracondylar ridges and also assess for any irregularity over the area. They can be simultaneously palpated by asking the child to flex the elbow to 90° and the examiner palpating from behind using the thumb along with the index/middle finger of both hands along the ridges (Figure 6.7).

6.5.3 Head of Radius

With the elbow in a flexed position, palpate the lateral epicondyle with the thumb and move downwards to identify the initial depression, which is the radiocapitellar joint, and immediately distal to that is the radial head. The radial head can be located easily by performing a simultaneous movement of supination and pronation and palpating the corresponding movements of the radial head. Tenderness may be elicited in acute trauma (radial neck fractures are common in children rather than head fractures).

If there is pain on the application of pressure at the radiocapitellar joint in addition to axial load, supination, and pronation of the forearm, it is suggestive of Panner's disease. It is osteochondrosis of the capitellum in preadolescent children.

6.5.4 The Proximal Ulna and Olecranon Process

Ulna palpation is easier as it is subcutaneous posteriorly. Palpate along the subcutaneous border of

the ulna to detect any bony irregularity or tenderness. If we suspect a proximal ulna fracture, the clinician should simultaneously palpate the radial head also to identify Monteggia fractures/ variants.

The olecranon is the most prominent bony landmark felt posteriorly in a flexed elbow and palpated by moving the fingers proximally along the subcutaneous border of the ulna. It may be tender in an olecranon fracture, and abnormal projection of the olecranon process posteriorly may be seen in an SC humerus fracture in children and posterior dislocation of the elbow in adults. Swelling resulting from olecranon bursitis (student's elbow) will be more distinct and sharply demarcated like a "goose egg" over the olecranon process. Olecranon apophysitis may present as a point of tenderness in the olecranon and along with triceps insertion due to overuse.

Examination of the posterior aspect of the elbow for any pathology can be done with the elbow in a 25–30° flexion position as it unlocks the olecranon process and humerus along with the relaxation of the triceps muscle. Palpate for any fullness and tenderness over the medial and lateral aspects on the posterior side of the olecranon fossa. Adolescents who play overhead throwing games may have tenderness along the superior and medial margin of the olecranon process following a valgus extension overload called posterior impingement.[10]

6.5.5 Three-Point Bony Relationship

The relationship can be demonstrated from the front or behind. When examined from the front, the child places both the palms over his/her head, which flexes the elbow slightly more than 90° and both the triangles can be compared side by side. The two epicondyles of the humerus and tip of the olecranon process are palpated with the thumb, middle finger, and index finger. Another way of doing this is to ask the child to place the palm on the waist, which flexes the elbow to 90°, and the triangles can be compared from behind. In a normal extended elbow joint, these three bony points lie on a straight horizontal line but on flexing the elbow to 90° they form a triangle. Confusion regarding the accurate interrelationship exists even in standard orthopedic books/literature, labeled by various authors as an isosceles triangle, equilateral type, or a different triangle. Dhillon et al. observed 200 normal elbows and found that this triangle is neither isosceles nor equilateral, but a scalene triangle of unequal sides.[11] Always compare with the opposite sound side in an identical position of the elbow to the deformed side (ideally 90° elbow flexion). The three-point bony relationship is maintained in malunited supracondylar humerus fracture, and lateral limb length is increased in lateral condyle humerus fracture (Figure 6.8).

Finally, palpate the epitrochlear lymph nodes in the subcutaneous connective tissue on the anteromedial aspect of the elbow (adjacent and posterior to the basilic vein and superficial to the brachial fascia and medial intermuscular septum), about 2 cm to 3 cm above the medial epicondyle in a semi-flexed elbow for any enlargement. Usually, epitrochlear nodes are not clinically palpable unless altered by a pathological process such as infection or malignancy.

6.6 MOVEMENTS

The humeroulnar joint allows flexion and extension movement, and movements of pronation and supination occur at the radio humeral and superior radioulnar joint level. The normal range of motion at the elbow in the flexion–extension plane is considered to be 140° for flexion and 0° extension to −10° for hyperextension, which is assessed in a supinated forearm. The normal range of motion for pronation is 80° and for supination is 90°. Movement of flexion and extension can be demonstrated in sitting as well as standing posture, while hyperextension is best demonstrated in the standing position of a supinated forearm (Figure 6.9).

First, get the child to sit on the chair and place the posterior aspect of the arm from shoulder to elbow on the table in front of the child. Keep the forearm in supination and wrist and fingers in extension. From this position, ask the child to reach the table with the posterior aspect of the hand without elevating the shoulder, which can be described as the position of zero-extension. Next, ask the child to move the forearm toward the upper arm, which can demonstrate the flexion arc of the elbow (Figure 6.10). Movements should always be compared to the other side. For daily living activities, a functional range of motion from 30° to 130° of flexion is needed with about 50° of both pronation and supination.

Axial rotation of the forearm is measured with the child's elbow flexed to 90° and held at the waist. Start with the thumb pointed upward, rotation of the palm to face the ceiling/roof is supination, and rotation of the palm to face the floor is pronation (child can be given a pen/pencil on both hands for

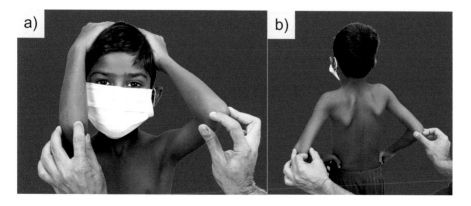

Figure 6.8 Three-point bony relationship.

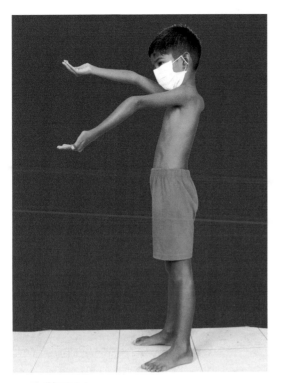

Figure 6.9 Hyperextension at the elbow in a case of malunited supracondylar humerus fracture.

comparison). The arc of movement is measured and compared simultaneously with the opposite side.

Forearm rotation can be demonstrated either by a passive or active method. The passive method can be best demonstrated by holding the lower end of the forearm to eliminate the carpal involvement in rotation and making the rotatory movement of pronation and supination. Active methods using the position of hand and thumb may result in over evaluation with regard to true forearm rotation due to the involvement of carpal rotation.

The increased internal rotation at the same side shoulder joint is noticed due to malunion of the distal humeral fragment in internal/medial rotation. It can be elicited by asking the child to abduct the shoulder joint to 90° and flexing the elbow to 90°; with the forearm acting as a lever arm, we can compare the shoulder joint rotation with the opposite side (Figure 6.11). Usually, in malunited SC humerus fracture, internal rotation at the shoulder increases with a decrease in external rotation (arc of motion range remains the same) when compared with the opposite sound side.

Yamamoto et al.[12] described a method to accurately measure the internal rotation of the shoulder joint. First, ask the child to bend forward, then ask him/her to keep their arm by their side and the shoulder joint in maximum extension while flexing the elbow to 90°. The examiner stands behind the child applying maximum internal rotation force to the child's upper limb around the long axis of the humerus. The angle formed between the horizontal plane of the back and the midline of the forearm is measured (Figure 6.12). Normally, the horizontal plane of the back and midline of the forearm lies parallel, and in case of internal rotation deformity because of cubitus varus, a certain abnormal angle will be formed, and this is termed the internal rotation angle. Remember that the hyperextension and internal rotation components are hallmarks of malunited supracondylar humerus fractures and differentiate it from cubitus varus due to malunited lateral condyle fractures.

6.7 MEASUREMENTS

Measurements will be taken with a flexed elbow to make the epicondyles prominent in a supinated forearm.

- The arm length should be measured starting from the acromion angle (posterolateral corner) to the lateral epicondyle of the humerus. Similarly, medial arm length can be measured from the angle of the acromion to the medial epicondyle of the humerus.
- The length of the forearm should be measured from the lateral humeral epicondyle to the distal point (tip) of the styloid process of the radius. The forearm length is shortened in the posterior dislocation of the elbow.
- *Three sides of the triangle* were measured after marking both epicondyles and the tip of the olecranon. Measurement should be done using a Vernier caliper and compared with the opposite side (Figure 6.13).

Measurement of the girth of the arm and forearm is done at the level of maximal muscle mass and compared with the opposite side for any wasting.

6.7.1 Measurement of Carrying Angle

Make the child stand with arms placed by the sides, elbow fully extended, and forearm in a supinated position.

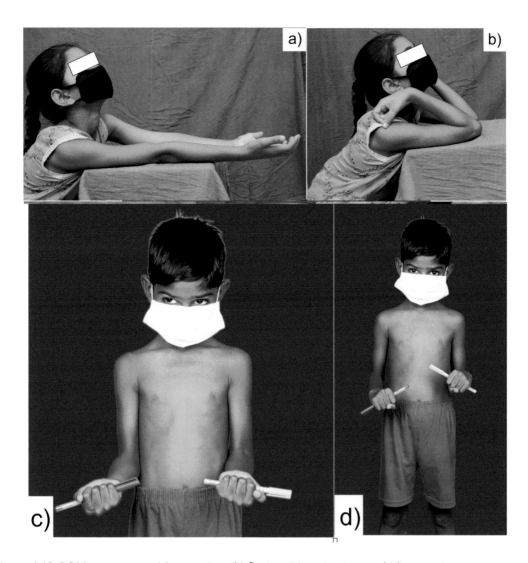

Figure 6.10 ROM assessment: (a) extension, (b) flexion, (c) supination, and (d) pronation.

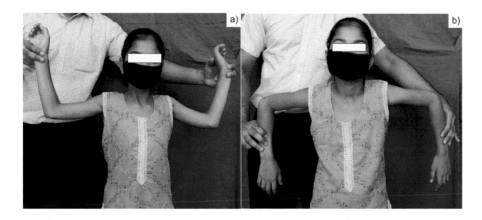

Figure 6.11 Shoulder rotation assessment in an abducted position of the shoulder.

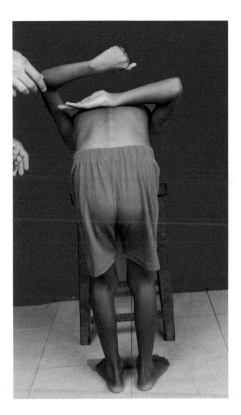

Figure 6.12 Yamamoto test for assessment of exaggerated internal rotation at shoulder joint.

First, draw a line from the anterior axillary fold to the lateral margin of the deltoid bulge. The center point of the line is marked as point A. The center point of the interepicondylar line in the distal humerus is marked as point B. Joining these two points, A and B, forms the long axis of the arm. Draw a line connecting the styloid process of the radius and styloid process of the ulna, which is called the interstyloid line. The center point of the interstyloid line is marked as point C. Joining points B and C forms the long axis of the forearm. The angle formed between the long axis of the arm and forearm will be the carrying angle and should be measured using a goniometer and compared with the contralateral side (Figure 6.14).

6.8 INSTABILITY TESTS

- *Valgus stress test.* To perform this test, place the elbow at around 30° flexion and the forearm in supination. Support the elbow on the lateral aspect with one hand. Next, using the other hand, give the valgus force from the medial side of the lower end of the forearm. Feel the medial collateral ligament (MCL) at the joint line medially while giving the valgus stress. The clinician should take note of the degree of medial joint line opening, nature of the endpoint, and perception of pain by the child. A positive test signifies medial collateral ligament tear (Figure 6.15).

- *Moving valgus stress test.* Keep the shoulder at 90° abduction along with full external rotation. The elbow should be kept in maximum flexion. In this position, apply valgus stress at the elbow while simultaneously extending the elbow to 30° flexion. This test assesses the integrity of the MCL. When pain is produced at the medial side of the elbow, particularly between 120° and 70°, it indicates a positive test. A positive test may be present in a partial tear of the MCL (Figure 6.16).

- *Modified milking maneuver.* To assess injuries to the MCL, the positioning of the shoulder should be in adduction and full external rotation. The forearm should be placed in supination along with 70° of elbow flexion. The clinician should then pull the patient's thumb with one hand to create valgus stress. The medial joint line is palpated using the other hand while the valgus stress is applied. Pain, laxity, and/or apprehension about the medial elbow by the patient reflects a positive test (Figure 6.17).

- *Varus instability test.* Keep the forearm in supination and the elbow at around 20–30° flexion. Stabilize the elbow on the medial side with one hand. Using the other hand, apply varus and adduction force from the lateral aspect of the lower forearm and examine the lateral collateral ligament at the joint line. Opening up of the joint line with excess laxity signifies lateral collateral ligament injury (Figure 6.15).

- *Posterolateral pivot shift test.* This is done to examine the stability of the posterolateral ligament complex at the elbow. The child is asked to lie down in the supine position, abduct the arm above the head, externally rotate the shoulder, extend the elbow, and supinate the forearm. The examiner should then apply valgus stress at the elbow together with axial load along the arm while at the same time flexing the elbow. When the elbow is flexed about 40°, a patient who has posterolateral ligament

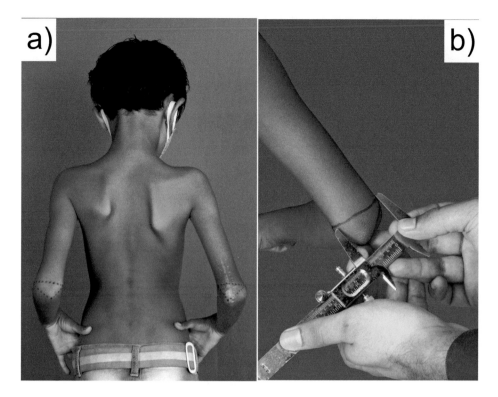

Figure 6.13 Three-point measurement with caliper.

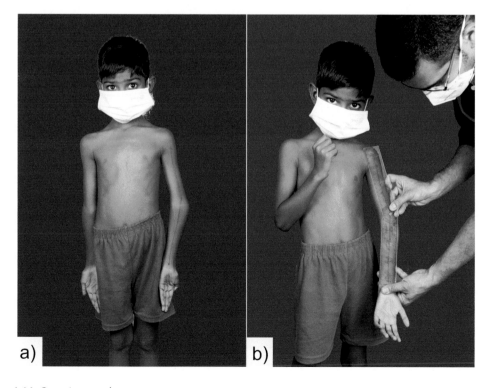

Figure 6.14 Carrying angle measurement.

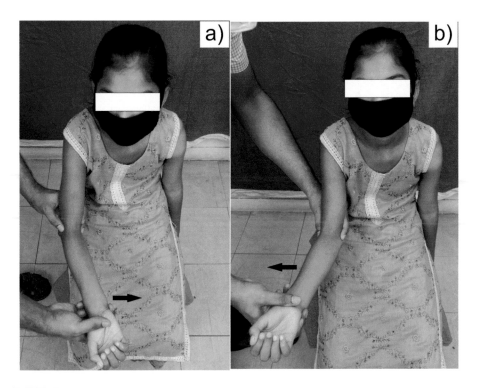

Figure 6.15 (a) Varus stress test and (b) valgus stress test.

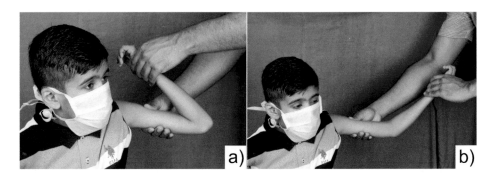

Figure 6.16 Moving valgus stress test.

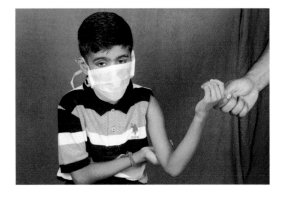

Figure 6.17 Modified milking maneuver.

instability experiences pain/uneasiness due to radial head subluxation posterolaterally, and a dimple can be seen proximal to the radial head. When the elbow is flexed further, the radial head bounces back to its place, and the patient can feel relieved. The test is considered positive with the subluxation of the radial head, followed by its reduction signifying posterolateral ligament instability (Figure 6.18).

These examination techniques are helpful for evaluating a certain group of chronic pathological conditions of the elbow, such as the

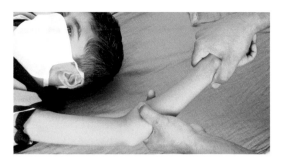

Figure 6.18 Posterolateral pivot shift test.

development of valgus instability following mal-union or non-union of a fracture at the medial epicondyle of the humerus. The development of posterolateral ligamentous instability follows certain conditions like dislocation of the elbow with injury to the lateral collateral ligament secondarily and also in cases with cubitus varus deformity following supracondylar humerus fracture in childhood.[10]

6.9 NEUROLOGICAL EXAMINATION

In children with acute as well as chronic elbow injuries, complete neurovascular assessment of the upper limb should be done. In the presence of neurological symptoms or signs in upper limb extremities, the entire upper limb along with the cervical spine, should be examined to distinguish the cause. Pain at the elbow without any local lesions could be referred pain from other sites such as the cervical spine, shoulder, or wrist. Therefore, an examination of these sites should also be done.

In acute scenarios, the examination should be started from the unaffected or normal area in a gentle manner as it helps reassure the child, and hence, they will be cooperative as it is not painful.

6.9.1 Motor Examination

Following any injury to an upper limb extremity, the motor function of the hand should be assessed by individually testing the function of the ulnar nerve, median nerve, and the radial nerve. In SC humerus fracture of the extension type, the most commonly injured nerve is the anterior interosseous nerve. It is a branch of the median nerve without any sensory component. The detailed examination of individual nerves is dealt with in Chapter 14.

One of the methods for examining a younger child includes playing the game called "rock-paper-scissors," in which rock assesses median nerve function, paper assesses the radial nerve, and scissors assesses the ulnar nerve. Most of the flexor muscles of the forearm and hand, along with the thenar muscles of the hand, are supplied by the median nerve. Roughly, the median nerve function can be tested by asking the patient to make a fist (indicates rock). The radial nerve that supplies the forearm and finger extensors can be grossly tested by asking the patient to show by hand gesture the paper shape (finger extension). Most of the intrinsic muscles of the hand, including the interossei and third/fourth lumbricals, are supplied by the ulnar nerve. The ulnar nerve can be tested by asking to show the scissors shape by hand gesture (active spreading of the extended index finger and middle finger) (Figure 6.19).[13]

6.9.2 Sensory Examination

A light touch is primarily tested by gently stroking the skin with a wisp of cotton and asking when the stimulus is sensed. Testing of the median nerve is done by gently touching the palmar side of the index finger and ulnar nerve by stroking the medial border of the little finger and radial nerve over the first dorsal web space.

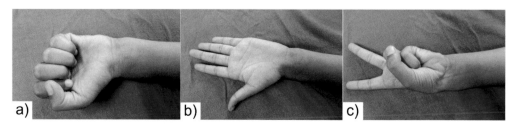

a) b) c)

Figure 6.19 (a) Rock, (b) paper, and (c) scissors test.

Detailed examination of distal limb perfusion – temperature (warmth/cold), finger perfusion (pink/pale), and radial pulse (palpable/ not palpable) – is very important in case of acute injuries around the elbow joint.

REFERENCES

1. Wingfield JJ, Ho CA, Abzug JM, Ritzman TF, Brighton BK. Open reduction techniques for supracondylar humerus fractures in children. *J Am Acad Orthop Surg.* 2015;23(12):e72–e80. doi:10.5435/JAAOS-D-15-00295
2. Larson AN, Garg S, Weller A, et al. Operative treatment of type II supracondylar humerus fractures: Does time to surgery affect complications? *J Pediatr Orthop.* 2014;34(4):382–387. doi:10.1097/BPO.0000000000000124
3. de Haan J, Schep NWL, Eygendaal D, Kleinrensink GJ, Tuinebreijer WE, den Hartog D. Stability of the elbow joint: Relevant anatomy and clinical implications of in vitro biomechanical studies. *Open Orthop. J.* 2011;5:168–176.
4. Card RK, Lowe JB. Anatomy, shoulder and upper limb, elbow joint. [Updated 2019 Jan 16]. In: *StatPearls* [Internet]. Treasure Island, FL: StatPearls Publishing; 2020. https://www.ncbi.nlm.nih.gov/books/NBK532948/
5. Aquilina AL, Grazette AJ. Clinical anatomy and assessment of the elbow. *Open Orthop J.* 2017;11:1347–1352.
6. Malagelada F., Dalmau-Pastor M., Vega J., Golanó P. Elbow anatomy. In: Doral M, Karlsson J, editors. *Sports injuries.* Berlin: Springer; 2014. https://doi.org/10.1007/978-3-642-36801-1_38-1
7. Morrey BF, An KN. Articular and ligamentous contributions to the stability of the elbow joint. *Am J Sports Med.* 1983;11(5):315–319.
8. Safran MR, Baillargeon D. Soft-tissue stabilizers of the elbow. *J Shoulder Elbow Surg.* 2005;14(1 Suppl S):179S–185S.
9. Schunk JE. Radial head subluxation: Epidemiology and treatment of 87 episodes. *Ann Emerg Med.* 1990;19(9):1019–1023. doi:10.1016/s0196-0644(05)82567-3
10. Varacallo M, Mody KS, Herman MJ. Physical examination of the pediatric elbow. In: Abzug JM et al. editors. *Pediatric elbow fractures.* Switzerland AG: Springer international publishing AG; 2018. pp. 13–21. https://doi.org/10.1007/978-3-319-68004-0_2
11. Dhillon MS, Gopinathan NR, Kumar V. Misconceptions about the three-point bony relationship of the elbow. *Indian J Orthop.* 2014;48(5):453–457.
12. Yamamoto I, Ishit S, Ogino T, Kaneda K. Cubitus varus deformity following supracondylar fracture of the humerus, a method for measuring rotational deformity. *Clin Orthop.* 1985;201:179–185.
13. Davidson AW. Rock-paper-scissors. *Injury.* 2003;34(1):61–63.

7

Examination of Pediatric Hand and Wrist

MOHSINA SUBAIR, SATYASWARUP TRIPATHY, AND RANJIT KUMAR SAHU

Accurate examination of the hand is necessary for deciding on appropriate diagnosis and treatment. It also ensures a good outcome in both acute and chronic conditions. General examination of the pediatric hand is similar to that of the adult, but it is more challenging depending on the child's age and cooperation.

7.1 SETTING UP HAND CLINIC AND ESTABLISHING RAPPORT WITH THE CHILD

Clinical examination of a child is a bit tricky as the child may not follow commands for various tests as described in adults. Hence, inspection and close observation play an important role in making the diagnosis. The child is often apprehensive and may not cooperate with a thorough examination. To overcome this, it is advisable to set up the clinic in a child-friendly manner. The use of colorful and familiar posters and toys to create a child-friendly environment is essential. Interacting with the child in the presence of the parents will further help establish rapport. This step is essential before proceeding to further examination of the child.

7.2 SURFACE ANATOMY OF THE HAND

Knowledge about the surface anatomy of the hand is essential for a thorough and systemic clinical evaluation of the hand.[1] A brief description of the important landmarks is covered in this chapter.

7.3 KEY TERMINOLOGIES

- Two surfaces:
  - Volar/palmar: Lined by glabrous skin in the palm region, flexor side.
  - Dorsal: Extensor side is referred to as the dorsal side.
  - Radial side: Side of the thumb.
  - Ulnar side: Side of little finger.
- Palmar surface (Figure 7.1a):
  - Thenar eminence: On the thumb side; formed by intrinsic muscles of the thumb.
  - Hypothenar eminence: On the little finger side, formed by intrinsic muscles of the little finger.
  - Palmar creases: Longitudinal and transverse creases are present.

- Kaplan's cardinal line: Transverse line from the apex of first web space to the pisiform bone running parallel to the proximal palmar crease.[2] Used as a surface guide during carpal tunnel surgery (Figure 7.2).
  - The intersection of Kaplan's line with a perpendicular line along the radial border of the middle finger corresponds to the recurrent motor branch of the median nerve and superficial palmar arch (Figure 7.2).
  - The intersection of Kaplan's line with a perpendicular line along the ulnar border of the ring finger corresponds to the distal margin of the transverse carpal ligament (Figure 7.2).
- Dorsal surface (Figure 7.1b):
  - Skin is thin and loose.
  - Extensor tendons and superficial veins are easily visible on the dorsum.
  - Knuckles: Formed by heads of metacarpal.

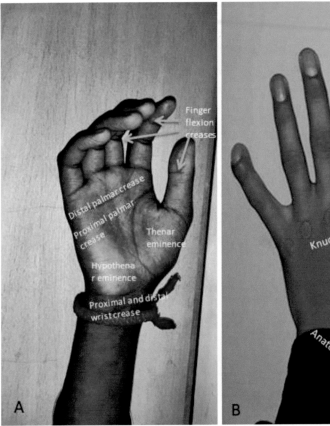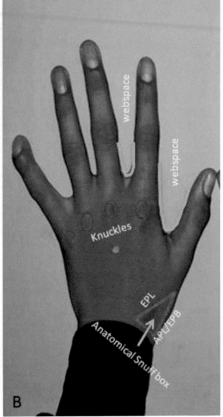

Figure 7.1 Surface anatomy of hand with key landmarks. (a) Palmar surface, (b) dorsal surface.

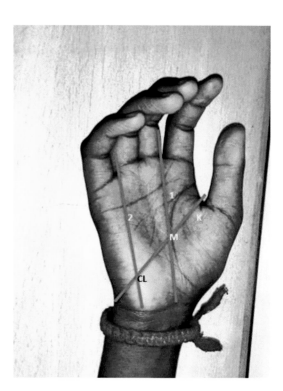

Figure 7.2 CL – distal margin of transverse carpal ligament, K – Kaplan's cardinal line, M – recurrent motor branch of median nerve and superficial palmar arch, 1 – perpendicular line along radial border of middle finger, 2 – perpendicular line along ulnar border of ring finger.

- Web spaces: Characteristic hourglass appearance.
- Intermetacarpal spaces formed by interossei muscles: Hollowing of these spaces indicates wasting of the muscles.
- Anatomical snuffbox: Triangular deepening bounded by abductor pollicis longus (APL) and extensor pollicis brevis (EPB) anteriorly and extensor pollicis longus (EPL) posteriorly.[3] The floor is formed by the scaphoid and trapezium.

7.4 HISTORY

A thorough history should include the following:

- General information such as age, sex, and hand dominance of the child.
- History regarding mode of onset – congenital or acquired.

- History of the duration of symptoms:
  - Acute: 7 days.
  - Subacute: 7–14 days.
  - Chronic: >14 days.
- Accurate history regarding the time and mechanism of injury and the environment and circumstances in which the injury was sustained in case of trauma.
- Various symptoms should be elucidated from the parents/proxy regarding pain, deformity, stiffness, weakness, and paresthesia.
- If congenital problem – antenatal history about drug intake, perinatal problems, details of mode of delivery, and post-natal period – developmental history needs to be elicited. History of similar problems in family (especially for disorders such as syndactyly or polydactyly).
- History of previous hand injuries.
- In older children, the child's activities, sports, music, etc. should be documented if relevant.

7.5 GENERAL EXAMINATION

Position yourself across from the patient with the patient's hand resting on the table. In the case of younger children, the child can be held comfortably by a parent to facilitate examination. Assess the nutritional status, growth, and developmental milestones, general appearance, and body proportions. In the case of congenital anomalies, other system evaluations such as cardiac, renal, vertebral, and examination of the cranium are important.

Instruments and materials required for a complete hand examination include:[4]

- Cotton and pin to assess soft touch and pain.
- Tuning fork to assess vibration (256 Hz).
- Goniometer to assess range of motions.
- Two-point discriminator/bent paper clip.
- Dynamometer.
- Hand-held Doppler.
- Materials such as a ball, bottle, card, and key to assess grasp and pinch.

7.5.1 Inspection

Inspection should be carried out after exposing the whole upper limb up to the shoulder girdle and neck.

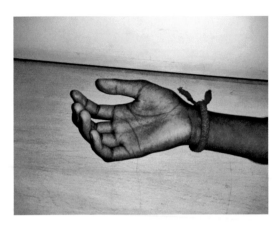

Figure 7.3 Normal digital cascade.

When unilateral, compare with the opposite side.

The following points need to be assessed in inspection:

- Assess how the child positions the hand and the resting posture of the hand:
  - Digital cascade: In a normal resting hand, all fingertips should face the scaphoid tuberosity with increasing flexion from index to little finger, with all nails in a plane parallel to the palm (Figure 7.3).
  - If there is any abnormality in the digital cascade, look for the following disorders:[5]
    - Bone: Metacarpal or phalangeal fractures.
    - Joints: Dislocation.
    - Tendons: Tendon injuries or deformity such as trigger finger, mallet finger.
    - Nerves: Claw hand in ulnar or median nerve injury, wrist, and finger drop in radial nerve injury.
- Skin discoloration and sweating pattern of the palm – loss of sweating and dryness can indicate chronic denervation.
- Swellings over hand:
  - Localized swellings such as paronychia, pulp or web space abscess, soft tissue, or bony lesions/tumors/vascular lesions/cysts.
  - Generalized swellings such as cellulitis or lymphangitis.
  - A few clinical examples are shown in Figure 7.4.
- Rule out signs of acute injury such as laceration/puncture wounds, redness, edema, hyperemia.
- Look for signs of chronic skin lesions, ulcerations, non-healing wounds, post-burn sequelae (Figure 7.5).
- Nail complex should be inspected:
  - Pitting/spots/brittle nails indicate systemic disease/nutritional deficiency/chronic nail infection.
- Trophic ulcers over the contact areas are indicative of nerve disorders.[6]
- Ask the child to flex fingers, oppose the thumb, and assess the hand's mass movements.

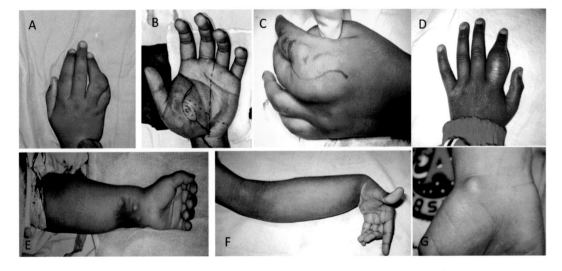

Figure 7.4 Hand swellings: (a) enchondroma, (b) vascular malformation, (c) vascular tumor, (d) tuberculous dactylitis, (e) hemangiopericytoma, (f) venous malformation of forearm, (g) ganglion of the wrist.

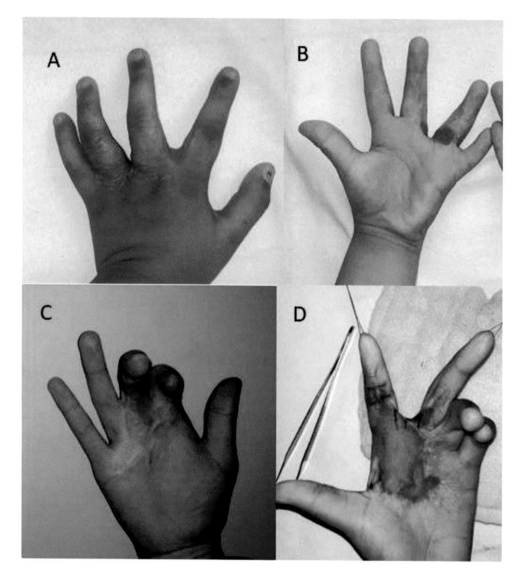

Figure 7.5 Post-burn sequelae in hand: (a) and (b) post-burn syndactyly, (c) post-burn flexion contracture, (d) post-burn web space contracture.

- Look at any signs of wasting:
  - Thenar muscle wasting – median nerve pathology.[6]
  - Hypothenar and interossei muscle wasting – ulnar nerve pathology.[6]
  - Forearm muscle wasting with flexion contracture of fingers – Volkmann ischemic contracture (Figure 7.6).
- Look for specific congenital abnormalities such as syndactyly, polydactyly, central hand deficiency, clinodactyly, Kirner's deformity, mirror hand, trigger thumb, thumb hypoplasia or duplication, club hand, constriction band syndrome, etc. (Figures 7.7 and 7.8).

7.5.2 Palpation

- Assess for temperature and tenderness.
- Localized increase in temperature – inflammatory condition; cold or decreased temperature – ischemic problems.
- Rub a pen/pencil against the palm of the child. A loss of resistance due to loss of sweating can indicate autonomic dysfunction.

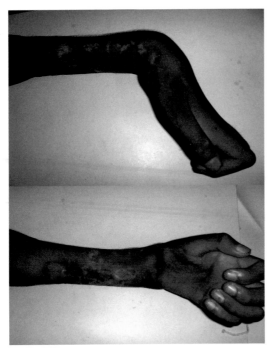

Figure 7.6 Volkmann ischemic contracture; forearm wasting with flexion contracture of wrist and fingers.

7.5.3 Functional Tests

Basic hand positions (Figure 7.9):

- Precision pinch: Holding a fine object between the tips of the thumb and index finger.
- Pulp pinch: Holding an object between the pulp of the thumb and index finger.
- Chuck grip: Holding an object between the tips of the thumb, index finger, and middle finger.
- Key pinch/lateral pinch: Holding a key between the thumb and lateral side of the index finger.
- Hook grip: Holding an object in a hooking motion with fingers.
- Span grasp: Span is the maximum distance attainable with active motion between the distal digital creases of the thumb and index finger.
- Power grasp: Holding an object with all four fingers and thumb.

7.6 SENSORY EXAMINATION

The hand can be divided into defined zones of sensory distribution:

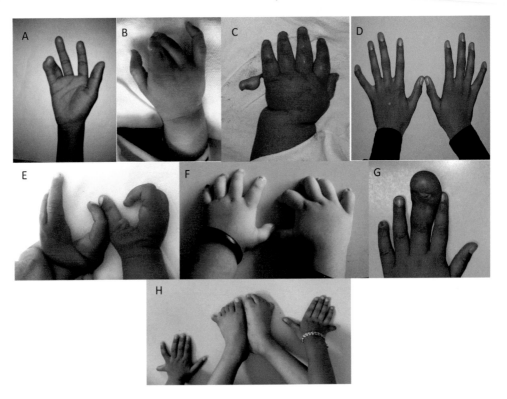

Figure 7.7 Congenital anomalies of hand: (a) and (b) syndactyly, (c) polydactyly, (d) Kirner's deformity, (e) cleft hand, (f) brachydactyly, (g) macrodactyly, (h) polydactyly of hand and feet.

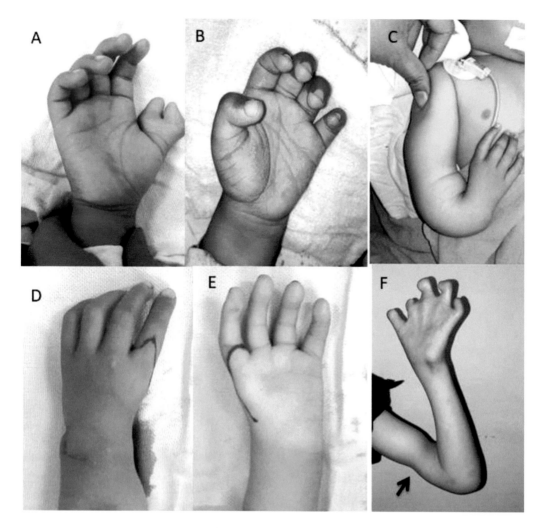

Figure 7.8 Congenital anomalies of hand: (a) thumb duplication, (b) trigger thumb, (c) radial club hand, (d) and (e) thumb hypoplasia, (f) auto-amputation of distal phalanges with constriction band syndrome (black arrow).

Palmar aspect: lateral 3½ fingers – median nerve; medial 1½ fingers – ulnar nerve.

Dorsal aspect: lateral 3½ fingers up to proximal interphalangeal (PIP) joint – radial nerve; distal to PIP joint – median nerve; medial 1½ fingers – ulnar nerve.

The sensory examination can be divided into two:

Tests for threshold – for sensations such as light touch, pain, temperature, and vibration:[4,7]

- This is carried out by providing stimulus to the sensory zones.
- Touch with finger or a fine object such as a cotton swab, pinprick for eliciting pain sensations, test-tube with warm and cold water for temperature, and a 256-Hz tuning fork for vibration can be utilized for examination.

Tests for innervation density – static and dynamic two-point discrimination:

- This can be done using a calibrated two-point discriminator or a bent paper clip.
- Perform the test from distal to proximal direction.
- The instrument points should be in a direction parallel to the longitudinal axis and carried out both on the ulnar and radial aspects of the finger. This will help prevent erroneous measurement of the adjacent digital nerve.

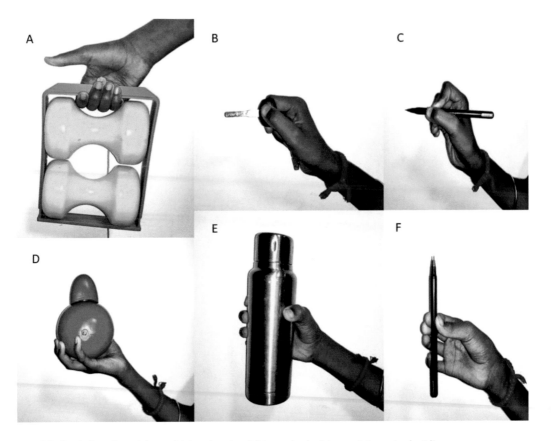

Figure 7.9 Basic hand positions: (a) hook grip, (b) key pinch, (c) precision pinch, (d) power grasp, (e) span grasp, (f) chuck grip.

- Static two-point discrimination: the two points are applied simultaneously, starting with 15 mm and sequentially brought together. The least distance the patient is able to discriminate is the measured value.[5,8]
- Dynamic two-point discrimination: move the caliper/paper clip along the borders of the digits.
- Reference values for static two-point discrimination for the hand are:
  - Distal to distal interphalangeal (DIP) joint 3–5 mm.
  - PIP joint to DIP joint 3–6 mm.
  - Metacarpophalangeal (MCP) joint to PIP joint 4–7 mm.
  - Palm 6–10 mm.
  - Dorsum 7–10 mm.

Examination of sensations is difficult to elicit in a younger child; pain can be evaluated by assessing the child's facial expression. The specific tests can be carried out in a cooperative older child.

7.7 MOTOR EXAMINATION

7.7.1 Power

This involves examination of the extrinsic and intrinsic muscles of the hand. Abnormal motor examination can occur due to musculotendinous problems or neurological problems. The tenodesis effect can be utilized to roughly differentiate between these two conditions.[9]

- Normal pattern of tenodesis – wrist extension produces finger flexion, and wrist flexion produces finger extension. This will be preserved in a purely neurological injury leading to loss of motion (Figure 7.10).
- Loss of normal tenodesis – indicates disrupted musculotendinous units.

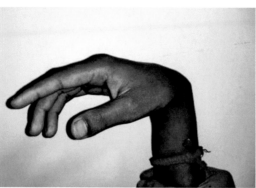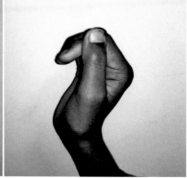

Figure 7.10 Normal pattern of tenodesis: (left) wrist flexion produces finger extension, (right) wrist extension produces finger flexion.

7.7.1.1 EXAMINATION OF TENDONS OF THE WRIST

- Wrist flexors: Ask the child to flex the wrist with fingers extended. Resistance can be provided by pressing the hand. Ask the child to flex in ulnar or radial deviated positions and palpate for the flexor carpi ulnaris (FCU) and flexor carpi radialis (FCR) tendons, respectively.
- Wrist extensors: Ask the child to extend the wrist with fingers flexed. Resistance can be provided by pressing the dorsum of the hand. Ask the child to extend the wrist in ulnar or radial deviated positions and palpate for extensor carpi ulnaris (ECU)/extensor carpi radialis longus and brevis (ECRL, ECRB) tendons, respectively.

7.7.1.2 EXAMINATION OF EXTRINSIC MUSCLES OF THE HAND

Place palm up, fingers extended while examining flexors, palm down while examining extensors and test the action on the joint on which tendon inserts:

- Flexor digitorum profundus (FDP): Block the PIP joint flexion and ask the child to flex the DIP joint (Figure 7.11).
- Flexor digitorum superficialis (FDS): Hold the DIP joints of the other fingers in extension and ask the child to flex the PIP joint of the finger being tested. The FDPs of the little, ring, and middle fingers have a common belly and hence will be eliminated by blocking the DIPs of the other fingers leading to the isolated action of the FDS (Figure 7.11).

- Testing the FDS of the index finger: Ask the child to touch the pulp of the thumb with pulp of index finger. If FDS is normal, there will be hyperextension of the DIP joint and flexion at the PIP joint. If FDS is weak/absent, there will be flexion at the DIP due to FDP action (Figure 7.11).
- Flexor pollicis longus (FPL): Block the MCP joint of the thumb and ask the child to flex the interphalangeal (IP) joint of the thumb against resistance (Figure 7.11).
- Extensor digitorum communis (EDC): Keep the wrist on the table with the IP joints flexed (to eliminate intrinsic action) and ask the child to extend the MCP joint. Resistance can be applied proximal to the PIP joint (Figure 7.12).
- Extensor indicis proprius and extensor digiti minimi: Ask the child to make a fist to nullify the action of EDC and instruct the child to extend the index finger and little finger, respectively (Figure 7.12).
- Extensor pollicis longus: Ask the child to lift the thumb from the table (Figure 7.12).
- Abductor pollicis longus: Ask the child to abduct the thumb away from the hand.
- Extensor pollicis brevis: Ask the child to extend the MCP joint of the thumb against resistance.

7.7.1.3 EXAMINATION OF INTRINSIC MUSCLES OF THE HAND

- Dorsal interossei: Keep the hand palm up on the table and try to push the index and ring finger toward the middle finger and instruct the patient to resist the action. For the middle

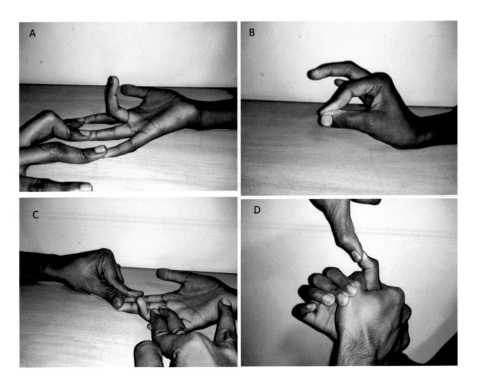

Figure 7.11 Examination of long flexors: (a) testing FDS of middle finger, (b) test for FDS of index finger, (c) testing FDP of ring finger, (d) testing FPL.

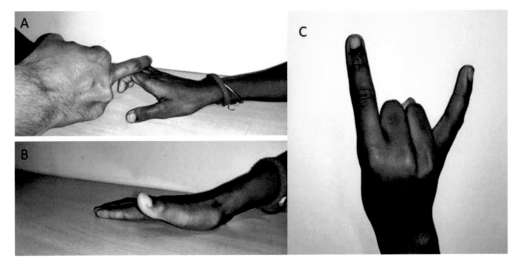

Figure 7.12 Examination of long extensors: (a) testing EDC, (b) test for EPL, (c) test for extensor indicis pollicis (EIP) and EDM.

finger, test against resistance when the patient tries to move it to either side.

- Palmar interossei: Ask the patient to hold a card between the extended and adducted fingers and try to pull it out (examiner should

also hold the card in the same position between the fingers) (Figure 7.13).

- Adductor pollicis: Ask the child to hold a card with the thumb against the palmar surface of the index finger and try to pull it out.

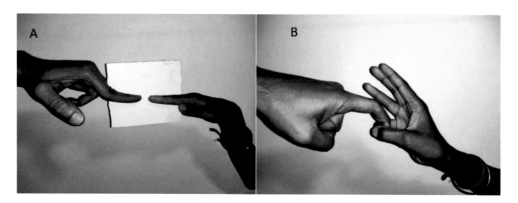

Figure 7.13 Examination of intrinsic muscles: (a) card test for palmar interossei, (b) test for opponens pollicis and opponens digiti minimi.

- Opponens pollicis and opponens digiti minimi: Ask the child to oppose the thumb and little finger in the form of an "o" and try to separate it while assessing the resistance (Figure 7.13).
- Abductor pollicis brevis: Keep the hand flat with palm up and ask the child to move the thumb perpendicular to the plane of the palm while applying resistance.
- Abductor digiti minimi: Ask the child to abduct the little finger against resistance and feel for muscle contraction.
- Intrinsic tightness: Bunnell test – compare IP flexion with the MCP joint flexed and extended. The test is considered positive and suggestive of intrinsic tightness if PIP flexion is limited with the MCP joint extended.[9,10]

7.7.2 Examination of Nerves

There are several named signs and tests for peripheral nerve examination. However, it is difficult to carry out these examinations on a younger child. In older children, these cannot be carried out unless the child is cooperative and follows commands.

The named tests pertaining to specific nerves are explained in the following sections.

7.7.2.1 MEDIAN NERVE

- Ape thumb deformity: the thumb lies supinated in the same plane as the palm as the thenar muscles are paralyzed, and opposition is lost.
- "O" test: Ask the child to make an "O" between the index finger and thumb and try to pull it apart. In median nerve injury, due to the paralysis of the FPL and FDP of the index finger, the DIP joint remains in extension and cannot form an "O."
- Ochsner's clasp test: Ask the child to clasp both hands with the fingers interlocked. The child will be unable to flex the index finger leading to a pointing index. This occurs due to paralysis of the long flexors of the index finger.
- Pen test: Keep the hand flat, palm up on the table. Keep a pen above perpendicular to the palm and ask the child to touch the pen with the thumb. The child cannot do this if the abductor pollicis brevis is paralyzed.

7.7.2.2 ULNAR NERVE

- Claw hand: Due to paralysis of intrinsic muscles, there is hyperextension of the MCP joint and flexion at the IP joints.
- Froment's sign: Ask the child to hold a card between the adducted and extended thumb and index finger and try to pull it out. If the adductor pollicis is paralyzed, the patient will try to hold by flexing the thumb IP joint using the FPL (supplied by the median nerve).
- Wartenberg's sign: Abduction of the little finger on extension of the fingers due to unopposed action of the extensor digiti minimi.
- Pitres–Testut sign: Inability to abduct the extended middle finger in either direction due to paralysis of the interossei.
- Jeanne's sign: Hyperextension of the thumb MCP joint during key pinch.
- Cross finger test: Inability to cross the index and ring finger over middle finger due to paralysis of the interossei muscles.

7.7.2.3 RADIAL NERVE

- Wrist and finger drop: Inability to extend the wrist and fingers at the MCP joint.

Birth brachial plexus palsy: It can be partial or pan brachial plexus injury. Erb's palsy is the most common type of partial injury characterized by the waiter's tip deformity (shoulder adducted, internally rotated, forearm pronated and wrist flexed; Figure 7.14).

7.7.3 Test for Ligament Stability

Compare with that of the opposite hand to assess laxity.

- Thumb, ulnar, and accessory collateral ligament. Stabilize the first metacarpal with one hand and use the other hand to hold the proximal phalanx and apply valgus stress. A valgus of >30° indicates a complete tear and <30° indicates a partial tear.
- Flexing the MCP joint to 30° and performing the test allows testing of the ulnar collateral ligament in isolation.
- Interphalangeal and metacarpophalangeal joint collateral ligament. Stabilize the hand proximal to the joint to be tested and apply the valgus and varus forces with the other hand to test the collateral ligaments.

7.7.4 Movements and Measurements

- Assess the passive and active range of movements at the shoulder, elbow, wrist, and small joints of the hand.
- The range of movements, such as flexion, extension, radial, and ulnar deviation, should be measured with a goniometer (Figure 7.15).
- For measuring movements at a particular joint, position the axis of the goniometer at the joint and the static arm on one bony axis. The

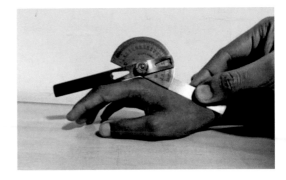

Figure 7.15 Measuring range of movements with goniometer.

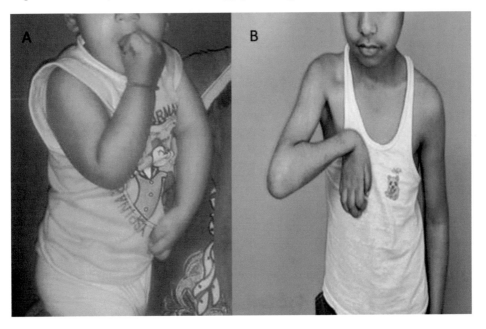

Figure 7.14 Birth brachial plexus palsy: (a) infant, (b) older child with untreated palsy.

Table 7.1 Normal Active Range of Motion in Fingers

Joint/Finger	Thumb°	Index Finger°	Middle Finger°	Ring Finger°	Little Finger°
CMC	−30 to 10	0	−10 to 0	−20 to 0	−30 to +10
MCP	−70 to 10	−90 to +20	−90 to +20	−90 to +20	−90 to +20
PIP	−90 to 0	−100 to 0	−100 to 0	−100 to 0	−100 to 0
DIP		−80 to 0	−80 to 0	−80 to 0	−80 to 0

Note: − indicates flexion and + indicates extension from neutral position.

moving limb measures the range of movements parallel to the other bony axis.

- The normal range of movements at various joints is shown in Table 7.1.[5,9]
- A passive range larger than the active range can indicate tendon adhesions/contractures.
- Assess passive tendon movements for flexor tendons:
  - Pressure on the forearm at the junction of the middle and distal third should cause flexion of the fingers through 1 cm and 2 cm.
  - This is particularly useful in younger children who do not cooperate for active movements.

7.7.5 Vascular Examination

Assess the pulse, capillary refill, and temperature:

- *Capillary refill*: Press the nail bed; blanching disappears, and color returns in 3 seconds. If a longer time is taken, suspect arterial problems.
- *Allen's test*: Palpate for the radial and ulnar pulses, obliterate both the pulses, and ask the child to carry out repetitive finger flexion until the palm is pale. Release one of the occluded vessels and assess for return of color. A delay of more than 6 seconds indicates a positive Allen's test. Repeat with the other vessel.[11]
- *Digital Allen's test*: Carry out in the same manner as the Allen's test by compressing the radial and ulnar aspect of the base of the fingers.

7.7.5.1 SKELETAL EXAMINATION

Look for areas of bony swelling/prominence/crepitus/abnormal mobility.

7.7.6 Investigations

Imaging modalities can be used as an adjunct to clinical examination to confirm the diagnosis. A brief overview is given in this chapter (Figure 7.16).

- X-ray for suspected bony and joint pathology (fractures, dislocations, bony swelling, to confirm the level of injury in traumatic amputations, congenital anomalies).
- Ultrasonography is useful for soft tissue injury and swellings such as cysts or abscesses. This can also be used to assess nerves and tendon sheaths.
- Audio/color Doppler is used to study the status of vessels in suspected vascular injury/compromise or in vascular lesions.
- Computed tomography is used for bony swellings, fractures, and joint dislocations.
- MRI is used for soft tissue injuries, tendon and ligament injuries, swellings, and brachial plexus injury.

7.7.7 Differential Diagnosis

The various hand pathologies in children can be broadly classified, as shown in Table 7.2. The common clinical findings and differential diagnoses are shown.

7.8 WRIST EXAMINATION

The wrist joint is formed of three joints – the radiocarpal, ulnocarpal, and distal radioulnar joint (DRUJ). It helps in placing the hand in the most appropriate position for a function. The wrist joint can be involved in children with trauma, inflammatory or infective arthritis, and metabolic conditions like rickets. It can also be involved in congenital conditions like Madelung's deformity,[12] hereditary multiple exostosis, radial club hand, etc. Madelung's deformity is a component of Leri–Weill syndrome (which is a dyschondrosteosis). It is seen more frequently in female patients, is often bilateral in involvement, and is inherited in an autosomal dominant fashion. Leri–Weill syndrome is characterized by mesomelic dwarfism, and assessment of stature in girls suspected of having this

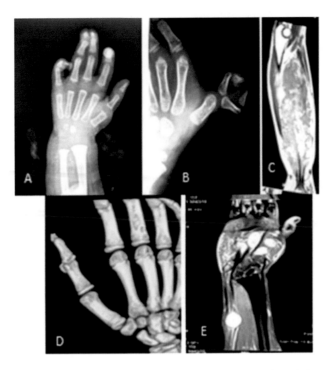

Figure 7.16 Investigations: (a) X-ray hand showing syndactyly, (b) X-ray hand showing thumb duplication, (c) MRI image showing venous malformation forearm, (d) CT scan demonstrating enchondroma of proximal phalanx of middle finger, (e) MRI showing multiple nerve sheath tumors along ulnar nerve.

Table 7.2 Classification of Pediatric Hand Anomalies, Relevant Examination Findings, and Differential Diagnosis

Hand Anomalies	Congenital	Traumatic	Inflammatory	Neoplastic
Relevant examination findings	Present since birth Family history+	History of trauma Signs of inflammation Altered digital cascade and tenodesis Abnormal mobility Tenderness Trophic ulcer	Pain Swelling Tenderness Warmth Edema Hyperemia	Swelling Pain
Common differential diagnoses	• Syndactyly • Polydactyly • Club hand • Trigger thumb, thumb hypoplasia • Birth brachial plexus injury (BBPI)	• Fracture or dislocation • Tendon, ligament, or nerve injuries	• Abscess • Cysts	• Enchondroma • Bony tumors • Vascular lesions • Vascular tumors

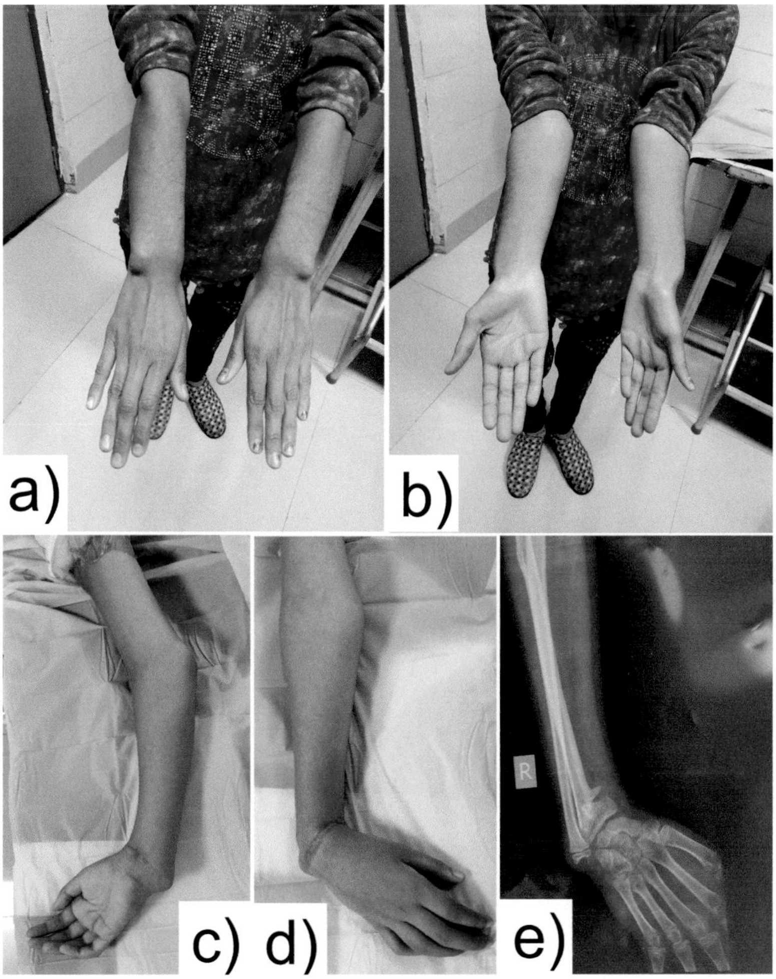

Figure 7.17 (a) and (b) Madelung's deformity, (c), (d), and (e) Post-traumatic physeal arrest with wrist deformation.

condition is thus essential. Patients usually present between the ages of 7 and 14 years with complaints of deformity, limitation of movements of the wrist, and pain. The pain is initially present on exertion and with sporting activities but can become a constant feature later.

Clinical examination of the wrist shows that the distal part of the radius to be tilted volar and ulnar with shortening of the radius. The ulna appears longer than the radius, is located more dorsally with a prominent ulnar styloid (Figure 7.17). This gives an appearance of relative subluxation of the carpus with the hand sitting out of the plane of the forearm. The range of motion is limited, especially the forearm supination, wrist dorsiflexion, and radial deviation. In some patients, the DRUJ

is unstable or even frankly subluxated. A positive ballottement test is seen in them. While the clinical features usually help in making a diagnosis, the examiner must however be aware of the possible other differentials that can mimic this pattern. They include hereditary multiple exostosis, sickle cell disease, post-traumatic or post-infectious growth arrests.

Children with hereditary multiple exostosis have variable involvement of forearm bones depending upon the localization of osteochondroma. There may be ulnar shortening with radial bowing, radial head dislocation, radial shortening, etc. The clinical findings depend upon the degree of involvement like forearm shortening, deformity, restriction of rotatory movements, etc.

REFERENCES

1. Rayan G, Akelman E. *The hand: Anatomy, examination and diagnosis*. Philadelphia PA: Lippincott Williams & Wilkins; 2011. pp. 1–160.
2. Vella JC, Hartigan BJ, Stern PJ. Kaplan's cardinal line. *J Hand Surg Am*. 2006;31: 912–918.
3. Hallett S, Ashurst JV. Anatomy, shoulder and upper limb, hand anatomical snuff box. In: *StatPearls* [Internet]. Treasure Island, FL: Stat Pearls Publishing; 2019. https://www.ncbi.nlm.nih.gov/books/NBK482228/
4. Kenney RJ, Hammert WC. Physical examination of hand. *J Hand Surg Am*. 2014;39:2324–2334.
5. Smith PJ, Lister G. *Lister's the hand: Diagnosis and indications*. London: Churchill Livingstone, 2002.
6. Elfar JC, Petrungaro JM, Braun RM, Cheng CJ. Nerve. In: Hammert WC, Calfee RP, Bozentka DJ, Boyer Mi, editors. *ASSH manual of hand surgery*. Philadelphia, PA: Lippincott Williams & Wilkins; 2010. pp. 294–342.
7. Gelberman RH, Szabo RM, Williamson RV, Dimick MP. Sensibility testing in peripheral nerve compression syndromes: An experimental study in humans. *J Bone Joint Surg Am*. 1983; 65:632–638.
8. Gellis M, Pool R. Two-point discrimination distances in normal hand and forearm: Application to various methods of fingertip reconstruction. *Plast Reconstr Surg*. 1977;59:57–63.
9. Wolfe SW, Hotchkiss RN, Pederson WC, Kozin SH. *Green's operative hand surgery*, 6th ed. Philadelphia, PA: Churchill Livingstone, 2011.
10. Hattam P, Smeatham A. *Special tests in Musculoskeletal examination: An evidence-based guide for clinicians*. London. Churchill Livingstone, 2010.
11. Higgins JP. Acute vascular injuries of upper extremity. In: Hammert WC, Calfee RP, Bozentka DJ, Mi B, editors. *ASSH manual of hand surgery*. Philadelphia, PA: Lippincott Williams & Wilkins; 2010. pp. 294–342.
12. Waters PM, Bae DS. Madelung deformity. In: *Pediatric hand and upper limb surgery: A practical guide*. Philadelphia, PA: Lippincott Williams & Wilkins; 2012. pp. 138–146.

8

Examination of a Child with Birth Brachial Plexus Palsy

SATYASWARUP TRIPATHY AND MOHSINA SUBAIR

Flaccid paralysis of the upper extremity due to stretching of the brachial plexus that occurs at the time of birth is defined as birth brachial plexus palsy (BBPP). This condition was earlier known as "obstetric brachial plexus injury." However, the term is not used anymore to avoid direct reference to obstetricians as the causative factor.[1] Broadly, BBPP is classified into two:[2]

- Early or infantile seen in less than 1 year of life.
- Late presentation is seen in children more than 1-year-old with sequelae such as secondary contractures or deformities.

8.1   KEY CLINICAL CLASSIFICATION

Before proceeding to examine a child with BBPP, one should be familiar with the common clinical presentations to rapidly and accurately identify the involved roots. The most common presentations of BBPP are shown in Table 8.1 .

Narakas has classified these common clinical presentations based on the roots involved, and this is the most commonly used classification.[5]

- Upper Erb's palsy, C5, C6.
- Extended Erb's palsy, C5, C6, C7.
- Total palsy without Horner syndrome, C5–T1.
- Total palsy with Horner syndrome, C5–T1.

8.2   HISTORY AND INITIAL EVALUATION

A detailed history should be obtained from the parents in the following categories:

- Maternal factors and antenatal history:[6]
  - Maternal age of more than 30 years.
  - High BMI.
  - High parity.
  - Gestational diabetes.
  - Pre-eclampsia.

Table 8.1 Clinical Presentation of BBPP According to the Roots Involved

	Roots Involved	Classic Clinical Presentations
Classic Duchenne Erb's palsy[3]	C5, C6	Shoulder internally rotated, adducted; elbow extended; forearm pronated; hand and finger preserved (Figure 8.1).
Upper-middle trunk BBPP	C5, C6, C7	Same as above; forearm pronated with palm facing backward. Classic waiter's tip deformity.
Klumpke's palsy[4]	C8, T1	Loss of function of small muscles of hand, sensory loss over medial arm and forearm.
Pan-plexus injury	C5–T1	
• Pre-ganglionic		Flail limb, Horner syndrome+
• Post-ganglionic		Flail limb, Horner syndrome−, serratus anterior and rhomboids function is preserved.

- Previous history of shoulder dystocia.
- Perinatal history:[6]
  - Breech presentation.
  - Shoulder dystocia.
  - Protracted active phase of labor.
  - Fetal distress can predispose the infant to hypotonia, which leads to a flail limb even with minimal traction.
  - Instrumental vaginal delivery.
  - Epidural anesthesia during labor.
- Post-natal or child factors:
  - High birth weight.
  - Lower head circumference than chest circumference.
  - Birth asphyxia.
- History regarding movements of the limb from the mother:
  - History of lack of movement of the upper limb and subsequent gradual recovery of movements since birth.
  - At the first visit, the parents should be counseled regarding the prognosis, such as the possibility of spontaneous recovery or the expected reconstructive procedures.
  - Often parents are asked to bring a video of the child's routine activities at home. They help in assessing the pattern of the involvement of the nerve roots and the progress in the pattern of the recovery.
  - Specific history regarding abnormal limb posture, which can be correlated with the key presentations mentioned in Table 8.1.

8.3 CLINICAL EXAMINATION

The child should be examined in a warm, quiet environment in the presence of the mother and father to make the child comfortable. The child should always be examined on a full stomach as children become irritable when hungry. Charming toys and dangling objects in the examination room often help in diverting the attention of the children. Observation is the key to examining a child with BBPP as these children are too young to

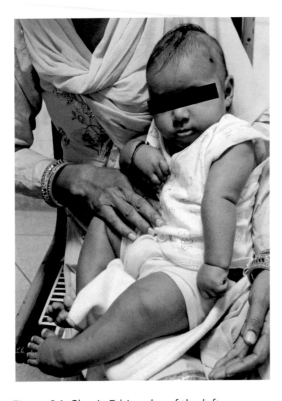

Figure 8.1 Classic Erb's palsy of the left upper limb. Notice the adducted and internally rotated shoulder, extended elbow, and pronated forearm leading to "policeman's tip" deformity.

understand and follow the routine commands for examination.

8.3.1 General Examination of the Child

- Note the skin for the presence of bruises, any swelling over the head region suggestive of the application of forceps, difficult labor, etc.
- Assess the general sweating pattern of the head and neck (anhydrosis or hypohydrosis).
- Eyes:
  - Conjugate eye movements.
  - Signs of Horner syndrome – ptosis, miosis, enophthalmos (suggestive of pre-ganglionic lesion)[7] (Figure 8.2).
- Neck:
  - Look for any swellings – assess size, shape, and position, e.g., swelling or fibrosis in the sternocleidomastoid muscle due to trauma (often called sternomastoid tumor).[8]

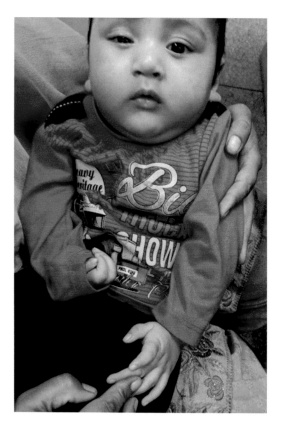

Figure 8.2 Pan-plexus injury with Horner syndrome; note the flail right upper limb with eye signs of Horner syndrome.

- Assess neck control in supported sitting and prone positions.
- Any favored laterality is suggestive of torticollis or traction injury to the sternocleidomastoid or scalene muscles.
- Chest:
  - Assess the respiratory pattern.
  - Assess symmetry of chest movement where asymmetry indicates the involvement of the phrenic nerve.
- Legs:
  - Assess the range of movements, tone, and movement patterns.
- Unaffected arm:
  - Assess the active and passive range of movements and strength.
- The natural, spontaneous reflexes present in infancy and early childhood are to be examined. Any deficit in eliciting them may suggest the presence of cerebral palsy or other neurological disorders.

8.3.2 Examination of the Affected Arm

Inspection and palpation:

- The affected arm should be inspected in the resting position.
- Note the attitude of the limb – look for any classical posturing as in Erb's palsy or Klumpke's palsy (Table 8.1).
- Look for atrophy of the muscles in the shoulder, arm, forearm, and hand. In an older child, the measurement of the girth around the arm and forearm may suggest the amount of musculoskeletal atrophy in the affected limb.
- Examine for contour irregularities around the clavicle, shoulder, and ribs to rule out possible fractures or dislocations; palpate for any bony irregularities.

Motor examination of the affected limb:

- The motor examination should start from the neck and continue to the shoulder, arm, elbow, forearm, wrist, and hand noting the movements and posture at rest.
- Look for abduction, external and internal rotation at the shoulder, flexion and extension at the elbow and wrist, and hand function.

- All movements should be assessed in supine as well as supported sitting posture.
- The examination should be like mentally walking through the plexus:
  - C5: Assess shoulder abduction and external rotation.
  - C6: Assess elbow flexion.
  - C7: Assess elbow and wrist extension.
  - C8: Assess thumb and finger flexion.
  - T1: Assess the intrinsic muscles of the hand. Dimpling on the dorsum of the metacarpophalangeal joint can indirectly indicate clawing.
- The passive range of movements at each joint has to be tested. Simultaneously palpate for the contraction of the corresponding muscle belly to accurately assess the involved nerve roots or muscles. For example, examine the biceps by putting a finger on it and feel for its contraction while flexing the elbow. One can have flexion at the elbow even with a paralyzed biceps; if intact, brachioradialis is present. Examining the biceps is important because it is supplied purely by upper nerve roots.
- In an older child, all these active and passive ranges of movements and power have to be examined when examining the upper limb. In smaller children, the natural voluntary movements of the shoulder and arm and hand movements are to be noted in response to toys, keys, or dangling objects to note the range of movements around each joint (Figure 8.3).

8.3.2.1 SPECIAL TESTS

These are carried out after 3 months of age to see the global functions rather than individual muscles. These tests help in sequentially assessing any recovery as well as playing a role in decisions regarding the timing of surgical intervention.

- Towel test:
  - Described by Bertelli and Ghizoni.[9]
  - The child's face is covered with a towel in a supine position and the unaffected arm is obstructed. The child will attempt to remove the towel using the unobstructed affected arm.
  - To remove the towel, shoulder flexion, elbow flexion and extension, and finger flexion and extension are needed, and hence these movements can be assessed.
  - If the child is able to remove the towel, it is considered a pass, suggestive of recovery of involved muscles, particularly elbow flexion.
- Eye obstruction test:

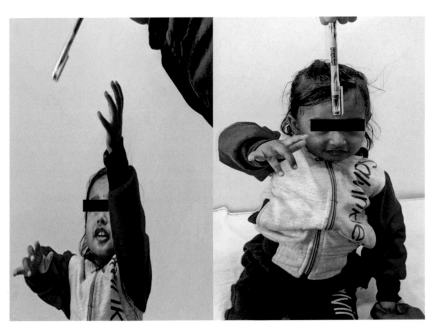

Figure 8.3 Assessing the movements at each joint in response to dangling objects. Left: comparison with the unaffected limb; right: assessment of affected limb by restricting the unaffected limb.

- Modification of towel test.[10]
- The eyes are covered using the examiner's hand instead of a towel. The child would immediately try to remove the hands with the action of the biceps and elbow flexion (Figure 8.4).
- Cookie test:
  - The child is given a cookie in the affected limb. The examiner holds the affected elbow adducted at the side to prevent compensation of the biceps function by arm flexion.
  - The child tries to take the cookie to the mouth. If the child is able to bring the cookie to the mouth without neck flexion >45°, it is considered a pass, thereby indicating the recovery of elbow flexors.[11]

8.3.2.2 SENSORY EXAMINATION OF THE AFFECTED LIMB

The sensory examination has to be carried out as for the regular upper limb examination in an older child. However, it is difficult to carry out in

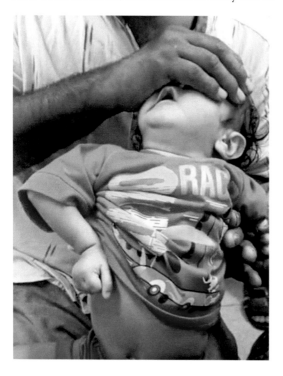

Figure 8.4 Modified towel test/eye obstruction test. The eyes are obstructed, and the unaffected limb is restrained to assess the elbow flexion of the affected limb.

infants, and hence surgeons often resort to indirect evidence.

- Look for the breakdown of the skin with the presence of inflammatory signs such as redness in the surrounding skin; repeated sucking and biting of the finger or arm are symptoms that may suggest the child might be having neuropathic pain. The repeated chewing and trauma may also be due to lack of sensation, which makes it painless for the child.
- The child's response to a pinch and the application of heat and cold is to be noted at regular intervals.

8.4 ASSESSMENT SCALES FOR MOTOR AND SENSORY FUNCTIONS IN BBPP

The classic Medical Research Council (MRC) grading for motor recovery is not applicable in infants.

- Modified MRC scale for BBPP by Gilbert and Tassin:[12]
  - M0: No contraction.
  - M1: Flicker or contraction without movement.
  - M2: Movement with gravity eliminated.
  - M3: Complete range of movements against gravity.
- Toronto Active Movement Score (AMS) by Curtis and Clarke:[13]
  - Power graded from 0 to 7.
  - 0–4 for movements with gravity eliminated; 5–7 for movements against gravity.
  - 0: No contraction.
  - 1: Contraction without movement.
  - 2: Movement <50% range of movements (ROM) with gravity eliminated.
  - 3: Movement >50% ROM with gravity eliminated.
  - 4: Full ROM with gravity eliminated.
  - 5: Movement <50% ROM against gravity.
  - 6: Movement >50% ROM against gravity.
  - 7: Full ROM against gravity.

The AMS scale is used more reliably than the MRC in the newborn with birth palsies.

- Mallet Shoulder Scale:[14]
  - Usually used to assess BBPP sequelae.
  - For children more than 4 years old.

- Assesses the upper plexus function in respect of the shoulder and elbow functions.
- 1: No function.
- 2–4: Progressive strength (Figures 8.5 and 8.6).
  - "Trumpet sign": The "hand to mouth" movement is graded, as shown in

Figure 8.5. In children with BBPP, the child tends to lift the shoulder into abduction to bring the hand to the mouth, which is known as the trumpet sign (Figure 8.6d). This term was coined due to the similarity to the position of holding a trumpet in a unit of the French army.

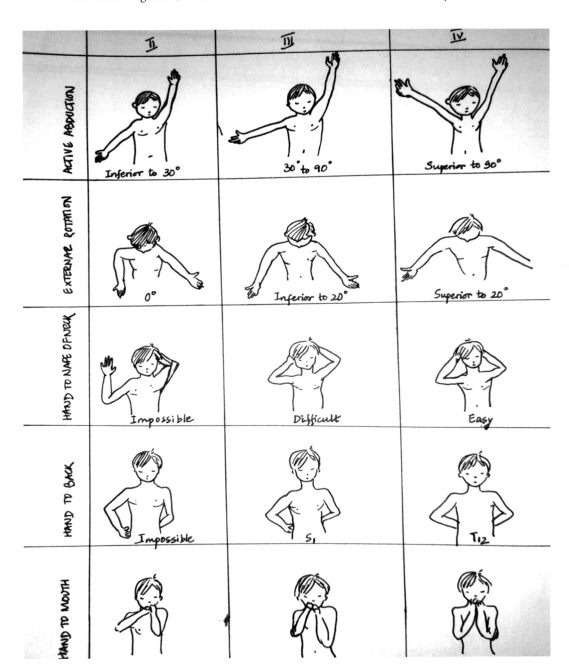

Figure 8.5 Mallet shoulder scale grade II–IV.

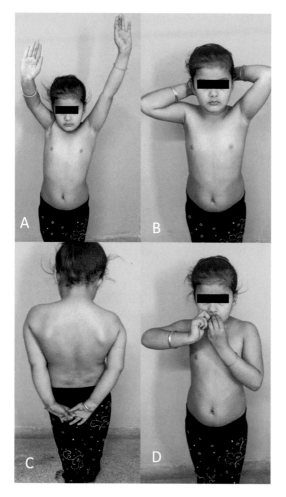

Figure 8.6 Clinical photographs showing the various Mallet shoulder scores: (a) abduction grade IV, (b) hand to neck grade II, (c) hand to back grade III reaching S1, (d) hand to mouth grade II (small clarion/trumpet sign).

- The grade II and III of this movement are referred to as trumpet sign and partial trumpet sign respectively.
  - 5: Normal function.
- Narakas sensory scale:[15]
  - S0: No reaction to stimulus.
  - S1: Reaction only to pain.

- S2: Reaction to touch.
- S3: Normal sensation.

8.5 SCALES TO ASSESS RECOVERY

Various scales have been described to assess the adequacy of spontaneous recovery. Proper documentation and close monitoring of recovery are essential for prognosis as well as in deciding the timing for surgery.

- Gilbert suggested the absence of elbow flexion at 3 months as an indication for surgery.
- The prognosis of shoulder recovery has been graded based on the biceps recovery by Gilbert and Tassin, as shown in Table 8.2.[16]

8.5.1 Gilbert and Raimondi Score for Elbow Function

The scoring system most commonly used for elbow function is shown in Table 8.3.[17]

8.5.2 Raimondi Score for Evaluation of Hand Function

- 0: Complete paralysis or functionally useless finger flexion.
- 1: Limited finger flexion, no extension.
- 2: Active wrist extension and use of tenodesis.
- 3: Complete active finger and wrist flexion, active thumb movement.
- 4: Complete active finger and wrist flexion, active wrist extension, weak finger extension, good opposition.
- 5: Same as 4 with active finger extension.[18]

8.6 CLINICAL EXAMINATION AND CORRELATION WITH TIMING OF SURGERY

Evaluating the extent of paralysis is important to decide an exploration and its timing.

Table 8.2 Correlation Between Age and Power of Biceps to Prognosis of Shoulder Recovery

Age	Power of Biceps	Interpretation of Shoulder Recovery
<1 month	Grade 5	Shoulder will recover
1–3 months	Grade 4	Shoulder should recover
>3 months	Grade 3	Shoulder recovery is insufficient

Table 8.3 Scoring for Elbow Function by Gilbert and Raimondi

Elbow flexion	None or some contraction	0
	Incomplete flexion	2
	Complete flexion	3
Elbow extension	No extension	0
	Weak extension	1
	Good extension	2
Extension deficit	0–30°	0
	30–50°	−1
	>50	−2

Note: 0–1, poor recovery; 2–3, average recovery; 4–5, good recovery and functionally useful.

The recommendation of the timing of surgery still remains controversial. However, the various recommended indications for surgery can be broadly described as follows:

- Gilbert's rule of three: Absence of active elbow flexion by 3 months.[12]
- Clarke and Curtis' recommend inability to perform cookie test by 9 months of age.
- Total palsy with Horner syndrome should be operated on by 2 months of age.
- Total palsy with the presence of finger flexion: Observe for additional 3 months, if no recovery by 6 months, then surgery.

8.7 COMMON SECONDARY DEFORMITIES IN BBPP

These occur in children later in age who fail to recover fully. The etiology of these deformities is a combination of muscle imbalance, co-contractions, and growth.

The common deformities that occur are as follows:

- Shoulder deformities:
  - Limited abduction with good external rotation.
  - Limited external rotation with good abduction.
  - Limited abduction and external rotation.
- Elbow deformities:
  - Elbow flexion contracture.
- Forearm deformities:
  - Pronation deficit.
  - Supination deficit.
  - Deficit in both directions of rotation.

These require secondary surgeries for correction to achieve optimum functions.

8.8 DIFFERENTIAL DIAGNOSIS FOR BBPP

Clinical differentiation in a newborn is very difficult and requires keen observation and clinical skills.

1. Fractured humerus, fractured clavicle: Palpable bony crepitus and deformity can help differentiate from BBPI.
2. Upper humeral epiphysiolysis: Usually follows septic pathology; a history of fever may be present.
3. Neonatal shoulder dislocation: Palpable bony deformity; immobile shoulder.
4. Pulled elbow: Rarely congenital, occurs during the post-natal period, passive range of movements may be painful.

REFERENCES

1. Vanheest A. Birth brachial plexus injury is the preferred terminology. *J Hand Surg Am* 2006;31:203.
2. Chuang DC, Mardini S, Ma HS. Surgical strategy for infant obstetrical brachial plexus palsy: Experiences at Chang Gung Memorial Hospital. *Plast Reconstr Surg.* 2005;116:132–142.
3. Erb W. Uber eine eigentumliche Lokalisation von Lahmugenim Plexus brachialis, Verhandl Naturhist Med Vereins. Heidelberg 'Carl Winters'. *Universitatas Buchhandlung* 1874;2:130–136.
4. Klumpke A. Contribution a letude des paralysies radiculaires du plexus brachial. Paralysies radiculaires totals. De la participation des filets sympathiques oculo-pupillaires dans ces paralysies. *Rev Med.* 1885;5:591–616.
5. Al-Qattan MM, El-Sayed AA, Al-Zahrani AY, et al. Narakas classification of obstetric brachial plexus palsy revisited. *J Hand Surg Eur.* 2009;34(6):788–791.
6. Bhat VR, Oumachigui A. Nerve injuries due to obstetric trauma. *Ind J Pediatr.* 1995;62:207–212.
7. Kanagalingam S, Miller NR. Horner syndrome: Clinical perspectives. *Eye Brain.* 2015;7:35–46.
8. Adamoli P, Pavano P, Falsaperla R, Longo R, VitalitiiG, Andaloro C et al. Rapid spontaneous resolution of fibromatosis colli in a 3-week-old girl. *Case Rep Otolaryngol.* 2014; Article ID 264940.
9. Bertelli JA, Ghizoni MF. The towel test: A useful technique for the clinical and electromyographic

evaluation of obstetric brachial plexus palsy', *J Hand Surg Br*. 2004;29(2):155–158.

10. Bhardwaj P, Venkatramani H, Sbapathy SR. A modified towel test for assessment of elbow flexion in children less than 9 months old with brachial plexus birth palsy. *J Hand Surg Eur.*.2011;36:707–708.

11. Clarke HM, Curtis CG. An approach to obstetrical brachial plexus injuries. *Hand Clin*. 1995;11(4):563–581.

12. Gilbert A, Tassin JL. Réparation chirurgicale du plexus brachial dans la paralysie obstétricale [Surgical repair of the brachial plexus in obstetric paralysis]. *Chirurgie*. 1984;110(1):70–75.

13. Curtis C, Stephens D, Clarke HM, Andrews D. The active movement scale: An evaluative tool for infants with obstetrical brachial plexus palsy. *J Hand Surg Am*. 2002;27(3):470–478.

14. Mallet J. Paralysie obstétricale du plexus brachial. II. Thérapeutique. Traitement des séquelles. Primauté du traitement de l'épaule. Méthode d'expression des résultats [Obstetrical paralysis of the brachial plexus. II. Therapeutics. Treatment of sequelae. Priority for the treatment of the shoulder. Method for the expression of results]. *Rev Chir Orthop Reparatrice Appar Mot*. 1972;58:166–168.

15. Narakas AO. Obstetrical brachial plexus injuries. In: Lamb DW, editor. *The paralysed hand*. Edinburgh: Churchill Livingstone; 1987. pp. 116–235.

16. Chuang DCC, Ma HS. Current concepts in the management of obstetrical brachial plexus injuries: The Taipei experience. *Semin Plast Surg*. 2004;18(4):309–317. doi:10.1055/s-2004-837257

17. Haerle M, Gilbert A. Management of complete obstetric brachial plexus lesions. *J Pediatr Orthop*. 2004;24:194–200.

18. Maillet M, Romana C. Complete obstetric brachial plexus palsy: Surgical improvement to recover a functional hand. *J Child Orthop*. 2009;3(2):101–108.

9

Examination of Hip Joint in a Child

NIRMAL RAJ GOPINATHAN, REET MUKOPADHYA, KARTHICK RANGASAMY, AND RAMESH KUMAR SEN

Hip ailments in a pediatric patient often result in significant morbidity affecting day-to-day activities. The importance of early diagnosis has been emphasized repeatedly as it is often missed in the early phases due to masquerading presentation. The examiner must be vigilant in localizing and diagnosing the pathology to facilitate early diagnosis and a better outcome. This chapter will focus on evaluating a child for disorders around the hip joint.

9.1 HISTORY

Certain hip disorders have a characteristic presentation, are common in particular age groups, and are to be kept in mind while evaluating a child. For example, developmental dysplasia of the hip (DDH) may be noticed when the child starts to walk and presents as a painless limp when it is unilateral. The same may present as a waddling gait in the case of bilateral involvement. Perthes' disease presents commonly in the age group of 4–8 years and is more common in boys. The parents usually notice a limp that is often aggravated by the end of the day. Slipped upper femoral epiphysis (SUFE) is again more common in boys and usually presents with sudden onset or progressive painful limp. It is common in the age group of 12–15 years in boys and 11–13 years in girls. In younger children, it may be associated with an endocrinopathy or a metabolic bone disorder. Although earlier literature suggests that a child with SUFE is usually a hypogonadal obese child, this may not be true all the time, and it may or may not be associated with endocrinopathy. The other diagnosis to be kept in mind in acute presentations are infections, transient synovitis

(common in boys of 3–10 years), idiopathic chondrolysis (common in adolescent girls), and at times an osteoid osteoma of the proximal femur, acetabular roof, or a myeloproliferative disorder like leukemia. All these conditions may present with hip or groin pain, demanding a detailed evaluation.

The history of trauma should be asked to rule out post-traumatic pathologies. Often the parents do state an antecedent trauma that may or may not be significant. The examiner should ask whether the trauma was witnessed by anyone to verify its authenticity. Also, it should be verified whether the child was able to get up, walk, and carry out day-to-day activities after the trauma or needed medical attention to identify the severity of the injury sustained.

The common complaints that bring the child to the clinic are pain, limp, swelling, or reduced range of motion affecting gait and day-to-day activities like squatting, sitting cross-legged, etc. A childhood history of intensive care therapy may indicate conditions like pneumonia with disseminated sepsis for which the child might have been treated. In such cases, hip joint sepsis might have been overlooked and might have settled with the systemic antibiotics administered. Such situations result in the child's presenting with post-septic sequelae without a recent history of fever or joint suppuration. It is also important to get a history of prolonged steroid use in conditions like bronchial asthma, dermatological, renal pathological conditions, and any hematological disorders/malignancies that may predispose the child to avascular necrosis. At times parents might give a history of a limp that is gradually worsening, indicating a progressive pathology.

Any childhood history of tuberculosis or infection among siblings, family members, and neighbors is important. It is also important to ask for loss of appetite and loss of weight in these patients. A tubercular patient might have night pain or a night cry, whereas a patient with inflammatory arthropathy might have early morning stiffness apart from pain in the joint. Remember that a painless limp may be seen every time the child walks in conditions like DDH, post-septic sequelae, or congenital femoral deficiency where there is a limb length discrepancy/instability. A painful limp may be seen in conditions like SUFE or arthritis (infectious or non-infectious). Also, note the use of aids for ambulation and restriction of activities of daily living like squatting, sitting cross-legged, ability to tie shoelaces, etc. Children with Perthes' disease might have waxing and waning of symptoms and symptom-free periods (occasionally painless limp) in between the initial phases. Also, a characteristic feature of Perthes' disease is the worsening of the limp after activities or by the end of the day after day-long exertion.

9.1.1 Why May Hip Pain Be Referred to the Knee?

Frequently, patients with hip pathology are missed for long durations without getting diagnosed as the hip pain is referred to other areas like the knee. The reason behind this being innervation of the hip from the obturator, femoral, and sciatic nerves. Hip pathology presenting as pain in the *anteromedial aspect of knee* is attributed to referral through the *anterior division of the obturator nerve*. Referral to the buttocks, thigh, groin, and even lower leg can occur in decreasing order of frequency with buttock pain and thigh referral being the most common combination.[1]

9.2 HEAD-TO-TOE EXAMINATION

It is important to examine the child from head to toe; 20% of patients with torticollis and 10% of patients with metatarsus adductus might have an accompanying DDH. Examination of the spine is imperative to pick up neurogenic hip pathologies. So, look for cutaneous lesions associated with

spinal dysraphism like hypertrichosis (tuft of hair), dimple, lipomas, acrochordons (true/pseudo tails), hemangiomas, aplasia cutis or scar, nevus, hyperpigmentation, etc.[2] Certain syndromic disorders are obvious and must be picked up in general examination. For instance, a child with arthrogryposis multiplex congenita (AMC) will demonstrate absence of normal creases and variable joint involvement like congenital talipes equinovarus (CTEV), congenital vertical talus (CVT), joint contractures, pterygium, etc., along with teratologic hip dislocation. Also, it is important to identify a child with hyperlaxity[3,4] as they might be associated with certain pathologies like DDH/pes planovalgus.

9.3 LOCAL PHYSICAL EXAMINATION

Prerequisites:

- The child must be comfortable and offered adequate privacy and the comfort of the parents/guardian nearby.
- Well-illuminated room.
- For proper evaluation, adequate exposure of both lower limbs, hips, and abdomen is required. The genitals are to be covered so that the child is comfortable.
- A hard couch is essential while examining the patient.
- Examine the sound, non-painful side first.
- Explain to the child and to the parent what are you going to do and the expected response.

The examination starts with a gait assessment, which has been dealt with in Chapter 3.

The patient can then be examined in a standing position from the front, back, and sides and in a supine and prone position.

9.3.1 Inspection of the Hip in Standing Position

9.3.1.1 INSPECTION FROM THE FRONT

In a standing position, it is imperative to first comment on both shoulders being at the same level or not. Also, note the position of the trunk and any increase in distance between the chest wall and upper arm, which may be a finding in cases with scoliosis (structural or functional) apart from other visible abnormalities like chest wall deformation. Note any prominent bony landmarks, and the presence of a pelvic tilt can be appreciated by comparing the position of the iliac crest on both sides. If the child has limb length discrepancy, the child will keep the shortened limb ankle in equinus or keep the opposite knee in a flexed position. Look for any rotational malalignment by looking at the position of the patella and where it is facing, and the position of the foot. Look for the presence of any swelling near the groin or thigh area. Quadriceps wasting, if present, is evident from the front.

9.3.1.2 INSPECTION FROM THE SIDE

Look for an increase in lumbar lordosis. The greater trochanter (GT) area should be inspected for any swelling, prominence, and any obliteration of hollowness of the area proximal to the GT. The presence of knee flexion deformity and ankle equinus is better appreciated from the side.

9.3.1.3 INSPECTION FROM THE BACK

Look for symmetry of the shoulders and look at the spine for any curvature or scoliosis. Look at the skin of the lower back for any tufts of hair/dimples/swelling. A pelvic tilt, if any, should be identified by comparing the position of the posterior superior iliac spine (PSIS) (dimple of venous) on both sides. The gluteal fold level and any sagging/atrophy should be compared with the opposite side.

Look at the skin from all sides for any scars, sinus, or swelling.

We will describe the rest of the local examination in the supine/prone position as it is the posture preferred for demonstration.

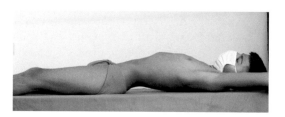

Figure 9.1 Exaggerated lumbar lordosis.

9.3.2 Inspection in Supine Position

The examination starts with a description of the lumbar lordosis and limb attitude. To start with, the resident must comment on the lumbar lordosis, whether it is exaggerated or not. The examiner will be able to make out exaggerated lumbar lordosis in individuals with flexion deformity of the hip joint (Figure 9.1). For attitude description, the patient lays supine, comfortable, and as straight as possible. Normally the limb is kept at a neutral flexion–extension, neutral adduction–abduction, or mild abduction and external rotation (patella facing out and foot rotated externally) at the hip joint. The knee is in extension, and the foot may be in gravity equinus (Figure 9.2).

Now compare both the medial malleoli and patellae in position and note if they are at the same level or at a higher or lower level. The limb may be kept in flexion; abduction and external rotation attitude at the hip in the synovitis stage, which is the position of maximum joint capacity, also leads to apparent lengthening. The hip adapts flexion, adduction, and internal rotation in true arthritis stage and may or may not be accompanied by true shortening. The hip is flexed, adducted, and internally rotated in posterior dislocation, along with true shortening. In anterior dislocation, the attitude is flexion, abduction, and external rotation.

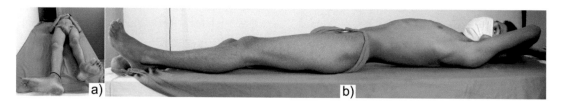

Figure 9.2 Attitude of the left lower limb. The attitude of the left lower limb is described as neutral flexion/extension, neutral adduction/abduction with reduced external rotation (in comparison to other side) of the hip joint, knee in extension, and ankle in gravity equinus.

9.3.2.1 INSPECTION FROM THE FRONT

The iliac crest and anterior superior iliac spine (ASIS) are visible in many children. At times it may be difficult to visualize them in obese children as they are localized beneath the abdominal fold at the waist. The examiner will be able to make out the ASIS on either side and must comment on whether they are at the same level or altered (Figure 9.3). Look for fullness or swelling, if any, in the anterior aspect. Apart from this, look for any erythema, scar (surgical or a puckered scar that has healed by secondary intention indicating suppuration), sinus, dilated veins, atrophy/spasm of nearby musculature, discoloration, etc. Asymmetry of the thigh folds can be seen in children with DDH (Figure 9.4) but is not pathognomonic of the disorder. Bilateral dislocations in syndromic disorders may be associated with widening of the perineum.

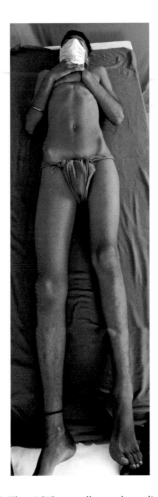

Figure 9.3 The ASIS, patella, and medial malleolus are at a higher level on inspection.

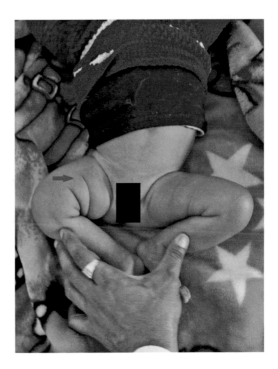

Figure 9.4 Asymmetry of thigh folds.

9.3.2.2 INSPECTION FROM THE SIDE

Normally in lean children, the examiner will be able to appreciate supratrochanteric hollowness (Figure 9.5). Look for its obliteration by swelling or fullness, if any. As already mentioned, in pathologies with fixed flexion deformity of the hip, a compensatory exaggeration in lumbar lordosis is present and needs to be looked for.

9.3.2.3 INSPECTION FROM THE BACK

From the posterior aspect, inspect the dimple of Venus and PSIS on both sides and their symmetry. The gluteal fold is a transverse crease formed at the junction of the buttock and posterior thigh and is formed by the gluteus maximus as it gets inserted into the proximal femur. Unilateral hip pathologies may lead to atrophy of the gluteus maximus, and the gluteal folds might look asymmetric (Figure 9.6). Remember to look for muscle atrophy in the region of proximity in joint involvement, so for hip pathology, look for more pronounced gluteal atrophy apart from vastus medialis wasting.

9.3.3 Palpation

Start palpation by assessment of local temperature and anterior joint line tenderness.

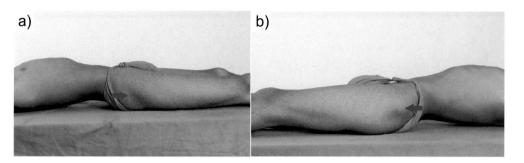

Figure 9.5 Supratrochanteric hollowness on the normal side (a) and its obliteration on the affected side (b).

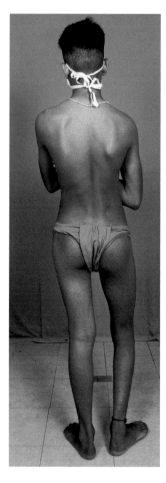

Figure 9.6 Gluteal atrophy on the left side in unilateral hip pathology.

9.3.3.1 ANATOMICAL LANDMARKS

It is imperative to clearly identify and mark the bony landmarks to avoid missing or misinterpreting an important clinical finding. The bony landmarks are fixed and can be marked without mistake by having a general knowledge of bony anatomy. The fixed bony landmarks are the ASIS, pubic tubercle, PSIS, greater trochanter, and the ischial tuberosity. Remember that the soft tissue and overlying skin can slide over the bony landmark and hence do not stretch or press hard while palpating or while marking as the mark may shift when the pressure is released. Also, the marks may vary with various joint positions, which should also be kept in mind.

The ASIS is the anterior end of the iliac crest and is marked by identifying the point where the finger starts dipping into soft tissue while palpating anteriorly along the iliac crest. The other way of marking ASIS is palpation along the inguinal ligament laterally and the first bony resistance that is felt is the ASIS. The pubic tubercle is a small bony prominence on the pubis just lateral to the pubic symphysis. The inguinal ligament is attached to both the ASIS and pubic tubercle. To locate the anterior joint line, the femoral arterial pulsation is localized medial to the midpoint of the inguinal ligament (Figure 9.7). The anterior joint line is palpable inferior and lateral (2 cm in an older child but less than that in younger children) to the point of palpation of the femoral artery.

The trochanteric tip is located by palpating down and lateral from the highest point of the iliac crest on the gluteus medius. It is felt as a sharp bony resistance (easily identified in the attitude of mild flexion, adduction, and internal rotation) or palpation along the lateral aspect of the femur proximally and is localized where the bony resistance offered by the femur is lost. The PSIS is localized in the same way as the ASIS except that the palpation is carried out posteriorly along the iliac crest. The sacroiliac (SI) joint is localized as a longitudinal bony prominence, it is overhung by the PSIS, and

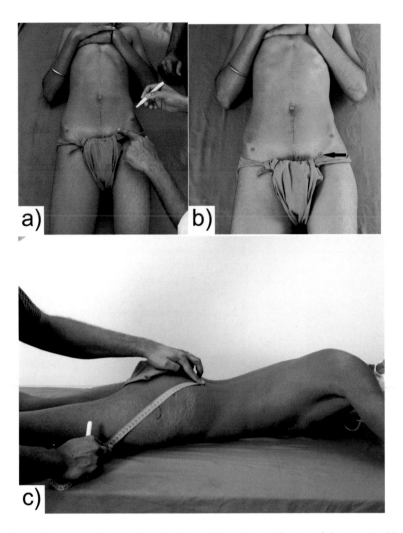

Figure 9.7 (a) Femoral artery pulsation localized medial to the midpoint of the inguinal ligament. (b) Anterior joint line localized below and lateral to femoral arterial pulse localization. (c) Posterior joint line at the junction of the lateral one-third and medial two-thirds of the line joining the greater trochanter and PSIS.

is continuous with it (PSIS). The posterior joint line (posterior lip of the acetabulum) is localized at the juncture of the lateral third and medial two-thirds of a line joining the PSIS and the greater trochanter (Figure 9.7). Ischial tuberosity is surface marked at the level of the gluteal fold in the middle of the buttock in prone position. If attempted in supine position, flexion of the hip facilitates localization by displacing the gluteus maximus muscle away from the bony prominence (Figure 9.8).

The examiner will be able to compare and confirm the symmetry or asymmetry of the ASIS levels. Also, assess and compare the volume of femoral pulsations at the base of the Scarpa's triangle. The femoral pulsation is weak or sometimes not palpable in conditions like posterior dislocation hip and excised or dissolved head and neck femur as the bony base against which the femoral arterial pulsation is felt is absent (vascular sign of Narath). On the lateral aspect, assess for an increase in temperature and tenderness over the trochanteric region. Tenderness on touch and deep pressure may point to localized pathology in the trochanter like bursitis, fracture, or a cyst. Thrust tenderness might be elicitable in conditions leading to inflammatory or secondary hip arthritis. Assessment for trochanteric thickening/trochanteric widening may be appreciated in longstanding localized trochanteric

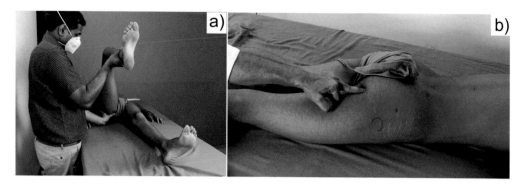

Figure 9.8 Palpation of ischial tuberosity. (a) Supine position with hip and knee flexed. (b) Prone position in the midpoint of the gluteal fold.

pathologies mentioned previously. Trochanteric proximal migration can be made out by the digital Bryant's assessment method (Figure 9.9). The tips of the thumbs are placed over the ASIS and the tips of the middle fingers are placed over the trochanteric tips while the tips of the index fingers over the imaginary point of intersection of perpendiculars, one dropped down from ASIS towards the bed and another from the trochanteric tips directed to the first line.

Posteriorly palpate and look for warmth and posterior joint line tenderness. A hard globular mass that moves with movements of the femur may be appreciated posteriorly in the gluteal region in the posterior dislocation of the femoral head.

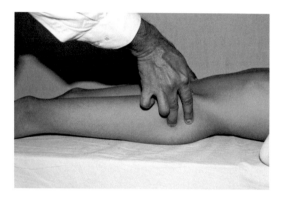

Figure 9.9 Digital Bryant's method to assess supratrochanteric shortening with thumb at ASIS, middle finger at the tip of GT, and index finger projected vertically downwards.

9.3.4 Movements

9.3.4.1 ASSESSMENT OF HIP RANGE OF MOTION

While assessing the range of motion, it is important to stabilize the pelvis in such a way that any movement of the pelvis is appreciated to document the true range of motion. The thumb can be placed over the ASIS and the middle finger can be placed over the PSIS to stabilize the pelvis.

9.3.4.2 MOVEMENTS

Certain disorders have characteristic movement restrictions that should be kept in mind while examining the child. In Perthes' disease, abduction and internal rotation are restricted, whereas flexion and extension remain relatively unaffected. The key finding in SUFE is the loss of internal rotation; it is a change in location of a relatively preserved arc of motion in SUFE rather than loss.

There is increased external rotation, extension, and adduction and limitation of internal rotation, flexion, and abduction.

In DDH, the restriction of abduction is a reliable sign and is best appreciated by abducting both hips simultaneously with the child being placed on a firm surface (Figure 9.10). There is a visible reduction of abduction on the affected side in comparison with the normal side. Also, remember that a painless range of motion usually rules out joint suppuration and should be useful in differentiating other conditions mimicking arthritis.

9.3.4.2.1 Flexion–Extension

In resting (zero) position, the posterior aspect of the thigh, calf, and heel must be in contact with the bed. In the lateral decubitus position, the long axis of the limb is parallel to the bed and is in line

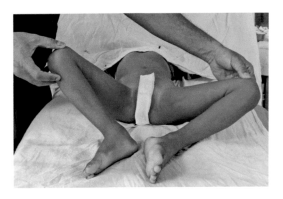

Figure 9.10 Limitation of abduction in unilateral DDH (right side affected).

with the trunk (zero position). Normally, the front of the upper thigh must touch the front of the lower abdomen in complete flexion.

9.3.4.2.2 Abduction–Adduction

The long axes of the limb are parallel to each other and to the axis of the trunk. It is marked by joining the ASIS, mid-patellar point, midpoint on the anterior aspect of the ankle joint (midpoint on a line connecting the prominent points of the two malleoli), and the second web of the foot. During adduction, the middle third of the contralateral thigh is crossed before the pelvis starts moving. A way of preventing pelvic movement while assessing abduction is to position the contralateral limb

in abduction and allow the leg to drop off the table, flexing the knee. This stabilizes the pelvis preventing any coronal movement after which abduction can be assessed. In the same manner, rotational movements are tested in hip flexion and extension; adduction–abduction can also be tested in flexed and extended positions of the hip joint (Figure 9.11).

9.3.4.2.3 Internal Rotation–External Rotation

Rotatory movements are described from the relaxed position of the lower limb and can be compared with the other side. For clarity, rotational movements are to be tested actively/passively in hip extension and in 90° flexion. With the hip in extension, rolling the limb out and in, holding the junction of the middle and lower third of the thigh gives an idea of the range (Figure 9.12). The hip and knee are flexed to 90° to measure rotation in hip flexion. With the hip as the fulcrum and knee fixed by one hand and the heel secured by the other hand, the leg is taken out and in to assess the internal rotation (IR) and external rotation (ER), respectively (Figure 9.12). After a certain range, there is a terminal catch, and if forced, the patient's buttock lifts. The examiner should stop short of this, and the angle made between the axis of the leg and the line drawn vertically downwards

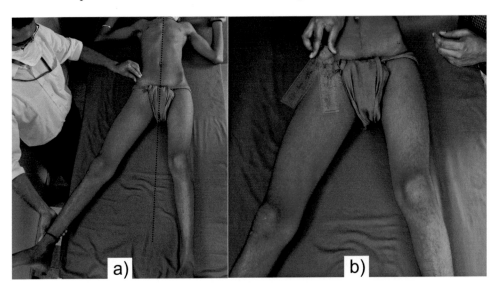

Figure 9.11 Normal abduction of the hip joint. (a) Examiner ensures to stop abduction just short of the movement of the pelvis. (b) Positioning goniometer with the center over the ASIS and one limb along the axis of the thigh and another limb parallel to the midline.

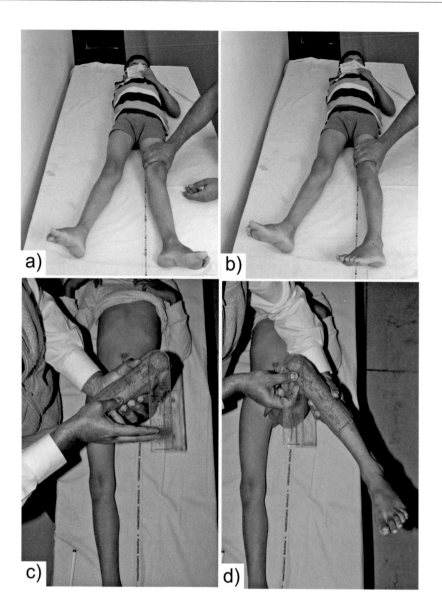

Figure 9.12 Rotatory movements in supine position. (a) External rotation with hip in neutral flexion/extension. (b) Internal rotation with hip in neutral flexion/extension. (c) External rotation with hip and knee flexed to 90° with leg acting as lever facilitating measurement. (d) Internal rotation with hip and knee flexed to 90°.

from the xiphisternum gives the value of rotatory movement. The rotation can also be tested in prone position with the knee flexed to 90° and the hip in neutral flexion–extension. The angle between the leg axis and a line drawn vertically upwards gives the value of IR and ER. Note: when the foot moves away from the midline, it is IR and vice versa for ER. The movements can be documented as active, passive, pain-free, and painful, accordingly (Figure 9.13); see Table 9.1.

Remember that pain/protective muscular spasm might be a reason for the restriction of the range of movements. A gentle examination reveals the true range of motion. The following characteristics are to be kept in mind:

- Synovitis: the range of movements is normal, but the terminal arc is painful.
- Arthritis: the range of movements painful and restricted.

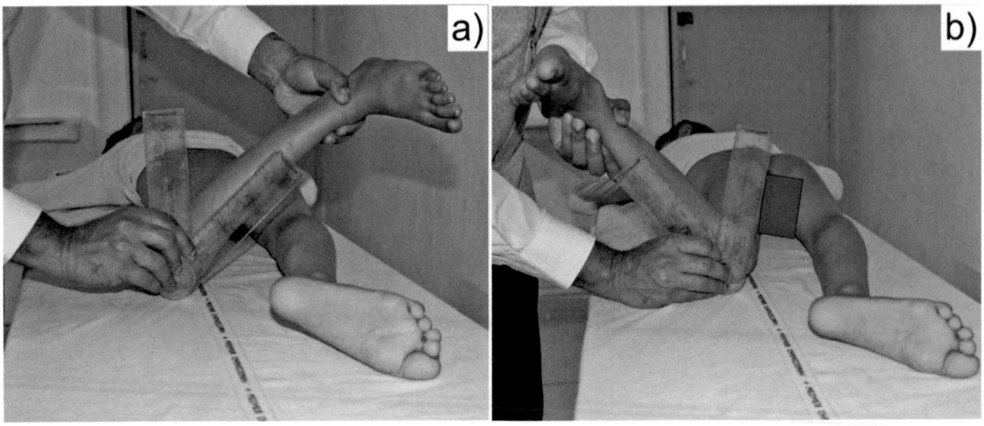

Figure 9.13 Rotatory movements in prone position with knee in 90° flexion and leg acting as a lever. The angle between the long axis of the leg and an imaginary vertical line is measured. (a) External rotation. (b) Internal rotation.

Table 9.1 Hip Range of Motion

Movement	Range (°)
Flexion	0–130
Extension	0–20
Adduction	0–35 to 45
Abduction	0–45 to 55
Internal rotation	0–30 to 40
External rotation	0–40 to 50

The range of movements may be exaggerated in a few cases of post-septic sequelae/Tom Smith arthritis with complete dissolution of the proximal femur.

9.3.5 Thigh Girth Measurement

Thigh girth should be compared equidistant from the medial knee joint on both sides. It is usually measured on the distal part of the thigh to include the vastus medialis obliquus. This is involved in the terminal extension of the knee and is the first quadriceps muscle to get wasted.

9.3.6 Deformity

9.3.6.1 FIXED DEFORMITY

A fixed deformity[5] is a particular fixed position of the joint from which the joint cannot be taken back to neutral position, but further movement may be possible on the same axis.

In case of a fixed deformity, there may be compensatory measures to:

- Conceal the deformity.
- Make up for limb length discrepancy.
- Shifting the center of gravity to maintain equilibrium.

To assess fixed deformities, it is essential to neutralize the postural compensatory mechanisms and reveal the actual deformity.

9.3.6.2 FIXED FLEXION DEFORMITY

The compensatory mechanism in flexion deformity of the hip is an exaggeration of lumbar lordosis, which needs to be obliterated to reveal the actual deformity for accurate measurement. The flexion deformity is quantified by the Thomas test,[6] first described by Hugh Owen Thomas in 1876, and discussed below.

9.3.6.3 THOMAS TEST

Prerequisites:

- Hard flat surface (on a soft couch exaggerated lordosis and its obliteration are not well appreciated).
- Sufficiently undressed patient in a well-illuminated room to visualize the lumbar lordosis and ischial tuberosity.

The original description is as follows. The undressed patient lies on a hard surface, and the clinician manipulates the sound limb and flexes it so that the knee joint touches the chest. By doing that, he/she ensures that the pelvis and spine are flat on the surface. With an assistant maintaining the knee chest position, the patient is asked to actively extend the limb as much as he/she can. The angle between the thigh and the hard surface gives an idea of the flexion contracture at the hip. But when you carefully examine the ischial tuberosity while positioning the patient with knee flexed on the chest, it starts raising beyond a certain limit, and the lumbar lordosis is well obliterated before this point is reached. The pelvis starts tilting anteriorly as the ischial tuberosity starts to move and thereby the flexion contracture is inappropriately exaggerated. Hence, it is enough to flex the sound limb until the lumbar lordosis is obliterated, which can be verified by the inability to insinuate the fingers between the back and table, and this reveals the flexion deformity by obliterating the compensatory exaggerated lumbar lordosis. In this position, the patient him/herself can hold the normal limb, and the affected limb is actively and then passively extended as much as possible without changing this position; the deformity is measured by the angle between the couch and the long axis of the thigh (Figure 9.14). Try to maintain the affected limb in neutral adduction–abduction position as abduction will conceal the severity of flexion contracture. The Thomas test is not useful in bilateral pathology, as the sound limb needs to be maneuvered, and patients with knee pathologies restricting flexion.

9.3.6.4 PRONE HIP EXTENSION TEST

The prone hip extension test[7] can be performed on a regular padded examination table. The patient is positioned prone with both hips flexed comfortably over the end of the examination couch. The child is adequately undressed to allow visualization of the back. The other limb can be held between the examiner's knees, can be kept on a stool, or can be hung from the edge of the table. The examiner slowly extends the thigh while placing the other hand over the pelvis. The point at which the pelvis begins to rise denotes the termination of extension at the hip joint and the beginning of movement at the spine. At this point, the angle between an imaginary horizontal line parallel to the trunk and thigh gives the value of hip flexion contracture. This test can be performed in patients with bilateral hip pathology (Figure 9.15).

9.3.6.5 FIXED ABDUCTION DEFORMITY

In patients with fixed abduction deformity, the pelvis is tilted downward on the affected side; the ASIS is lower when compared to the sound side. To quantify the amount of fixed abduction deformity, the involved limb is abducted until the ASIS on the

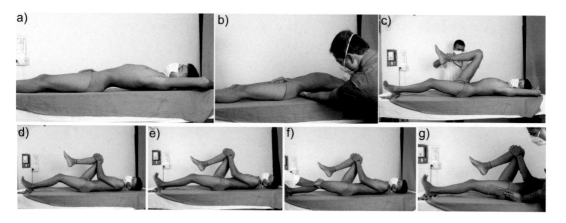

Figure 9.14 Thomas test. (a) Exaggerated lumbar lordosis. (b) The examiner is able to insinuate a hand between the patient's back and the couch. (c) Normal limb flexed until the exaggerated lumbar lordosis is obliterated. (d) The patient maintains the normal limb in this position. (e) The patient actively extends the involved limb as much as possible. (f) Examiner ensures by passively extending the involved limb without losing the position. (g) Flexion deformity measured with one limb of goniometer parallel to the examination table and the other along the long axis of the thigh.

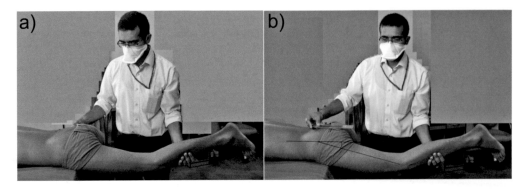

Figure 9.15 Staheli prone hip extension test. (a) The patient is positioned with hip projected over the edge of the examination table, and the hip extends just short to induce pelvic movement. (b) The angle is measured between a line parallel to the back and another along the long axis of the thigh.

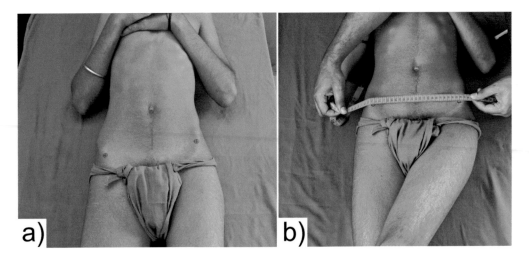

Figure 9.16 Perkins' method of squaring pelvis. (a) ASIS of the left side at a higher level due to fixed adduction deformity. (b) Limb adducted until both ASIS are at the same level.

involved side is in the same horizontal line as that of the opposite side. When the line joining the two ASIS intersects the midline at right angle or when both ASIS are at the same distance from the xiphisternum, the pelvis is considered to be squared up (Perkins' method) (Figure 9.16). With the limb kept in this position, a vertical line is drawn from the ASIS and the angle subtended between this line or the midline of the body; the long axis of the thigh denotes the fixed abduction deformity.

9.3.6.6 ALTERNATIVE METHOD

Keeping the affected limb in a position of maximum comfort, join both ASIS. From either side of this line, drop perpendicular lines toward the midline. The angle subtended between the two lines quantifies the angle of fixed abduction deformity which was described by ML Kothari (Kothari's method is not useful in bilateral cases).

Kothari's method does not require squaring of the pelvis (Figure 9.17). Rule out spinal deformities during these evaluations, e.g., in a child with a fixed scoliotic deformity in the spine, ASIS will be at a different level and the limbs will still be parallel.

9.3.6.7 FIXED ADDUCTION DEFORMITY

Here, a reversal of the maneuver carried out for fixed abduction deformity is performed. In fixed

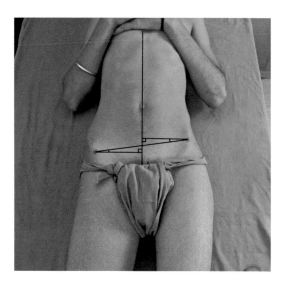

Figure 9.17 Kothari's method of assessing fixed coronal plane deformations.

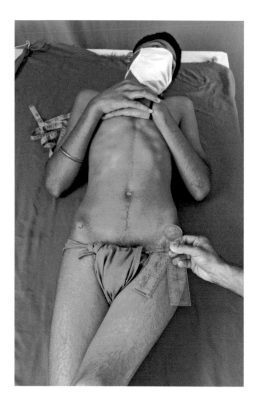

adduction deformity, the ASIS is at a higher level in comparison to the other side. The pelvis is squared by adducting the limb until both the ASIS are at the same level. With the limb kept in this position, an imaginary vertical line is drawn from the ASIS; the angle subtended between this line or midline of the body and the long axis of the thigh quantifies the fixed adduction deformity. Squaring is not possible in fixed scoliosis due to fixed pelvic obliquity (Figure 9.18).

Figure 9.18 Measuring fixed adduction deformity in a squared pelvis with one limb of a goniometer along the long axis of the thigh and another line parallel to the midline with the center over the ASIS.

9.3.6.8 FIXED ROTATIONAL DEFORMITIES

To quantify the fixed rotational deformities in an extended hip, note the angle subtended between the imaginary perpendicular line drawn over the center of the patellar anterior surface and a plumb line drawn vertically upwards over from the same point (Figure 9.19). This assessment can be augmented by positioning the patient with knees flexed and dangling over the edge of the table. The leg is used as a lever to quantify the amount of rotational deformity. This is similar to prone rotation assessment with the hip in neutral position and knee in flexion. The rotational deformities can also be quantified by the method shown in section 9.5 in a 90° flexion in the hip and knee in supine position. The rotational deformation range may differ between flexed and extended hip in pathologies altering the femoral head morphology (sphericity of the femoral head).

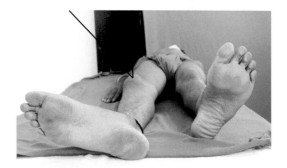

Figure 9.19 Measurement of rotational deformity between a line perpendicular to the anterior surface of the patella and another line drawn vertically upwards.

9.3.7 Measurements

As we discussed, there are compensations that can conceal the real discrepancy and so the examiner should measure the apparent and true discrepancy to quantify the compensation.

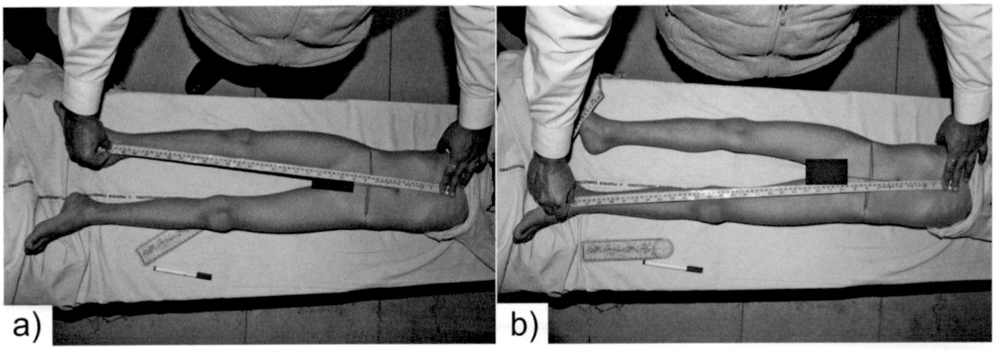

Figure 9.20 Apparent length measurement from a fixed midpoint like the xiphisternum to the tip of the medial malleolus.

9.3.7.1 APPARENT MEASUREMENT

The patient lies supine with the body as straight as possible (affected limb in line of the trunk). For apparent length measurement, the lower limbs are to be parallel and the measurement can be obtained by handling the unaffected side. Measure from a fixed central point on the trunk (midpoint of suprasternal notch, xiphisternum) to the distally sharp bony point of the malleolus (medial) and this denotes the functional length of the lower limb (Figure 9.20).

9.3.7.2 TRUE MEASUREMENT

In a squared pelvis, it is measured from the ASIS to the tip of the medial malleolus while both lower limbs are kept identical, as explained in the following.

9.3.7.3 TRUE MEASUREMENT IN SUPINE POSITION

The patient is adequately exposed, and bony points are marked with a skin marker. The bony landmarks are the ASIS, central point of the knee joint line (medial or lateral), distal sharp bony point on the medial malleolus (inferoposterior aspect), sharp point on the posterosuperior aspect of the GT, and sharpest point on the ischial tuberosity marked by flexing the hip and knee at 90°. The concealed fixed coronal plane deformation must be unmasked by squaring the pelvis. The limbs are kept in an *identical* position. Manipulate *the affected limb to square the pelvis and manipulate the normal limb to bring it to a position identical to the affected one.* The actual measurements are done

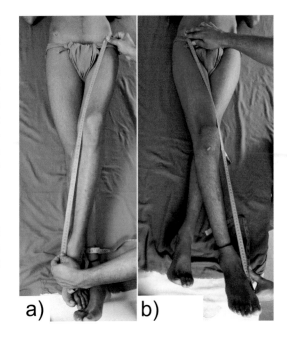

Figure 9.21 True length measurement in a patient with fixed adduction deformity on the left side after squaring the pelvis and the right lower limb positioned similar to the left during measurement.

first at the normal side from the ASIS to the tip of the medial malleolus (Figure 9.21).

- True shortening = apparent shortening – no compensation.
- True shortening > apparent shortening – part of shortening compensated by tilting of pelvis

downwards, which results in fixed abduction deformity.

- True shortening < apparent shortening – fixed adduction deformity apart from shortening without any compensation.

9.3.7.4 SEGMENTAL MEASUREMENTS

Once limb length discrepancy is identified, it is important to assess the origin of the discrepancy. The following landmarks are useful for segmental measurement.

9.3.7.4.1 Thigh Length

- Supratrochanteric: Measurement for length of neck and head of the femur.
- Infratrochanteric: Tip of GT to knee joint line.

Leg length is measured from the central point on the medial knee joint line to the tip of the medial malleolus.

9.3.7.4.2 Supratrochanteric Measurement

The disparity in supratrochanteric lengths can be measured by constituting a geometrical Bryant's triangle. It is drawn in a *squared* pelvis. A line is dropped from the ASIS perpendicular to the bed or couch. The base of the triangle is a line drawn up from the GT, and it is perpendicular to the first line. The hypotenuse is drawn connecting the ASIS and the tip of the trochanter. In comparison with the other side, if the base of the triangle is shortened, it indicates the proximal migration of the trochanter (Figure 9.22).

9.7.3.4.3 Femoral Versus Tibial Discrepancy (Alternate Method)

To find out whether the femur or tibia contributes to the limb length discrepancy, the patient is asked to lie down supine on the examination table, and the hips and knees are flexed to 90° (Figure 9.23). The patient's knees are to be at the same level in this position and if they are of different lengths, the level of the longer one is higher and the shorter one is lower. This is also a method of identifying a child with suspected DDH (the Galeazzi test/Allis sign). To find out the tibial length discrepancy, the patient lies prone with knees flexed to 90°. The soles of the patient rest at different heights from the table if the tibia is contributing to the limb length discrepancy (Figure 9.23). Shortening of the hindfoot, that is, the talus or calcaneum, can also present a similar picture and is differentiated by assessing the resting position of the malleoli, which are at the same level when the tibial lengths are equal.

9.3.7.4.4 Block Method (Performed on a Standing Patient)

In this method, blocks of various thicknesses are placed under the shortened extremity of the standing patient. The examiner places blocks to eliminate the pelvic obliquity, and an imaginary line drawn between the iliac crests is made parallel to the floor. The thickness of the blocks gives a fair estimate of the limb length discrepancy (Figure 9.23).

9.3.7.4.5 Pelvic Obliquity

While discussing limb length discrepancy (LLD), it is very important to understand pelvic obliquity.

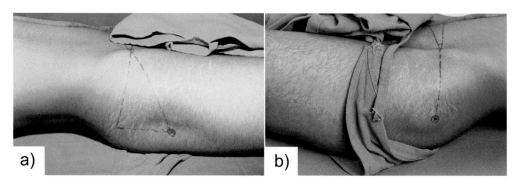

a) b)

Figure 9.22 Bryant's triangle and interpretation. (a) Normal side. (b) Complete obliteration of the triangle in a patient with significant trochanteric proximal migration.

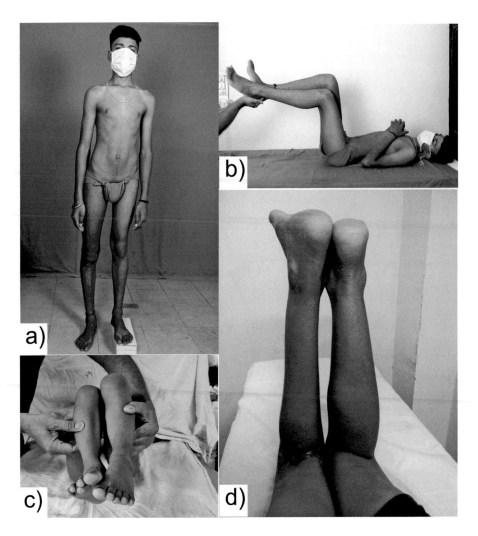

Figure 9.23 (a) Quantification of LLD by the block method. (b) By flexing hips and knees to 90. (c) Galeazzi/Allis test in a child with DDH. (d) Tibial contribution to limb length discrepancy demonstrated in prone position.

In a normal standing patient, the two sides of the pelvis must be level with each other. To check it, the examiner stands behind the patient. The patient should not be wearing footwear and should keep both feet together with the knees extended. The examiner imagines a line drawn between both iliac crests by placing a finger or two on both iliac crests. If this imaginary line is not parallel to the floor, then pelvic obliquity is present, and it may be either true LLD or apparent (functional) LLD.

True LLD is caused by the altered anatomy of one or more of the lower limb bones, which results in it being shorter or longer than its counterpart.

Functional LLD may be caused by spinal abnormalities like scoliosis, coronal plane contractures of the hip, or knee flexion contracture, etc. Secondary scoliosis caused by LLD disappears when the patient is asked to sit or when the LLD is compensated, whereas structural scoliosis and pelvic obliquity (see Figure 12.15) persists even when the patient is made to sit or on compensation of LLD.

9.3.7.5 LINES

The altered trochanteric position can also be verified by the following lines.

9.3.7.5.1 Nelaton's Line

The patient lies lateral decubitus on the normal side, and the affected limb is moderately flexed at the hip and knee. A line is drawn from the ASIS to the sharpest bony point marked on the ischial tuberosity. Normally, the tip of the trochanter is at the level of this line; in proximal migration, it is above this line (Figure 9.24).

9.3.7.5.2 Shoemaker's Line

In a supine patient, a line is drawn from the tip of the trochanter to the ASIS and is projected medially. A similar line is drawn on the other side, and these two lines should meet in the midline at or above the umbilicus. When the trochanteric tip is migrated up, the line on the affected side will intersect the other line below the level of the umbilicus and will be away from the midline toward the normal side. It may not be of much use in obese individuals with a pendulous abdomen.

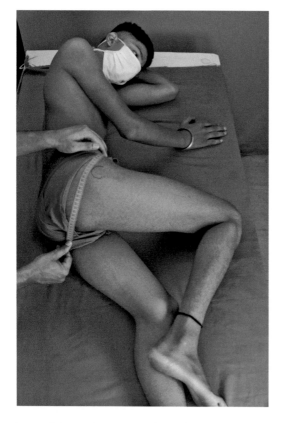

Figure 9.24 Nelaton's line from the ASIS to ischial tuberosity in a flexed hip with the tip of the GT not crossing the line in a normal hip.

9.3.7.5.3 Chiene's Test

The lines drawn between the two ASIS and the tips of the GT must be parallel; in case of proximal migration of GT, it will be convergent on that side.

9.3.7.5.4 Morris Bi-Trochanteric Test

The distance from the pubic symphysis to the tip of the trochanter should be equal on both sides. It will be increased if the limb is rotated externally or if the trochanter is displaced back and vice versa. Usually, it is measured with graduated calipers.

9.4 SPECIAL TESTS

9.4.1 Standard Trendelenburg Test

The Trendelenburg test[8] commonly denotes an abductor deficiency but can be positive in a variety of conditions involving the hip, knee, and ankle.
Prerequisites:

- Pain-free hip with flexion possible to at least 30°.
- Absence of fixed coronal deformity as the hip has to abduct and adduct freely for the test to be possible.

The examiner stands behind the patient and observes the angle made between the line joining the iliac crests (pelvis) and the ground. The patient raises the foot on the opposite side being tested with the hip kept between neutral and a flexion of 30°. The position of the pelvis is noted. On the weight-bearing side, a supporting stick can be given, or the examiner may support both the shoulders to maintain balance.

Once the patient attains balance, he/she is now advised to raise the non-weight-bearing side of the pelvis as high as he/she can. The examiner may hold the arm on the stance side for support. If the patient leans too far to the side of the stance hip, the examiner can correct this to get the vertebra prominens approximately over the center of the weight-bearing hip by gentle pressure on the shoulders.

9.4.1.1 INTERPRETATION

- Negative test: when the pelvis on the non-weight-bearing side raises as high as possible and is capable of maintaining it for 30 seconds with the vertebra prominens centered over the hip and foot.

- Positive test: if the patient is not able to do said maneuver and this also includes cases where the pelvis is elevated on the non-weight-bearing side above the stance side, but the elevation is not maximal. Also, if the pelvis can be lifted on command but cannot be maintained for 30 seconds, this is a positive test (Figure 9.25).

9.4.2 Telescopy Test

This test is done to evaluate the stability of the hip joint. The patient is positioned supine on the examination table, and this is better done with the examiner standing on the side that is to be examined. The hip and knee are flexed to 90° and the hip kept in mild adduction. The pelvis is supported with one hand by placing the thenar eminence over the ASIS and the fingers on the greater trochanter. The knee/distal thigh is held with the other hand, and a gentle push and pull force is applied along the long axis of the thigh. If the hip is unstable, an up and down trochanteric excursion can be felt with the other hand (Figure 9.26). When the excursion is more than that compared to the other side,

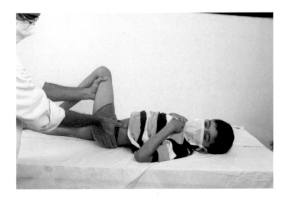

Figure 9.26 Telescopy test done with hip flexed, adducted, and with fingers over GT to feel the instability movements while the other hand holds the distal thigh, and push and pull forces are applied.

think of conditions like a femoral neck fracture nonunion, hip dislocation, etc.

9.4.3 Sectoral Sign

The sectoral sign or axis deviation test implies sectoral involvement of the femoral head in pathology

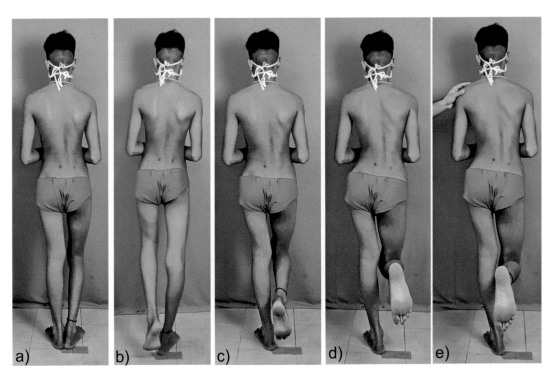

Figure 9.25 Standard Trendelenburg test. (a) Both limbs on ground. (b) Weight bearing on normal side with normal elevation of pelvis on non weight bearing side. (c), (d), (e) Weight bearing on affected side with drop in pelvis on opposite side indicating positive test.

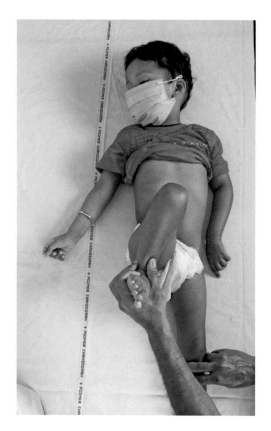

Figure 9.27 Sectoral sign: normal flexion of the hip with the knees pointing toward the opposite shoulder. It is considered positive with knee drifting toward the ipsilateral shoulder.

like avascular necrosis and is accompanied usually by important clinical signs like loss of internal rotation of the hip. It is also seen in conditions like SUFE. When the hip is flexed, it usually points to the opposite shoulder (Figure 9.27), and if it deviates toward the same shoulder, it is considered to be positive.[9] It is equivalent to the Drehmann sign

seen in SUFE with impingement, which is obligatory external rotation happening on flexion of the hip.[10]

9.4.4 Impingement Test

Children with femoroacetabular impingement[11,12] are usually adolescent children with a history of gradual onset groin or buttock pain. The range of hip joint motion may be reduced in certain positions. The internal rotation is restricted, with the hip flexed to 90°. In severe cases, obligatory external rotation with hip flexion can be seen.

9.4.4.1 ANTERIOR IMPINGEMENT SIGN

The anterior impingement sign is a controlled recreation of cam and pincer femoro-acetabular impingement (FAI) pain. The patient is positioned supine on the examination table with the hip flexed to 90°, adducted and internally rotated. If the patient feels pain or demonstrates apprehension, the test is positive, and this is due to the direct contact of the femoral neck with the acetabular rim or labrum (Figure 9.28).

9.4.4.2 POSTEROINFERIOR IMPINGEMENT SIGN

This maneuver is useful to elicit pincer FAI pain. The patient is positioned supine on the edge of the examination couch. With the hip in extension and knee flexed, the hip is gradually externally rotated. The test is positive if the patient demonstrates apprehension or feels pain as it loads the posteroinferior aspect of the hip (Figure 9.28).

9.4.4.3 GEAR-STICK SIGN

The gear-stick sign is useful in differentiating trochanteric impingement from other sources of hip

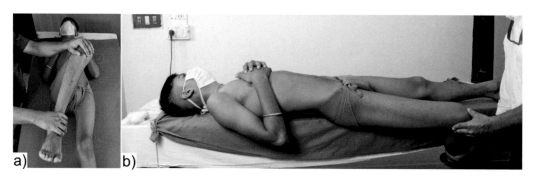

Figure 9.28 (a) Anterior impingement test. (b) Posterior impingement test.

pain. The child is placed in a lateral decubitus position with the symptomatic hip up. The limb is passively abducted in extension at the hip from the adducted position. The test is considered positive with the reproduction of the patient's symptoms implicating that hip pain is extra-articular and arises from trochanteric impingement (proximally migrated trochanter like Perthes' sequelae).

9.4.5 Modified Schober's Test

The Schober's and modified Schober's test[13] are used to diagnose the restriction of lumbar spine flexion in patients with inflammatory arthropathy, particularly ankylosing spondylitis. We will describe the modified Schober's test. With the patient standing, the examiner marks the level of the lumbosacral junction. Then mark two points, one 10 cm above (a) and the other 5 cm below (b) the level of the lumbosacral junction (distance between the two points (a and b) being 15 cm). The patient is asked to bend forwards and attempt to touch their toes with the knees kept straight. Measure the distance between the two points, a and b, and if the distance does not increase by at least 5 cm, the test is said to be positive, indicating restriction of lumbar spine flexion (Figure 9.29).

9.4.6 SI Joint Tests

9.4.6.1 PATRICK'S TEST

Patrick's test is a provocative indirect stress test for the assessment of inflammation of the sacroiliac joint. It is known by the acronym FABER, which stands for flexion, abduction, and external rotation, resulting in a figure of 4 position. The limb on the side of examination is gradually positioned into the figure of 4 position. The ankle of the side to be tested rests on the opposite thigh proximal to the knee joint. The examiner presses down on the knee with counterpressure applied on the contralateral ASIS using the other hand (Figure 9.30). If the patient experiences *posterior hip pain*, sacroiliitis must be suspected. Remember, an arthritic hip or an iliopsoas pathology might produce an anterior groin pain, which should be differentiated from the one resulting from sacroiliitis.

9.4.6.2 GAENSLEN'S TEST

This maneuver stresses the sacroiliac joint and is performed by positioning the patient supine with the buttock on the side of examination, projecting over the edge of the table. Both knees are actively drawn toward the chest by the patient. Maintaining the contralateral limb in this position, and the

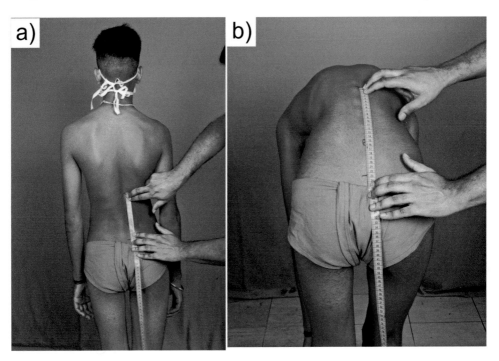

Figure 9.29 Modified Schober's test.

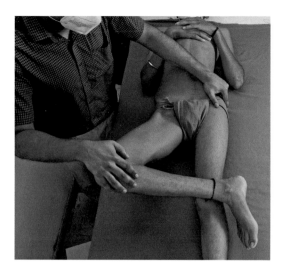

Figure 9.30 Patrick's test for sacroiliitis.

patient stabilized by the examiner, the ipsilateral thigh is dropped off the edge of the table, thereby completely extending the hip. If this maneuver induces pain, sacroiliac pathology must be suspected (Figure 9.31).

9.4.7 Examination of Lymph Nodes

Regional examination is not complete without examining the draining lymph nodes. Deep inguinal nodes drain the anterior aspect, while the medial and posterior aspects drain into the internal iliac nodes. They are examined in the following locations.[14]

9.4.7.1 DEEP INGUINAL LYMPH NODES

These lymph nodes are about four to five in number and lie medially to the upper part of the femoral vein. The most proximal node of this group is the gland of Cloquet or of Rosenmuller and is situated in the femoral canal.

9.4.7.2 EXTERNAL ILIAC NODES

There are eight to ten of these nodes, and they lie along the external iliac vessels, either medial, lateral, or anterior to the vessel. They receive afferents from the inguinal lymph nodes. The surface-marking of the external iliac artery is as follows. Mark a point 1.2 cm below and lateral to the umbilicus (at the level of vertebra L4). The external iliac artery is denoted by the lower two-thirds of a line drawn from the first point to the mid-inguinal point. Palpation is feasible only in thin patients.

Do not forget to palpate the base of the iliac fossa inferiorly. Tenderness elicited in this region will help differentiate abdominal pathologies like psoas abscess masquerading as hip pathology. Tubercular cold abscess can present as swelling at the iliac fossa, Scarpa's triangle base, gluteal region, and above the trochanter and mid-thigh (anteromedial aspect even up to the knee joint). The examination is never complete without an examination of the spine, contralateral hip, and both knees and ankles for any secondary changes or else primary pathology.

9.4.8 Tests Specific for DDH

9.4.8.1 ORTOLANI TEST

With the child in supine position, the hips are flexed to a right angle and slightly internally rotated with the knees flexed.[15] The knees are held in the palms of the hands, and the thumbs are placed on the inner aspect of the knees. From this position, the hips are abducted and externally rotated, and simultaneously, the fingers press the

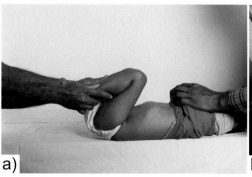
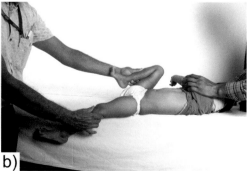

Figure 9.31 Gaenslen's test for sacroiliitis.

greater trochanters medially. This is usually not painful and easily performed when the child is relaxed. The examiner might feel a snap, which indicates that the head of the femur has returned to the acetabular cavity, and the restriction of the abduction of the thigh is released. The head comes to jump over the labrum, which produces the sensation of snapping (Figure 9.32).

9.4.8.2 BARLOW'S TEST

The infant is placed supine position and the examiner stands at the patient's legs.[16] The knees are fully flexed while the hips are flexed to 90°. The examiner examines each hip individually while the other hand is used to stabilize the opposite femur and pelvis. The examiner places the middle finger over the greater trochanter and the thumb adjacent to the inner side of the knee and thigh opposite the lesser trochanter on either side. The hip is gradually abducted with the examiner applying forward pressure behind the greater trochanter with the middle finger. If the femoral head slips forward within the acetabulum with a click, clunk, or jerk, the test is positive, and the hip was dislocated. This part of the test is like Ortolani's test.

Now the examiner uses his/her thumb to apply pressure on the inner thigh backward and outward. If the head slips out over the posterior lip of the acetabulum and then reduces again with the removal of pressure, then the hip is unstable. The hip is dislocatable but not dislocated. The procedure is repeated on the other side. This is used in children up to 6 months of age and should not be repeated often to avoid damaging the articular cartilage of the head of the femur (Figure 9.33).

9.4.8.3 KLISIC TEST

The examiner places the middle finger over the greater trochanter and the index finger on the ASIS.[17] An imaginary line is drawn between the fingers and in a normal child should point toward the umbilicus, and in the case of a dislocated hip, the more proximal greater trochanter results in the line pointing approximately halfway between the umbilicus and the pubis (Figure 9.34).

9.5 TORSIONAL ASSESSMENT OF THE LOWER LIMB

9.5.1 Femoral Version

When the neck of femur neck angulates forward in relation to femoral shaft, greater than 8–15°, the patient has increased femoral anteversion.[18] A patient with increased femoral anteversion stands with the limb in internal rotation, producing intoeing. When an individual is standing normally in a relaxed position, the feet should point outward

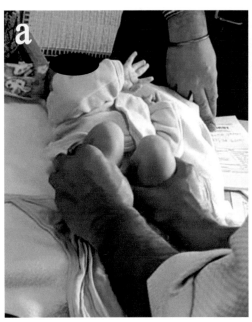
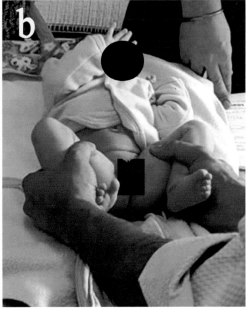

Figure 9.32 Ortolani's test.

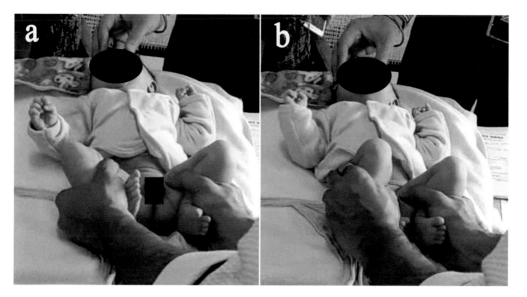

Figure 9.33 Barlow's test.

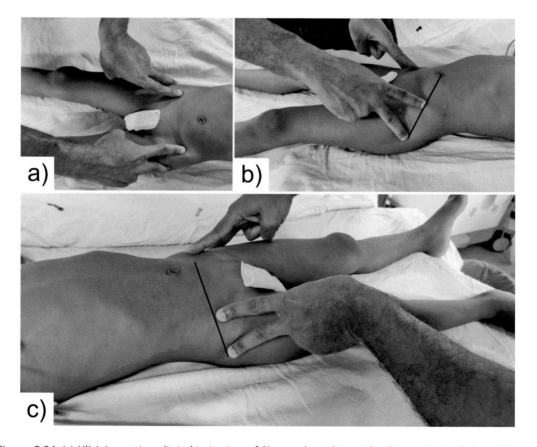

Figure 9.34 (a) Klisic's test is a digital imitation of Shoemaker's line with a line projected along the middle finger on the GT and index finger on the ASIS. (b) Crossing midline normally at or above the umbilicus. (c) Crossing midline below the level of the umbilicus.

approximately 10–20° from the straight-ahead position. A patient with femoral retroversion will have out-toeing due to a tendency to stand with limbs externally rotated.

9.5.1.1 CRAIG'S TEST/RYDER METHOD

This test is commonly performed to estimate the amount of femoral anteversion. The patient is positioned prone with the ipsilateral knee flexed to 90°. The examiner palpates the lateral prominence of the GT with one hand while controlling the rotation of the limb using the leg as a lever with the other. The reference for this test is an imaginary vertical line. The limb is rotated internally (away from the midline) until the lateral prominence of the GT is felt to be maximal. At 90° flexion at the knee, the leg is positioned perpendicular to the posterior aspect of the femoral condyles, and hence the angle between the imaginary vertical line and the leg gives a measure of the femoral neck anteversion.

9.5.1.2 TIBIAL TORSION

Refer to the tibial torsion assessment in Chapter 13.

REFERENCES

1. Lesher JM, Dreyfuss P, Hager N, Kaplan M, Furman M. Hip joint pain referral patterns: A descriptive study. *Pain Med.* 2008;9:22–25.
2. Taj FT. Cutaneous markers of spinal dysraphism: A cross sectional study. *Ind J Paediatr Dermatol.* 2018;19:215–219.
3. Wynne-Davies R. Acetabular dysplasia and familial joint laxity: Two etiological factors in congenital dislocation of the hip. A review of 589 patients and their families. *J Bone Joint Surg Br.* 1970;52:704–716.
4. Beighton P, Solomon L, Soskolne CL. Articular mobility in an African population. *Ann Rheum Dis.* 1973;32:413–418.
5. Pandey S. Hip. In: Pandey S, Pandey AK, editors. *Clinical orthopaedic diagnosis*, 4th ed. New Delhi: Jaypee Brothers Medical Publishers (P) Ltd; 2018. pp. 347–391.
6. Rang M. *Anthology of orthopaedics*. Edinburgh and London: E & S. Livingstone Ltd, 1968. pp. 137–138.
7. Staheli LT. The prone hip extension test: A method of measuring hip flexion deformity. *Clin Orthop Relat Res.* 1977;123:12–15.
8. Hardcastle P, Nade S. The significance of the Trendelenburg test. *J Bone Joint Surg Br.* 1985; 67:741–746.
9. Babhulkar S. Osteonecrosis of femoral head: Treatment by core decompression and vascular pedicle grafting. *Indian J Orthop.* 2009;43:27–35.
10. Kamegaya M, Saisu T, Nakamura J, Murakami R, Segawa Y, Wakou M. Drehmann sign and femoro-acetabular impingement in SCFE. *J Pediatr Orthop.* 2011;31:853–857.
11. Zebala LPS, Clohisy JC. Anterior femoroacetabular impingement: A diverse disease with evolving treatment options. *Iowa Orthop J.* 2007;27:71–81.
12. Parvizi J, Leunig M, Ganz R. Femoroacetabular impingement. *AAOS.* 2007;15:10.
13. Macrae IF, Wright V. Measurement of back movement. *Ann Rheum Dis.* 1969;28:584–589.
14. Garg K. *BD Chaurasia's human anatomy - regional and applied, dissection and clinical*, 4th ed. New Delhi: CBS Publishers and Distributors; 2004. pp. 133, 317, 401.
15. Rang M. *Anthology of orthopaedics*. London: E & S. Livingstone Ltd; 1968. p 144.
16. Magee DJ, *Hip. orthopedic physical assessment*, 6th ed. St. Louis, MO: Elsevier Saunders; 2014. pp. 689–764.
17. Herring JA. Developmental dysplasia of hip. In: Herring JA, editor. *Tachdjian's pediatric orthopaedics: From the Texas Scottish Rite hospital for children*, 5th ed. Philadelphia: Elsevier Saunders; 2014. pp. 485–535.
18. Mortell JM. Pelvis, hip and thigh. In: Reider B. *The orthopaedic physical examination*, 2nd ed. Philadelphia: Elsevier Saunders; 2005. pp. 161–200.

Examination of Knee Joint in a Child

ANIL AGARWAL

10.1 INTRODUCTION

The knee is a complex joint, and its evaluation can be a challenge even to the most experienced. The main components of a complete knee examination are a detailed history, followed by a systematic clinical examination. Relevant imaging and laboratory investigations, as suggested by the history and clinical examination, may be obtained to arrive at a diagnosis.

10.2 HISTORY

Pain, swelling, limitation of movement, deformity, and gait abnormalities are the most common knee complaints. History-taking is chiefly elaborating on these symptoms and the terminology used by the patient in detail. It is, therefore, necessary to characterize pain in terms of onset (rapid or insidious), distribution (generalized or local), location, duration, severity, and nature (e.g., dull, excruciating). Identify the factors aggravating and relieving the pain. If pain followed an injury, the injury characteristics should be identified in detail. Take a note of the position of the foot during the incident, location of the blow, if any, to the knee (e.g., anterior in dashboard injury), or whether the injury resulted from twisting or decelerating forces. If possible, inquire whether the patient was up and able to walk after injury.

The sequence of the appearance of effusion (swelling) and its amount provides important clues in the differential diagnosis of knee pathology. Bursal swellings are localized, whereas trauma and effusions resulting from generalized disease, such as rheumatoid disease, are diffuse. In traumatic situations, a large effusion with onset within a few hours indicates rupture of cruciate ligaments or intra-articular fractures, whereas a mild to moderate effusion with delayed appearance is more suggestive of meniscal damage.

Often, the patient uses terms such as "locking" and "giving way" in his/her own perception of symptoms. The ambiguity should be removed by discussing the exact sequence and description of complaints with the patient, e.g., are the movements less than full extension or are there none at all? Similarly, the symptoms of giving way should also be deciphered clearly. The patient's daily routine and hobbies (sedentary, dance, athletics, contact sports, scouting, cycling, hiking, skating, etc.) should also be requested and noted.

Other details such as past history (e.g., involvement of other joints), rheumatoid arthritis, multifocal infections, and systemic signs of illness (i.e., fever, rash), personal history (e.g., recent travel to a high-risk area with a prevalence of tuberculosis, brucellosis, Lyme disease, exposure to ticks), medical history (e.g., previous injury, instability, or surgery on the joint, coexisting chronic illness such as lupus, inflammatory bowel disease), drug history (e.g., use of over-the-counter, herbal, or prescription medication), family history (e.g., family history of autoimmune or rheumatologic

disease), and use of walking aids should also be inquired.

10.3 EXAMINATION

10.3.1 Gait Examination

The examiner observes for any gait abnormalities, and the knee position during stance and swing phase is noted. Any instability noted during walking is recorded. For example, a patient with genu varum might have a varus thrust gait, and painful pathologies of the knee can result in an antalgic gait pattern.

10.3.2 Position of Examination

Ideally, the patient should be examined in an upright position, supine lying down position, prone position, and sitting position with legs hanging down. The contralateral knee serves as a control for the examined knee, if unaffected. Ensure that it is exposed and available for comparative examination. The hip joints and distal extremity to the toes should also be exposed.

10.3.3 Inspection

The inspection of the knee should comprise of assessing for any asymmetry, swellings, limb length inequality, and malalignments.

10.3.3.1 ATTITUDE

Normally, the anatomical femoral and tibial axes meet at the knee (170–175°, obtuse laterally) to form the physiological valgus angle of 5–10° of the knee joint (Figure 10.1).

Variations in the anatomical angle lead to genu valgum (<165°) or genu varum (>180°). The valgus or varus attitude at the knee is best observed in the standing position. In the sagittal plane, there may be hyperextension at the knee resulting in genu recurvatum, which may be physiological in hyper lax children or pathological as seen in children with congenital knee dislocation (Figure 10.2a).

The genu varum and valgum can be quantitatively measured as an intercondylar and intermalleolar distance, respectively. The child is instructed to stand erect with the patella pointing

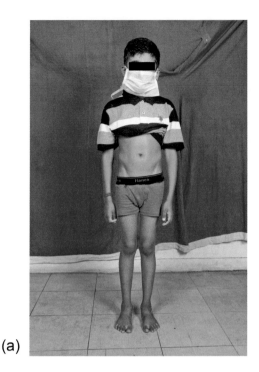

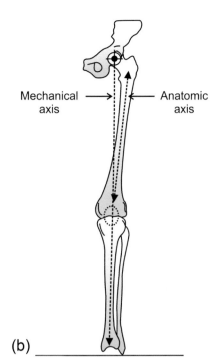

Figure 10.1 (a) and (b) Anatomical femoral and tibial axes meet at the knee to form the physiological valgus angle of 5–10° of the knee joint.

forward. The knees or ankles are adjusted such that the condyles or malleoli are just touching (no overlap!) each other. The horizontal distance between the bony landmarks can be measured using a non-stretchable measuring tape. Physiological variations exist between different ages, sexes, and ethnic groups. It is, therefore, necessary to match the obtained measurements with the standard reference values. Sagittal plane malalignment may be seen in the form of recurvatum, which is hyperextension to gross dislocation in a condition like congenital knee dislocation (Figure 10.2b).

In Indian pretext, squatting and sitting crosslegged is common practice and the ability to do so indicates significant preserved motion at the hip and knee joints.

The patellar size, shape, and location are inspected in standing and supine positions. Further examine the knee for wasting, particularly of vastus medialis muscle, changes in skin color, ecchymosis, bruises, presence of any scars, sinuses, rash marks, or healed surgical incisions. Examine for any swelling or lumps in the knee region. In the posterior aspect of the knee, look for any swelling, varicose veins, and abnormal pulsations.

10.3.4 Palpation

A systemic physical examination of the knee should include an examination of the knee from anterior, medial, lateral, and posterior aspects. The knee palpation should include evaluation for warmth, point tenderness, quadriceps contraction, patellofemoral articulation, bursal swellings and effusions, range of movement, muscle power, neurological assessment, instability (including patellofemoral instability), and ligament/ meniscal injuries. The examination may be inaccurate if there is muscle spasm and guarding. Therefore, at most, an attempt should be made to keep the child relaxed. It is sometimes beneficial to examine the unaffected knee before the affected knee as it makes the patient less apprehensive by preparing the patient for the repeat maneuver. Also, it secondarily provides the examiner with an inherent control as regards the presence and degree of asymmetrical observations.

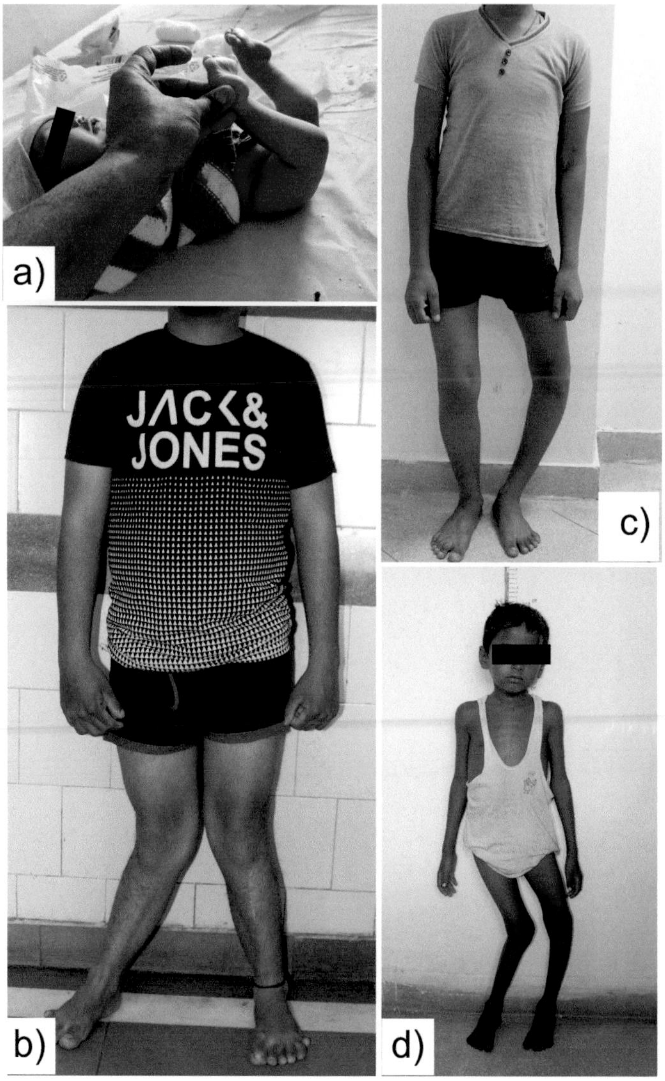

Figure 10.2 (a) Sagittal plane deformation in a case of congenital knee dislocation. (b), (c), and (d) Coronal plane deformation – genu valgum, genu varum, and windswept deformity.

10.3.5 Evaluation for Warmth

Always use the back of your fingers as the temperature assessment tool. The palmar surface of the hand can be less sensitive to temperature because of the thickened skin. In wintery climates, ensure that the hands are warm enough before touching the patient to feel any temperature differences. Begin by comparing both knees. Make accommodations for the temperature difference in the exposed part when compared with the covered part, e.g., wrapped with blankets, stockings, etc. An overall increase in temperature signifies a generalized disease such as rheumatoid disease or infection. A localized increase in temperature may also be evident in pathologies such as blunt injuries, fractures, or bursal inflammations. A temperature gradient may arise in the same limb between the knee region and distal extremity because of vascular derangements such as Buerger's disease or diabetic affections. Always feel and compare the distal and popliteal pulse under such circumstances.

10.3.6 Evaluation of Point Tenderness

Point tenderness should be specifically sought. The sensitivity of this finding to localize the site of pathology may be as high as 75%. The joint line can be easily identified if the knee is moved slightly along a short arc. The medial and lateral knee joint lines are perpendicular to the long axis of the tibia and can be felt as depressions as one moves up along the proximal portion of the tibia. Palpate both joint lines. Place both your thumbs on the anterior aspect of the knee on either side of the patellar tendon and then move gradually along the joint line from front to back (e.g., tenderness from injuries of the meniscus, collateral ligaments, or inflammation of an arthritic joint). If in doubt, compare with the opposite knee. You may start by feeling the prominent bony structures on the medial side of the limb, e.g., the medial tibial plateau, medial femoral condyle (e.g., tenderness may be present in osteochondritis dissecans), and adductor tubercle followed by those on the lateral aspect, e.g., the lateral tibial plateau, lateral femoral condyle, lateral femoral epicondyle, and head of the fibula. The medial ligament of the knee is attached to the medial epicondyle of the femur and on the medial aspect of the tibia. Occasionally, a valgus injury of the knee is followed by hematoma formation and subsequent calcification in the upper attachment of the medial ligament. They may be responsible for sharp localized pain over the ligament on palpation (Pellegrini–Stieda disease). Another sign is Bassett's sign indicating reduced medial patellar stability. There will be tenderness on palpation of the adductor tubercle and medial femoral epicondyle resulting from injury to the medial patellofemoral ligament (MPFL).

The infrapatellar pad of fat forms a thin layer beneath and on either side of the patellar tendon. Surgery or infection in the region may restrict the mobility of this fat pad, which may get pinched during knee extension and become painful. The site of insertion of the patellar tendon and tibial tuberosity is also palpated for any tender lumps (e.g., Osgood–Schlatter's disease).

In the flexed position of the knee, feel for the two heads of the gastrocnemius originating above their respective femoral condyles; they are prominent when the patient flexes the knee against resistance. Also, feel for the biceps femoris tendon laterally and medial hamstrings medially. Gently palpate the common peroneal nerve as it swirls over the posterolateral aspect of the fibular neck.

10.3.7 Evaluation of Quadriceps Mechanism and Patellofemoral Articulation

The quadriceps muscle is the main knee extensor, and its vastus medialis portion is the most important component responsible for achieving the last degrees of extension. This portion of the quadriceps muscle rapidly undergoes wasting in pathologies of the knee, leading to extensor lag.

The patellofemoral joint is part of the quadriceps mechanism. The patella lies between the quadriceps muscle superiorly and the patellar tendon distally, which anchors it to the tuberosity of the tibia. The quadriceps angle (Q angle) is formed by the intersecting lines formed by the pull of the quadriceps mechanism and patellar tendon. Clinically, the angle is calculated in an extended knee position (standing patient). A straight line is drawn from the anterior superior iliac spine to the center of the patella and another line from the center of the tibial tuberosity to the patella's center (Figure 10.3). A significant variation in the Q angle (normal is approximately 6°) indicates altered quadriceps pull. This may predispose to patellar subluxation.

Begin by comparing the quadriceps muscle in both limbs. The musculature should be symmetrical bilaterally. Variations may be obvious in affections, e.g., chronic post-traumatic affection of the extremity, chronic osteomyelitis femur, etc. The muscle girth can be recorded by measuring it in reference to a fixed bony landmark such as the upper pole of the patella or above the knee joint line. Look at and palpate any gaps or defects in the rectus femoris muscle and patellar tendon that feel as soft yields in these otherwise firm structures. Examine the tone of the quadriceps muscle by palpating it after asking the patient to actively contract it. The patient can be helped in this maneuver by placing a hand or rolled towel in the posterior knee region and instructing the patient to press against it. The vastus medialis component can be selectively examined by asking the patient to dorsiflex the inverted foot while attempting a knee extension. Surface electromyography (EMG) studies

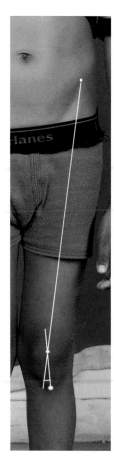

Figure 10.3 The Q angle is formed by the line of pull of the quadriceps mechanism and that of the patellar tendon as they intersect at the patella's center.

Patellofemoral tracking is assessed by instructing the patient to move the knee from the flexed position to extension. Observe the patellar movements while the patient performs the above maneuver. During normal tracking, the patella moves in a straight line as the knee starts extending. Later, during terminal extension, there is a slight lateral shift and tilt. An excessive lateral shift and tilt is indicative of patellar instability. When shifting is excessive, the patella topples over the lateral femoral trochlea edge during every active knee extension in habitual patellar dislocation. Check the apparent height of the patella (e.g., high patella in patella alta) and watch if the patella deviates medially or laterally in knee flexion or extension.

10.3.8 Evaluation for Bursal Inflammations and Effusions

There are several bursae around the knee (Figure 10.4). The semimembranosus bursa lies between the medial head of the gastrocnemius muscle and the knee joint capsule. The overlying gastrocnemius and semimembranosus muscle may compress the communication of this bursa to the joint resulting in a one-way valve mechanism. The resulting enlargement of this bursa in diseases such as rheumatoid arthritis presents as a lump in the popliteal region (Baker's cyst), which cannot be pushed into the joint. The suprapatellar bursa lies beneath the deep surface of the quadriceps muscle and the anterior surface of the lower femur. It may extend up to approximately 5 cm or more above the upper margin of the patella with the knee in extension. It has communication with the knee joint. The prepatellar bursa (sometimes called housemaid's knee bursa) covers the anterior surface of the lower patella and upper patellar tendon. The infrapatellar bursa is present between the skin and the lower part of the tibial tuberosity. The bursa may get enlarged and inflamed in children who keep their knees flexed and have predominant floor-sitting. The pes anserine (also known as subsartorial) bursa is present on the medial aspect of the tibial tubercle beneath the tendinous insertion of the sartorius, gracilis, and semitendinosus.

have shown that the muscle is facilitated by knee extension in an inverted dorsiflexed ankle. Much of the patella's articular surface is accessible to palpation if the patella is first pushed medially and then laterally in a relaxed knee. The undersurface of the patella may be tender in chondromalacia patellae or retropatellar arthritis. Point tenderness should also be sought over the quadriceps tendon (e.g., quadriceps tendinitis), anterior surface of the patella (e.g., fractures), and lower pole (e.g., Sinding–Larsen–Johansson disease), patellar tendon (e.g., strains), and tibial tubercle (e.g., Osgood–Schlatter disease in children and adolescents).

Move the patella up and down and side to side while pressing it lightly against the femur (the friction test). Ensure a relaxed quadriceps before eliciting this test. Painful grating or crepitus is felt in retropatellar arthritis or advanced chondromalacia.

In a minimal effusion, the first sign is the disappearance of normal knee "dimples" lying by the side of the patella (Figure 10.5).

The "bulge test" is useful with smaller effusions. The fluid is milked from the medial to the

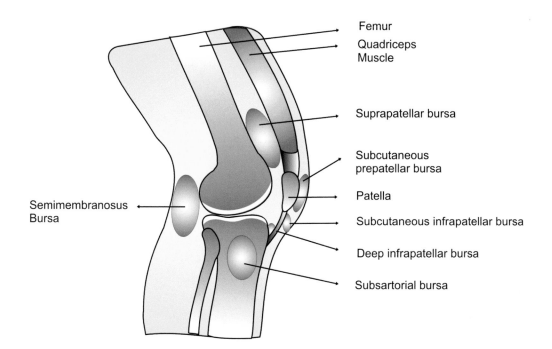

Figure 10.4 Important bursae around the knee joint.

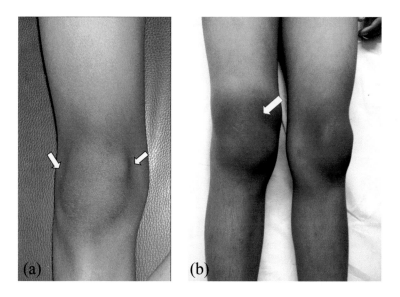

Figure 10.5 The dimple on both sides of the patella and its obliteration in a child with effusion.

lateral side using the thumb on one side of the patella and then quickly pressing the lateral side with the opposite thumb. The medial parapatellar region "fills out" after pressure on the lateral parapatellar region (positive "bulge sign"). This is indicative of knee effusion. With larger effusions, the suprapatellar space is filled up and "suprapatellar fullness" is felt. The patella is pushed anteriorly by the fluid. In a straight knee position, the fluid in the suprapatellar pouch can be pushed down by one hand into the lower compartments. With the opposite fingers, the elevated patella can be pushed against the femoral condyles and a palpable bounce can be felt. This test is known as the patellar ballottement test or patellar tap test.

Another test possible with a large amount of fluid in the knee joint is the "cross fluctuation test" between the suprapatellar and infrapatellar region

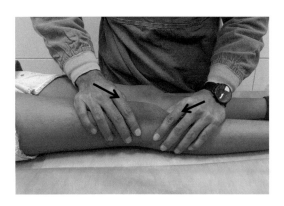

Figure 10.6 The cross fluctuation test is possible when there is a large amount of fluid in the knee joint.

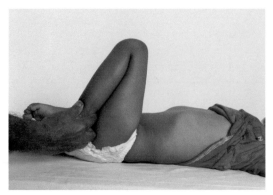

Figure 10.7 The flexion range at the knee joint from full extension is usually about 0–150°.

(Figure 10.6). The left thumb and index finger embrace the suprapatellar pouch while the right thumb and index fingers are placed on either side of the infrapatellar region. Fluid thrill can be felt on the other end by squeezing either hand. In large and tense effusions, fluid displacement tests would be negative.

Sometimes, the fluid present in the knee joint has its own characteristics, e.g., a hemarthrosis presents with a doughy feel. Feel for any bursal inflammation in their respective regions. About 2 cm proximal to the superior border of the patella, the synovium becomes superficial and is only covered by skin and subcutaneous fat. The layers of synovium roll back upon themselves in this region. It is, therefore, easy to feel the synovial thickening in the medial suprapatellar region (e.g., in chronic inflammatory conditions of the knee and villonodular synovitis). Carefully examine the posterior aspect of the knee for any swellings and tenderness. Note particularly for any pulsatile lumps present in the posterior knee region (e.g., popliteal aneurysms).

10.3.9 Range of Movement

The knee joint is a modified type of hinge joint. Flexion and extension take place around a variable transverse axis. Flexion is leg movement in the posterior direction until the calf meets the posterior aspect of the thigh. Extension is leg movement in the anterior direction leading to straight alignment of the thigh and leg in the sagittal plane. Full extension is usually recorded as 0°. From the

position of 0° extension, the flexion range is usually about 0–150° (Figure 10.7).

A few degrees of hyperextension at the knee is normal in view of the stability achieved in standing. Pathological hyperextension is encountered in conditions such as Ehlers–Danlos syndrome, ligamentous injury, etc. The knee flexion should preferably be measured with the hip flexed to avoid any restriction by a tight rectus femoris and vice versa; full flexion at the hip should be avoided during measurements of knee extension to avoid interference by the hamstring muscles. The variable axis of flexion and extension is determined by the shape of the medial femoral condyle. As the leg moves the full arch from full flexion to extension, the peculiar elongated shape of the medial femoral condyle ensures that the tibia glides as well as rotates on the femur, and as a result, the tibia rotates outwards with respect to the femur (assuming the thigh is fixed and the leg moves) (Figure 10.8).

In the fully extended position, the tibial tubercles are in close proximity to the femoral intercondylar notch, the menisci are tightly wedged between the tibial and femoral articular surfaces, the collateral ligaments are tight, and all together lead to a "locked" position of the knee with no further rotation of the tibia possible on the femur. This ensures adequate mechanical stability at the knee joint enabling the child to stand erect even when the quadriceps are weak. During the initiation of flexion, the tightening is reversed by the inward rotation of the tibia (assuming the thigh is fixed again) aided by the popliteus muscle.

The range of movement at the knee should be noted both passively and actively. Special attention should be given to the presence of any extensor lag,

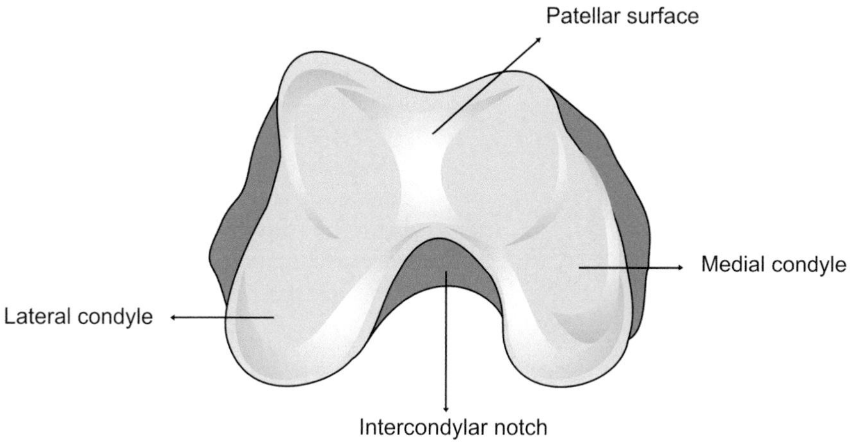

Figure 10.8 The elongated shape of the medial femoral condyle plays an important role in locking of the knee joint.

i.e., inability to extend the leg actively fully. In such circumstances, the passive extension at the knee might be complete. If the knee cannot be extended fully, even passively, assess the nature of resistance to full extension. In arthritic conditions, the resistance may be bony, whereas in meniscal tears, a springy block may be encountered. Similarly, note whether there is any restriction of flexion (e.g., in conditions like arthritis, cellulitis, and contusion). The range of movement in the knee is usually recorded in the following formats, e.g., for 10° terminal loss of extension on both active and passive examination, the range of movement can be recorded as 10–150° (range of movement); loss of 10° of extension, 140° flexion; 10° of flexion deformity, further flexion to 150°.

10.3.10 Muscle Power and Neurological Assessment

The main extensor at the knee is the quadriceps muscle (L2, L3, L4), and flexion is carried out by the hamstring group comprising of the semimembranosus (L5), semitendinosus (L5), and biceps femoris muscle (S1).

- Testing for quadriceps femoris. The patient is seated on the edge of the table, with both legs hanging. The examiner stabilizes the thigh against the table. Ask the patient to extend the knee without rotating the thigh. Exert counterpressure against the leg just above the ankle to oppose extension.

- Medial (semimembranosus and semitendinosus) and lateral hamstring (biceps femoris) group. The patient is in prone position on the table. The examiner stabilizes the thigh against the couch. For the medial group, instruct the child to flex the knee to 50–70° with the thigh in slight medial rotation, and the leg medially rotated on the thigh. For the lateral group, the thigh is rotated slightly laterally, and the leg laterally rotated on the thigh. In both situations, apply pressure against the leg above the ankle in the direction of knee extension.
- Sensation testing. The knee is covered by L2, L3, and L4 on the anterior aspect and S2 on the posterior aspect (Figure 10.9).

10.4 EVALUATION OF INSTABILITY

The knee is a complex joint, and many static and dynamic stabilizers contribute to its stability. The literature describes a number of physical examination tests for assessing knee stability. For the purpose of simplicity, knee stability can be attributed to four main stabilizers – the anterior cruciate ligament (ACL), posterior cruciate ligament (PCL), the medial collateral ligament (MCL) along with posteromedial stabilizers, and posterolateral stabilizers. It is to be understood that there is significant overlap between these stabilizers, with one component contributing to each other in different knee positions and vice versa.

Knee cruciates are strong cord-like structures present in the intercondylar region of the tibia

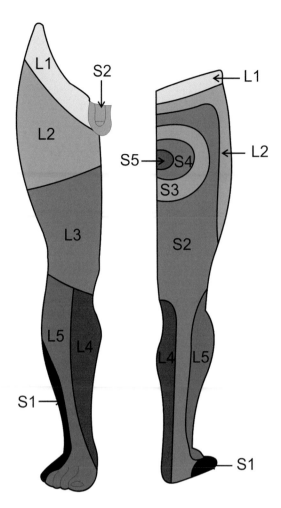

Figure 10.9 Dermatomes around the knee joint.

and femur, preventing their movements on each other in the anteroposterior direction. The ACL passes backward and outwards from the anterior intercondylar region of the tibia to attach to the posterior medial aspect of the lateral condyle of the femur. The PCL, however, originates from the posterior intercondylar region and adjacent popliteal surface of the tibia and passes inwards and forwards to insert on the anterior aspect of the lateral surface of the medial condyle of the femur. With an acute injury, the child may be in pain and muscle guarding may be present. The knee may be swollen because of hemarthrosis. In such circumstances, the various physical examination tests for anterior and posterior instability may be of less value. These tests have a greater value for chronically deficient knees.

10.4.1 Anterior Instability

The ACL is the primary ligament preventing anterior translation of the tibia relative to the femur. The main tests for detecting anterior instability are Lachman's test, the anterior drawer test, and the pivot shift test. In all these tests, it is necessary to ensure that there is no guarding by the patient and the hamstring muscles are sufficiently relaxed.

10.4.1.1 LACHMAN'S TEST (SENSITIVITY 75–90%, SPECIFICITY 80–95%)

The test is performed with the patient in supine position (Figure 10.10). The knee is held between full extension and 15° of flexion. The anterolateral distal femur is stabilized with one hand. The examiner uses the other hand to produce anterior displacement of the proximal tibia by applying firm pressure to the posterior aspect of the leg. Ensure that there are no tibial rotations while performing this test. This is to avoid action by secondary stabilizers and also that it is not posteriorly subluxated prior to initiation of the physical test (as occurs in a PCL-deficient knee).

In a concurrent PCL injury, the knee can be posteriorly subluxated at the beginning of the test. This may result in a false-positive pseudo-Lachman test for the ACL. The error can be appreciated if the contralateral knee is examined first and compared to the injured knee. The normally palpable prominences of the anteromedial and lateral tibial plateau in the flexed-knee position are not felt if the knee is PCL deficient and there is posterior subluxation. An abnormal contour or sag may be evident at the proximal anterior tibia when viewed from a lateral position.

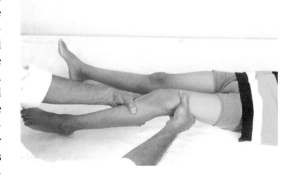

Figure 10.10 Lachman's test.

In a heavier patient with bulky thighs, the patient can be examined prone by the side of the couch with the thigh supported on the couch. The knee is flexed 30°, and both hands are now used to hold the tibia, which is pushed anteriorly. The result is appreciated in comparison to the contralateral normal knee. The feeling and/or visible anterior translation (obliteration of the normal slope of the infrapatellar tendon when visualized from the lateral aspect) of the proximal tibia relative to the distal femur with a spongy (soft/mushy/indefinite) endpoint is a positive test. The endpoint with an intact ACL is hard in comparison to the softer one in an ACL-deficient knee. The test can be false-negative in the presence of a concomitant bucket handle tear or adhesions of a torn ACL with PCL preventing anterior translation of the tibia over the femur.

10.4.1.2 THE ANTERIOR DRAWER TEST (SENSITIVITY 40–80%, SPECIFICITY 80–90%)

The test is performed in a supine patient position (Figure 10.11). The knee is held at 90° flexion. The examiner places the thumbs on the tibial plateau with the fingers of both hands holding the proximal tibia. Ensure relaxed hamstrings while palpating them with the index fingers. The feet point straight, and the examiner steadies them by sitting close to the patient's feet (the original description is examiner sitting on patients' feet, which may not be feasible in a child). The examiner pulls on the posterior aspect of the proximal tibia in an attempt to produce forward displacement. Ensure the tibia's neutral rotation to avoid action by secondary stabilizers [e.g., medial collateral ligament (MCL)] and that it is not posteriorly subluxated prior to initiation of the physical test (as occurs in a PCL-deficient knee). The results appreciation is always in comparison to the contralateral normal knee. The feeling and/or visibly obvious anterior translation of the proximal tibia relative to the distal femur with a soft endpoint is a positive test. The menisci, especially the lateral menisci, can give a false-negative anterior drawer test when they engage in the joint space under the femoral condyles in a "doorstop manner" during the anterior dislocation movement. A marked displacement is usually indicative of combined injuries of ACL and MCL ± posterolateral corner (PLC) ligament complex.

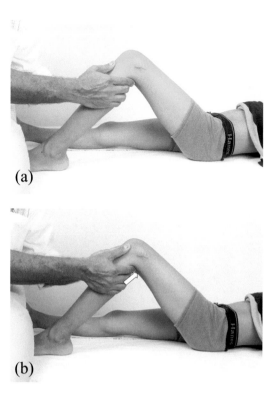

(a)

(b)

Figure 10.11 Anterior drawer test. (a) With thumb over tibial plateau. (b) Another way of placing the thumb over the joint line and femoral condyles to feel movement.

10.4.1.3 PIVOT SHIFT TEST (SENSITIVITY 85–100%, SPECIFICITY 95–100%)

With an ACL injury, provided the PCL and PLC structures are relaxed, the lateral tibial plateau subluxates anteriorly in knee extension and valgus stress (Figure 10.12). As the knee flexion increases (≥30°) with a change in relation to the knee axis, the iliotibial band, previously a knee extensor, becomes a knee flexor and pulls the subluxated lateral tibial plateau into a reduced position (axis located about the MCL). The sudden reduction of the joint is perceived as a palpable clunk and provides a positive pivot shift test. Slight hip abduction and flexion at the initiation of the test relaxes the iliotibial band and therefore enhances the test results.

In ACL deficiency, the femur falls posteriorly due to gravity. This results in apparent anterior dislocation of the tibia with respect to the femur. The pivot shift test demonstrates relocation of the internally rotated tibia about the MCL when the knee is moved with the application of a sustained

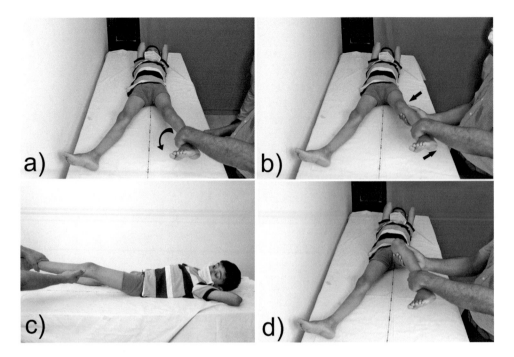

Figure 10.12 Pivot shift test.

valgus torque. It is demonstratable in chronic ACL deficiency, and as for any stability test, the prerequisite is a completely relaxed patient.

The test is performed in supine position. The hip is slightly abducted and flexed. The examiner supports the ankle with one hand and distal thigh with the other. Ensure that the limb is in slight internal rotation while it is being lifted off the table and in an extended position. Subsequently, the knee is flexed, and simultaneous valgus stress is applied with pressure over the upper aspect of the leg. In an ACL-deficient knee, the lateral tibial plateau is posteriorly subluxated over the femur at the initiation of the test (knee flexion 0° to >30°), and subsequently, with an increase in flexion to 30° or beyond, the displaced lateral tibial plateau reduces suddenly, producing a palpable and sometimes audible clunk, indicating a positive pivot shift test. The best site to observe this reduction is at the tubercle of Gerdy. The pivot shift test will be inaccurate if knee extension is not possible because of pain, swelling, or displaced meniscal tear.

A false pivot shift test may be present in generalized ligament laxity, iliotibial band injury, or a buckle handle tear of the meniscus. Carefully palpate the margin of the lateral tibial plateau in relation to the distal femoral condyle to avoid confusion with the anteromedial tibial subluxation. The jerk test of Hughston, the Losee test, the side lying test of Slocum, and the flexion rotation drawer test are variations of the pivot shift test and based on the secondary function of the ACL to prevent excessive internal rotation of the tibia on the femur (i.e., testing anterolateral stability).

10.4.2 Posterior Instability

The PCL is the primary ligament holding back posterior translation of the tibia over the femur. The secondary restraints are ligaments of the posterolateral corner (PLC) and MCL. The most important physical examination that demonstrates posterior tibial translation is the posterior drawer test. The quadriceps active test is based on the patient's quadriceps contraction. Other tests for the demonstration of posterior translation are the posterior Lachman test and the posterior sag test.

10.3.2.1 POSTERIOR DRAWER TEST (SENSITIVITY 90%, SPECIFICITY 99%)

Before initiation of the test, ensure that there is a normal anatomical relationship between the medial tibial plateau and medial femoral condyle in a knee in a 90° flexed position (Figure 10.13). In

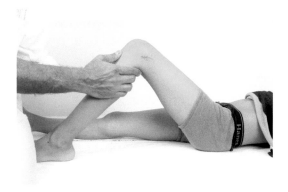

Figure 10.13 Posterior drawer test.

normal circumstances, the medial femoral condyle is 1 cm posterior to the palpable margin of the medial tibial plateau. In PCL insufficiency, when the tibia subluxates posteriorly with respect to the femur, the tibial tubercle is less prominent and the patella appears more prominent when both knees are inspected in profile (drop back phenomenon). The test is performed with the child in supine position. The hip is flexed 45° and knee to 90°, and the foot is in neutral position. The examiner takes the proximal tibia with both hands while the thumbs feel the anterior joint line. The examiner steadies the patient's feet by sitting close to them. The anterior aspect of the proximal tibia is pulled backward to produce posterior displacement. The feeling and/or visibly obvious posterior translation of the proximal tibia relative to the distal femur is a positive test and suggestive of a partial or complete tear of the PCL.

An internal rotated position of the foot may tighten the uninjured deep medial collateral ligament or arcuate ligament and provide false-negative results.

10.3.2.2 THE QUADRICEPS ACTIVE TEST (SENSITIVITY 50–98%, SPECIFICITY 97–100%)

In a normal knee, flexed 90°, the patellar tendon lies posteriorly oriented and active pull of the quadriceps does not result in an anterior shift of the tibia (Figure 10.14). In a PCL-deficient knee, there is posterior subluxation of the tibia over the distal femur in a flexed-knee position. The patellar tendon in such situations is directed more anteriorly, and active quadriceps contraction will result in anterior shift of the tibia.

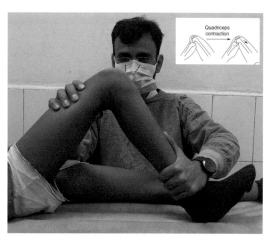

Figure 10.14 Quadriceps active test.

The test is performed with the patient in supine position. The hip is flexed 45°, knee 90°, and the foot is in neutral position. The patient is instructed to try sliding his/her fixed foot anteriorly to initiate a quadriceps contraction. A reduction of the posteriorly subluxated tibia is felt in a PCL-deficient knee.

10.4.3 Medial and Posteromedial Instability

The medial side of the knee is frequently injured from valgus force acting on the lateral aspect of the knee when the foot is stabilized on the ground. Often a part of multiligament injury, it is essential to check and document the neurovascular status of the limb as the associated knee dislocation gets spontaneously reduced at the time of presentation to the clinician. The MCL is the primary medial stabilizer of the knee joint against valgus stress. It, along with posteromedial corner (PMC) structures, provides protection against external rotation forces acting on the leg (Table 10.1). The medial aspect of the knee joint can be anatomically divided into anterior, middle, and posterior thirds (Figure 10.15). The structures in the medial aspect are given in the table.

Thus, the middle third (MCL) is a major restraint against valgus stress. Secondary restraints to valgus stress are the PMC and ACL.

The stability of the knee is assessed by applying *valgus stress* to an extended knee and one that is flexed 30° (Figure 10.16). The posteromedial capsule is an important structure that protects against valgus stress in the knee-extended position; when

Table 10.1 Medial Structures of the Knee Joint

Anterior third	Capsular ligaments
	Extensor retinaculum of quadriceps
Middle third	Fascia, superficial medial collateral ligament (MCL) (tibial collateral ligament), and deep MCL (meniscofemoral and meniscotibial components)
Posterior third	Posterior oblique ligament (POL), the oblique popliteal ligament, the attachment of semimembranosus tendon, and the posteromedial meniscus

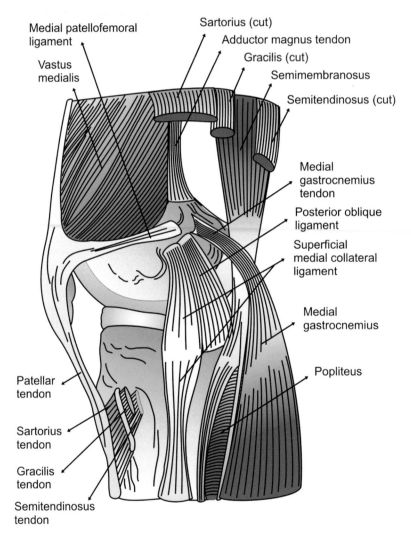

Figure 10.15 Anatomy of the medial aspect of the knee.

the knee is flexed, the posteromedial capsule is relaxed and does not participate in restraining valgus stress. Both tests are performed in supine position. A 30° test is typically for MCL and performed first. Keep the hip slightly abducted and flexed. The examiner stabilizes the leg between the waist and elbow. With one hand, feel the medial joint line opening and with the opposite hand, support the leg while the valgus stress is being exerted. In a bulky patient, the thigh may be rested on the table while the ankle and foot are supported by the examiner. Valgus stress in full extension is

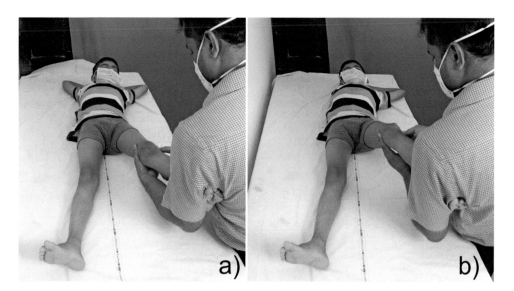

Figure 10.16 Valgus stress testing.

then applied. Opening of the medial joint line in full extension is suggestive of complete MCL rupture (grade III) and PMC damage. ACL injury, PCL injury, or patellar instability may also be associated.

Slocum's modified anterior drawer test differentiates between an isolated MCL and PMC injury (Figure 10.17). The test determines the degree of anterior translation of the tibia in the knee flexed to 90° and 15° external rotation of the tibia. When the tibia is externally rotated, the PMC should tighten and allow less anterior translation than testing in neutral position. In a positive test representing PMC injury, anterior translation of the medial tibial condyle in relation to the medial femoral condyle can be felt when compared with the contralateral knee.

10.4.4 Posterolateral Instability

The most common mechanism of injury for this type of instability is a high energy trauma involving a combined varus stress and hyperextension of the knee. The main static restraints in the posterolateral corner (PLC) of the knee are the fibular collateral ligament (FCL), arcuate ligament, fabellofibular ligament, popliteofibular ligament, joint capsules, and the coronary ligaments (Figure 10.18). The FCL forms a part of the PLC and

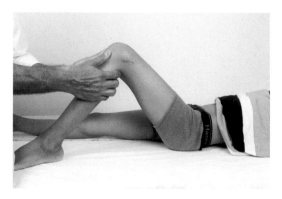

Figure 10.17 Slocum's modified anterior drawer test.

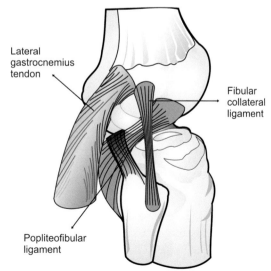

Figure 10.18 Anatomy of the lateral aspect of the knee joint.

both the FCL and PLC are usually evaluated in a combined manner with numerous tests, including the DIAL test, external rotation posterior drawer test, and external rotation recurvatum test.

10.4.4.1 DIAL TEST (TIBIAL EXTERNAL ROTATION TEST)

The test is typically performed with the patient in prone position. The knee is kept at 30° and 90° of flexion. In the test, the tibia is externally rotated relative to the femur, and it is positive if the external rotation of the tibia is increased by 10° or more compared to the contralateral normal side. A positive dial test at 30° of flexion is suggestive of injury to the PLC. A positive dial test at both 30° and 90° of knee flexion is suggestive of combined injury of the PLC and PCL (Figure 10.19).

10.4.4.2 OTHER TESTS FOR PLC INJURY

- External rotation posterior drawer test. The test is carried out with the knee in 90° flexion and the tibia in 15° external rotation. It assesses the amount of posterior translation of the anteromedial tibial plateau margin. In a positive test with a PLC injury, there will be a medial step off of the medial tibial condyle when compared with the contralateral knee.

- External rotation recurvatum test. The examiner picks up the big toe of the injured limb in full extension to perform this test. A positive test is observed when there is a tear of the PLC, ACL, and PCL. With a positive test, the tibia moves into asymmetric external rotation and recurvatum relative to the distal femur.

10.4.5 Patellofemoral Instability Assessment

- Patellar tracking (passive and active). The patient is seated comfortably with legs hanging down and arms behind extended to assume a tripod position. This relaxes the hamstrings by tilting the pelvis posteriorly. The examiner extends the knee from 90° of flexion to complete extension. Normally, the patella tracks in a relatively straight line or it moves slightly medial at the beginning of extension and then back slightly lateral upon terminal extension of the knee to assume the original position. Excessive gliding indicates tightness of the superficial retinacular fibers, and excessive tilting indicates pathology of the deep retinacular fibers. When the patient actively extends the knee, carefully observe the knee between 30° flexion to full extension. An abrupt lateral

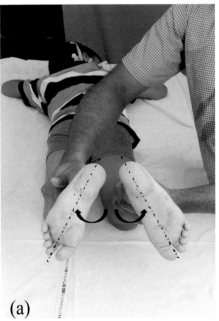
(a)

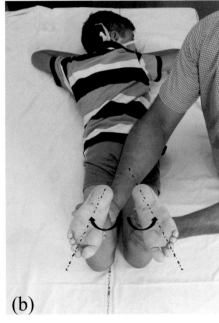
(b)

Figure 10.19 The DIAL test.

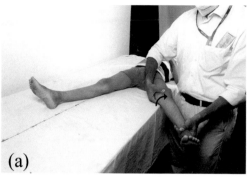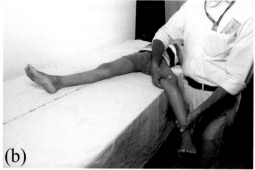

(a) (b)

Figure 10.20 Patellar apprehension test.

deviation/lateral J sign upon terminal extension indicates vastus medialis obliquus dysfunction.

- Patellar apprehension test. The examiner tries to subluxate the patella laterally with the fingers placed over the medial aspect of the patella, in a knee relaxed at 30° flexion (Figure 10.20a). The test is positive if it reproduces the patient's pain or an immediate leg extension (quadriceps contraction), preventing the patella from subluxating. A positive patellar apprehension test is indicative of patellofemoral instability and is often a sign of recurrent patellar dislocation.
- Patellar quadrant shift/patellar glide. The test is conducted with the patient in supine position. The patient should be relaxed with no muscle guarding. The knee is flexed 30°. The examiner moves the patella medially and laterally. To determine shift, the patella is divided into four quadrants. A glide greater than or equal to three quadrants indicates excessive patellar mobility and the possibility of instability.

10.5 EVALUATION OF MENISCAL INJURIES

The medial and lateral menisci are cresenteric fibrocartilaginous structures interposed between the intercondylar region of the femur and tibia. The medial meniscus is C-shaped, while the lateral meniscus is circular. Both menisci are firmly attached at the anterior and posterior horns near the intercondylar eminence. Further menisci are attached to the peripheral joint capsule via coronary ligaments. The medial meniscus has attachments to the deep MCL and therefore is less mobile when compared to the lateral meniscus. Anteriorly,

both menisci are connected via the transverse ligament.

A meniscal injury usually presents with delayed swelling. There is a history of twist injury to the knee. Several hours later, the patient may report painful popping and a catching sensation in the knee or a true locking, i.e., restriction of terminal 20–30° of extension.

The most important physical tests for menisci are joint line tenderness, McMurray's test, and Apley's grind test. There is a lot of controversy in the literature regarding the efficacy of these tests to predict the meniscal injury and several metanalyses have been undertaken for this purpose. These studies have taken arthrotomy, arthroscopy, or MRI as their reference benchmark for comparison. Most studies conclude that the various physical tests for menisci or even their combination are not very helpful in making clinical diagnosis or negation. Yet, the clinical tests continue to be part of the clinical examination armamentarium.

10.5.1 Joint Line Tenderness (Sensitivity 55–85%, Specificity 29–67%)

Rest your palm on the patella and place your thumb and index finger along the joint line. Carefully palpate the joint line for tenderness. Knee flexion facilitates palpation of the anterior half of the menisci. The medial edge of the medial meniscus moves forward with internal rotation of the tibia, making palpation easier. Similarly, palpate the anterior portion of the lateral menisci by performing an external rotation.

10.5.2 McMurray Test (Sensitivity 16–58%, Specificity 77–98%)

The test is performed with the patient supine (Figure 10.21). The examiner holds the patient's heel with one hand and stabilizes the knee with the other. The joint lines are palpated with the examiner's thumb and fingers. The patient's knee is then flexed maximally. To test the lateral meniscus, the tibia is rotated internally, and the knee is extended from maximal flexion to about 90° and vice versa. The examination of the whole of the posterior part of the menisci, beginning from the middle to their posterior attachment, is permitted by this gradual maneuver of flexion and extension. Added compression to the lateral/medial meniscus can be produced by placing valgus/varus stress, respectively, across the joint line while the knee is being extended. The occurrence of a click accompanied by a previously experienced sensation of pain as occurred when the knee gave way is indicative of a meniscal tear.

Before describing Apley's test, there are two things that are to be kept in mind. One is that it is a provocative test that can cause pain and should be avoided when other clinical findings suggest a particular diagnosis. Another thing is that it is not possible for the examiner to place himself/herself over the child's thigh and is better avoided.

10.5.3 Apley's Grind Test/Apley's Compression Test (Sensitivity 13–16%, Specificity 80–90%)

The test has three components (Figure 10.22). The test is best performed with the patient in prone position on a low examination couch. First, the examiner holds one foot in each hand and maximally rotates them externally. He/she then flexes both knees together completely. The examiner then changes grasp, internally rotates the feet, and extends the knees together again. Compare the asymmetrical rotation or occurrence of pain. This preliminary examination provides an estimation of limited and painful rotation and the precise angles of knee flexion at which these occur. This is useful later in the examination. Different knee flexions test different parts of the meniscus. A knee flexed more than 90° impinges more of the posterior horn, a knee at 90° flexion tests the central portion of the meniscus, and a knee closer

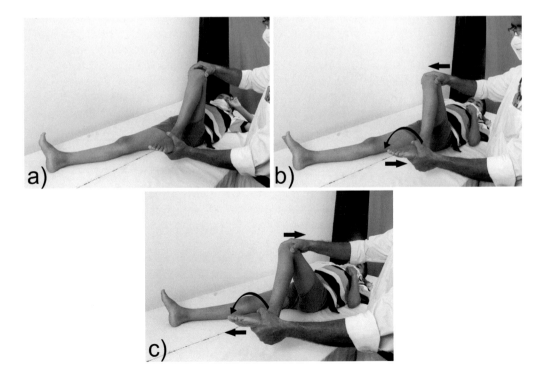

Figure 10.21 McMurray test.

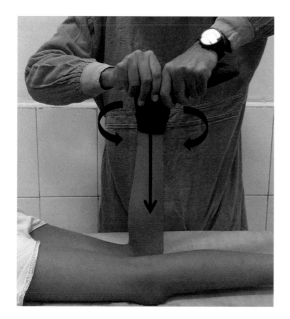

Figure 10.22 Apley's grind test.

to extension tests the anterior horn (<90° of knee flexion).

In the second step, each limb is individually tested. The patient's thigh is stabilized by the examiner's knee, and the examiner leans over the patient using their body weight to compress the tibia downward onto the couch. Then the foot is grasped in both hands and rotated forcibly externally with the knee in a 90°-flexed position. If this additional compression produces severe sharp pain, it is indicative of medial meniscal damage. The test may be repeated with the foot forcibly internally rotated for the detection of lateral meniscal injuries.

The third component of the test is Apley's distraction test. With the patient's thigh remaining stabilized, the patient's leg is pulled strongly upward, and in this distracted position, forcible external rotation of the foot is repeated. This distraction test produces increased pain only if there is ligament (ACL and MCL) damage. The test can be similarly repeated in the internal rotation position for ligamentous injuries on the lateral aspect of the knee.

10.6 TEST FOR OSTEOCHONDRITIS DISSECANS

10.6.1 Wilson Test

This maneuver is used to diagnose an osteochondritis dissecans lesion, which is usually located adjacent to the intercondylar notch on the lateral aspect of the medial femoral condyle. The patient lies supine on the couch with the knee flexed. The foot is first passively rotated internally, and subsequently, the knee is extended. This causes impingement of the ACL against the osteochondritis dissecans lesion. A positive test is one when there is pain on internal rotation and in extended knee position. The pain is relieved when the internal rotation at the knee is removed.

10.7 REGIONAL EXAMINATION

In the case of knee pathology, it is essential to examine the foot and ankle distally and the hip and spine proximally to detect referred and associated disorders.

BIBLIOGRAPHY

Malanga GA, Andrus S, Nadler SF, McLean J. Physical examination of the knee: a review of the original test description and scientific validity of common orthopaedic tests. *Arch Phys Rehabil.* 2003;84:592–603.

Lubowitz JH, Bernardini BJ, Reid JB. Comprehensive physical examination for instability of knee. *Am J Sports Med.* 2008;36:577–594.

Torg JS, Conrad W, Kalen V. Clinical diagnosis of anterior cruciate ligament instability in the athlete. *Am J Sports Med.* 1976;4:84–93.

Smith TO, Davies L, O'Driscoll ML, Donell ST. An evaluation of the clinical tests and outcome measures used to assess patellar instability. *Knee.* 2008;15:255–262.

Examination of Foot and Ankle in a Child

NIRMAL RAJ GOPINATHAN, MANDEEP SINGH DHILLON, AND
PRATIK M. RATHOD

11.1 INTRODUCTION

The foot provides a stable platform for the upright position and plays an important role in weight transmission and ambulation. Various pathologies related to the foot and ankle may be classified to those related to anatomical/morphological variations and the altered biomechanics that may result from neurological/musculoskeletal disorders. Sometimes, deformities in the foot and ankle provide a valuable clue for an underlying disorder like spinal cord anomaly/spinal dysraphism.

11.2 BRIEF ANATOMY

Thorough knowledge of normal anatomy is essential for the examination, and a brief review is presented here. The foot consists of 26 bones and 31 joints.[1] The ankle works like a hinge joint, with almost unidirectional motion between the talar dome and ankle mortice.

The components of the ankle mortise are:

- Distal articular surface of the tibial plafond.
- Medial articular surface of the lateral malleolus.

- Lateral articular surface of the medial malleolus.

These need to be stabilized and the soft tissue stabilizers of the ankle mortise are (Figure 11.1):

- Anterior inferior tibiofibular ligament (ATFL).
- Posterior inferior tibiofibular ligament (PTFL).
- Interosseous inferior tibiofibular ligament.
- Inferior deep transverse ligament, which is the inferior lower and deep portion of the posterior tibiofibular ligament.

It is important to be clear about the components of the medial collateral or deltoid ligament and the lateral collateral or lateral ligament, which contribute significantly to the stability of the ankle joint. On the lateral side, the lateral ligament complex consists of the anterior talofibular, calcaneofibular, and posterior talofibular (strongest) ligaments and are blended with the capsule of the ankle joint. The

deltoid ligament is attached to the tip of the medial malleolus proximally and is fan-shaped and attaches inferiorly to the following structures from the front backwards: tuberosity of the navicular, spring ligament, neck of the talus, sustentaculum tali, and the tubercle and body of the calcaneus. Thus, it has two components: superficial (tibionavicular, anterior tibiotalar, and tibiocalcaneal) and deep (posterior tibiotalar) (Figure 11.2a and b). The structures that traverse beneath the flexor and extensor retinaculum and the division of the foot are given in Table 11.1 and Table 11.2.

The medial and lateral longitudinal arches are located between the heel and the forefoot and the transverse arch between the first and fifth metatarsal heads. The arches function as shock/energy absorbers and play a vital role in weight transmission. The medial longitudinal arch is formed by the tuberosity of the calcaneus, talus, navicular, three cuneiforms, medial three metatarsals, and the corresponding phalanges, and the lateral longitudinal

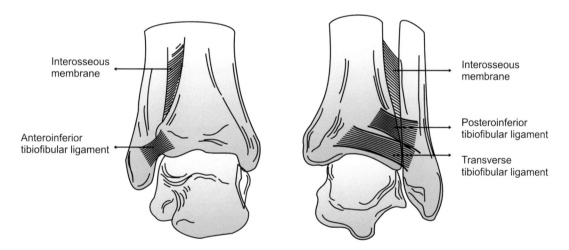

Figure 11.1 Soft tissue components of the ankle joint anterior and posterior.

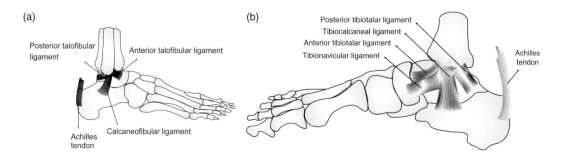

Figure 11.2 (a) Lateral collateral ligament. (b) Deltoid/medial collateral ligament.

Table 11.1 Structures Beneath Flexor and Extensor Retinaculum

Flexor retinaculum	Tibialis posterior, flexor digitorum longus, posterior tibial vessels and nerve, flexor hallucis longus
Extensor retinaculum	Tibialis anterior, extensor hallucis longus, anterior tibial vessels and deep peroneal nerve, extensor digitorum longus, and peroneus tertius

Table 11.2 Division of the Foot and the Corresponding Deformities

Part	Component Bones	Possible Deformations
Hindfoot	Talus and calcaneum	Equinus, calcaneus, varus, and valgus
Midfoot	Rest of the tarsal bones	Cavus, planus, rocker bottom feet
Forefoot	Metatarsals and phalanges	Adductus/abduction of metatarsals, claw foot, etc.

arch is formed by the calcaneal tuberosity, cuboid, lateral two metatarsals and the corresponding phalanges. The two muscles that have a role in maintaining the arches are the tibialis posterior and the peroneus longus. The collapse of the medial longitudinal arch results in a planovalgus or flatfoot and accentuation of the arch results in a cavus foot.

It is important to remember that the synovial reflection of the ankle joint communicates with other joints of the foot up to the tarsometatarsal joints. Also, it should be kept in mind that multiple small joints of the foot with their communicating synovial reflections result in the spread of diseases (for example, tuberculosis and inflammatory arthritis may affect multiple joints of the foot simultaneously).[2]

Common complaints related to the foot and ankle that make parents bring their children to the clinic are deformation, pain, swelling, limp, and abnormalities in gait. Sometimes, children are brought to the outpatient clinic with a deformation present since birth (congenital) (Figure 11.3 and 11.26). The deformity may be unilateral or bilateral. Bilateral involvement should always make the

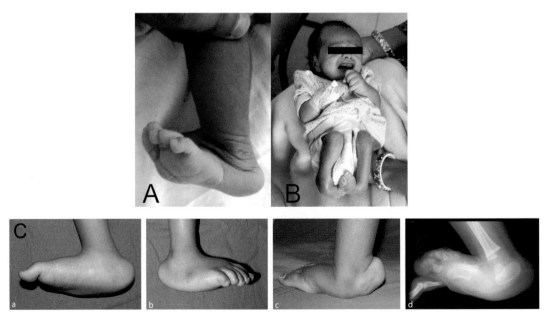

Figure 11.3 Congenital anomalies of the foot: (a) Calcaneus foot, (b) CTEV, (c) congenital vertical talus. Reproduced with permission from Nayagam S (2020). Congenital vertical talus. In: Joseph B, Nayagam S, Loder R, Torde I, editors. *Paediatric Orthopaedics: A System of Decision-Making* (2nd ed., 44), Taylor & Francis.

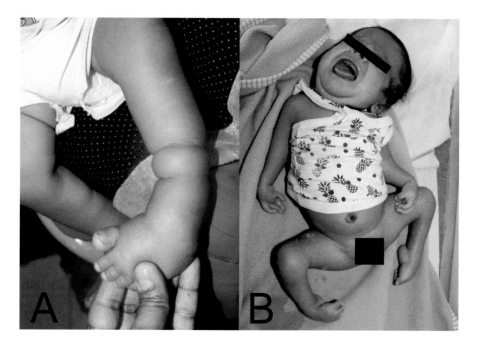

Figure 11.4 (a) Streeter's dysplasia and clubfoot deformation, (b) AMC (arthrogryposis multiplex congenita) with bilateral foot deformation.

examiner think of a congenital/syndromic/neurological disorder like arthrogryposis multiplex congenita or a case of spinal dysraphism (Figure 11.4). The congenital foot deformation might give a clue to the associated syndromic disorder; for example, the absence of lateral rays may be associated with congenital fibular and femoral deficiency. A painless progressive deformation may indicate an underlying neurological disorder. Remember that a neurological disorder can result in a symmetrical or asymmetrical involvement of both the foot and ankle.

For children with pain, the following questions need to be asked: determination of location, onset, duration, relation to gait, movements, and activities, and relieving factors, if any, are important, and the parents often play an important role in answering these. A note is to be made regarding the distance covered before pain begins. Pain, along with longstanding deformation, may indicate secondary arthritis and is often associated with reduced range of motion. Certain conditions like Freiberg's disease (osteochondritis second metatarsal head) have characteristic localization of pain, giving a clue to the diagnosis.

The child must undergo a general physical examination (head to toe). Equinocavovarus in a child with a midline scar or swelling (meningomyelocele) in the back is neurogenic and needs further neurological evaluation (Figure 1.1). Remember that progressive foot deformation may be due to a progressive neuromuscular disorder like cavus deformation in Charcot–Marie–Tooth disease (CMTD) (Figure 11.5), equinus in muscular dystrophies, or progressive planovalgus in cerebral palsy. One of the most important things to do is to examine the footwear of children who are walking, as this gives important clues based on the wear pattern (Figure 11.6). Barefoot walking on a foot that is not plantigrade leads to abnormal pressure distribution and callosity formation (Figure 11.7). A painless ulcer on the foot is a sign of neurological involvement (trophic ulcers) (Figure 11.8).

As foot and ankle pathologies affect the posture and gait, the *regional examination starts with close observation of the patient's posture and gait.* Observe how the patient walks and then ask the patient to do heel and toe walking and observe whether he/she can do it without difficulty. Make a note whether weight-bearing is done normally or on the lateral or medial border of the foot, signifying a static or dynamic deformity. A static deformity persists every time, irrespective of the phase of gait or weight-bearing, which is not passively

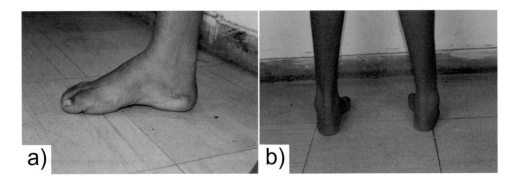

Figure 11.5 Cavovarus deformity in CMT.

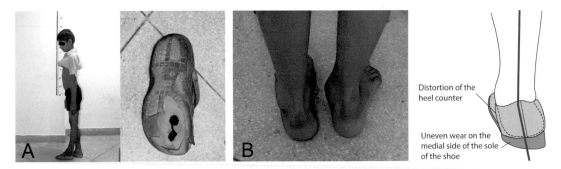

Figure 11.6 Footwear examination and clinical condition correlation in (a) equinus foot deformation and the characteristic wear pattern, (b) planovalgus foot and the associated wear pattern. Reproduced with permission from Joseph B (2020). Planovalgus deformity. In: Joseph B, Nayagam S, Loder R, Torde I, editors. *Paediatric Orthopaedics: A System of Decision-Making* (2nd ed., 50), Taylor & Francis.

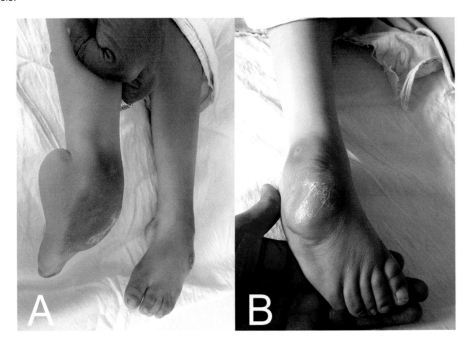

Figure 11.7 Callosity.

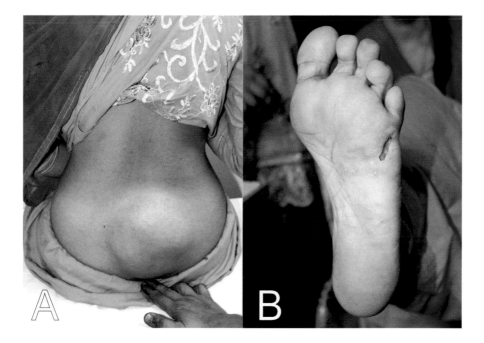

Figure 11.8 Trophic ulcer in a child with meningomyelocele.

correctable, whereas a dynamic deformity appears specifically at a certain phase of gait or activity and is passively correctable. Any abnormalities should be compared with the normal side, which can be taken as a reference.

11.3 LOCAL PHYSICAL EXAMINATION

11.3.1 Inspection

It is important to adequately expose the lower limbs for examination, respecting the child's privacy, or the examination may be carried out in an examination room in case of a busy clinic. The authors have found that it is always helpful to expose up to at least the middle of the thigh so that the knee, foot, and ankle can be simultaneously inspected. It is important to assess both the ankle and feet simultaneously in identical positions as far as possible. It is better to sit low so that the eyes are level with the knees of the child. The ankle and foot are visualized from the front, back, and the sides for any abnormalities in the skin like a scar, swelling, sinus, engorged veins, etc. The sole is examined for callosities, trophic ulcer, sinus, etc. In the case of varus, supination deformation, weight-bearing occur through the lateral border of the foot, and there may be callosities along the lateral border; in severe deformation, callosities may be seen in the dorsolateral aspect through which weight-bearing occurs.

11.3.1.1 ATTITUDE DESCRIPTION

The child is asked to stand with both feet identically placed, and the examiner inspects them from the back to look for heel alignment with the rest of the leg and ankle, which may be neutral, valgus, or varus. The midsagittal axis of the calcaneus is normally lateral to the midsagittal axis of the talus and tibia, and the foot is in slight valgus alignment[3.] (Figure 11.9) (valgus is the heel directed away from the midline, and varus is the heel directed toward the midline). Usually, the varus and valgus pertain to the subtalar joint; in rare circumstances, the valgus or varus might be due to ankle conditions like physeal arrest. Also, note the relation of the foot to the ankle, whether it is in equinus or calcaneus, in the sagittal plane.

Note: the ankle joint is in valgus orientation to the anatomic axis of the tibia in all normal neonates. In normal children, the distal fibula and lateral distal tibia grow relatively faster than the medial distal tibia until about 3–4 years of age. This results in the ankle joint or tibial plafond orienting itself perpendicular to the tibia, and this

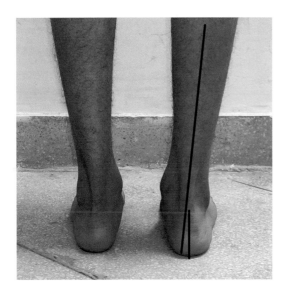

Figure 11.9 Normally line bisecting the calcaneus passes laterally in comparison to the midsagittal line on leg/valgus alignment.

anatomic alignment is maintained through skeletal maturity.[4]

Next, examine the malleoli; normally, the lateral malleolus is about a centimeter lower and posterior to the medial malleolus. If both malleoli are at the same level, it indicates an ankle valgus alignment (Figure 11.10). Ankle pathologies with gross effusion present with swelling all around the ankle joint. Tendon sheath swellings are usually longitudinal and appear along the long axis of the leg and foot, extending along the sheath beyond the joint level. Also, look for the fossae in front of the malleoli, which get obliterated in case of an ankle swelling. Posteriorly, look for the normal shallow concavity on either side of the tendoachilles. Inspect for any swelling along with the insertion of the tendoachilles into the calcaneal tuberosity, indicating enthesitis. Compare the calf muscle bulk with the normal side and inspect for the prominence of the tendoachilles. The heel should be observed for the following findings and should be compared with the normal side to find out whether it is broadened enlarged, or high riding.

Medially, the tibialis posterior lies just adjacent to the posteroinferior margin of the medial malleolus; look for its prominence, if any. Laterally the peroneal tendons lie just behind the distal fibula and lateral malleolus, and it is important to observe for their prominence if any.

From the medial aspect of the foot, the examiner evaluates the medial longitudinal arch, which usually should be present. It is obliterated in conditions causing flatfoot; this may be flexible or rigid,

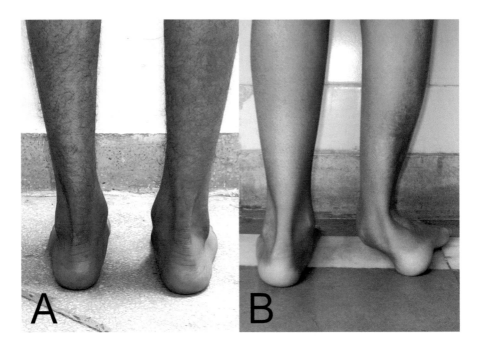

Figure 11.10 (a) normal relation of malleoli (lateral malleolus is lower than medial malleolus). (b) Both malleoli at the same level, indicating valgus originating from the ankle.

and an exaggerated arch is seen in a cavus foot. The examiner stands behind the child, and when the child is asked to raise both heels simultaneously with or without support, the medial arch appears (if it was obliterated on weight-bearing) and the heel swirls into varus due to the windlass effect, which is normal; this is used to differentiate between flexible and rigid pes planovalgus. The conditions that can lead to a rigid flatfoot are congenital vertical talus, tarsal coalition, or in a child with subtalar arthritis and deformation.

Note: in toddlers, a fat pad is present underneath the medial longitudinal arch, obliterating the arch and giving the appearance of a flat foot. This fat pad resolves between the ages of 2 and 5 years as the arch of the foot gradually appears.[5] When the children start walking, they are invariably flatfooted due to intrinsic laxity and lack of neuromuscular control.[6] Most flexible flatfeet are physiologic, and the medial longitudinal arch appears within the first 10 years of life.[7]

The anatomical alignment of the foot and toes and any abnormal alignment of toes or overriding is noted (Table 11.3, toe deformities). For example, in juvenile hallux valgus (Figure 11.11), the big toe deviates outwards away from the midline at the metatarsophalangeal joint. Also, in longstanding disorders, there may be continuous footwear irritation over the prominent distal medial metatarsal aspect leading to callosity formation (bunion).

The nailbeds are also inspected for abnormalities. In neurogenic cases, a trophic ulcer may be present on the weight-bearing aspect. Certain conditions of the foot like tuberculosis and mycetoma (Madura foot) presents with multiple sinuses (especially important in tropical regions, see Figure 11.13). In pes planus, as the foot is abducted/externally rotated, more toes are visualized from the posterior aspect, which is known as the "too many toes" sign[8] (visibility of more than one and a half toes, i.e., fifth and part of the fourth toe from behind along the lateral border of the foot) (Figure 11.14).

11.3.2 Palpation

Palpation starts with an assessment of the local increase in temperature if any. Ankle joint line tenderness must be assessed anteriorly; look for tenderness, thickening, or irregularity of the malleoli and define the relationship between the two malleoli by palpation. Note tendinous thickening if any and palpate for soft to firm swellings about the tendoachilles, confirming if it is anterior or posterior to the tendoachilles. A child with accessory

Table 11.3 Toe Deformations (see Figure 11.12)

Nomenclature	Components	Remarks	Etiology
Hammer toe	Flexion deformity PIP (proximal interphalangeal) joint, extension at MTP (metatarsophalangeal), and DIP (distal interphalengeal) joints	Commonly seen at the second toe	Rheumatoid arthritis, Charcot–Marie–Tooth disease, Psoriatic arthritis
Mallet toe	Plantarflexion deformity at DIP joint		Axially loaded hyperflexion injuries
Claw toe	Hyperextension of MTP joint, flexion of PIP and DIP joints		Synovitis, missed compartment syndrome of deep posterior compartment
Bunionette deformity	Painful osseous prominence of the fifth metatarsal head	Tailor's bursitis/bunion	Common in patients who put constant pressure on the lateral aspect of the foot
Curly toe	Flexion and varus of IP (interphalangeal) joints	Third and fourth toes frequently affected	Minor to moderate deformities resolve by 6 years of age

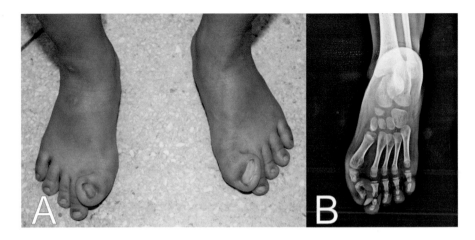

Figure 11.11 Hallux valgus in a child with radiograph showing bracket epiphysis proximal phalanx.

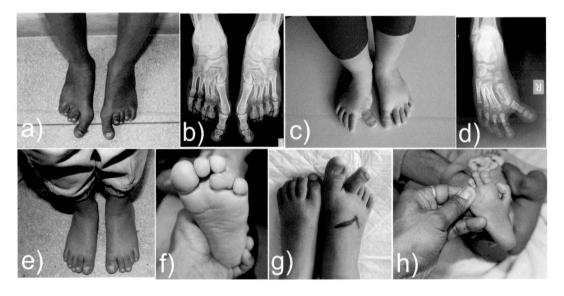

Figure 11.12 Toe deformations. (a), (b) Brachydactyly and radiograph. (c), (d) Hallux varus and radiograph. (e), (f) Curly toe. (g) Macro lipodystrophy. (h) Polydactyly.

navicular may have bony swelling and tenderness on the medial aspect in the region of the navicular, which is usually bilateral (Figure 11.15). Tenderness at the back of the calcaneal tuberosity in a child may be due to Sever's disease (calcaneal apophysitis) and is usually seen in boys around 10 years of age. Tenderness beneath the heel may be due to inflammation of the plantar fascial attachment at the calcaneal tuberosity (plantar fasciitis) or due to the presence of a bony spur underneath the calcaneal tuberosity. Tenderness may be localized to the base of the second metatarsal in case of a stress fracture[9] or at the second metatarsal head in case of Freiberg's infarct (osteochondritis/avascular) or

at the navicular in case of Kohler's disease. Any infection or inflammation in the ankle joint can lead to effusion (collection of synovial fluid) in the ankle joint. Vague pain in the region of the intermetatarsal space between the third and fourth metatarsal that is aggravated by squeezing the metatarsals together may be caused by Morton's metatarsalgia, but is rarely seen in patients less than 20 years of age.[10] Pulsation of the anterior tibial artery is felt between the tendons of EHL (extensor hallucis longus) and EDL (extensor digitorum longus). If it is not palpable, compare with the other side and remember that it may be absent in 2% of individuals.[11] The posterior tibial artery is

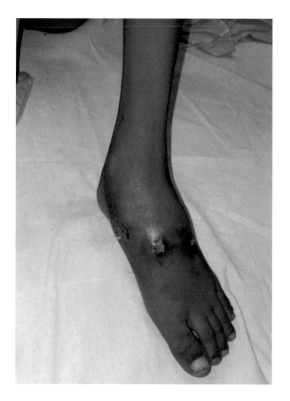

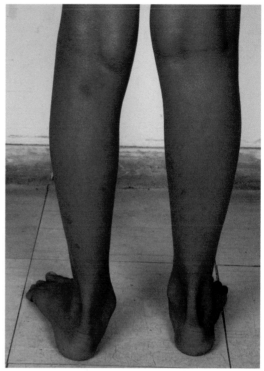

Figure 11.13 Tuberculosis midfoot with multiple sinuses.

Figure 11.14 Too many toes sign.

felt about one fingerbreadth posterior to the medial malleolus behind the tendon of the flexor digitorum longus. Any effusion or synovial swelling in the ankle is seen as outpouchings around the ankle in the posterolateral, posteromedial, anterolateral, and anteromedial aspects, and if present, is soft and doughy to palpation.

Tendoachilles rupture is rare and almost always traumatic in childhood, unlike the degenerative ruptures that occur in middle age and older individuals.[12] Even with complete rupture, plantarflexion is not completely absent due to the action of muscles like the tibialis posterior, long toe flexors, and the peronei and the range of dorsiflexion increases compared to the other side. A complete tear presents with a palpable defect in the tendon.

11.3.2.1 THOMPSON'S TEST

With the patient in prone position and feet hanging over the examination table or kneeling upon a stool/chair with the foot projected, the examiner squeezes the calf to compress the muscle.[13] If the tendoachilles is intact or even partially torn, the foot goes into plantarflexion. When the tendon is completely ruptured, plantarflexion movement in the ankle does not occur (Figure 11.16).

11.3.2.2 TIBIALIS POSTERIOR TENDON TENOSYNOVITIS

The child is asked to invert the plantarflexed foot while the examiner resists the inversion movement. The child will feel pain behind the medial malleolus, and at the same time, the examiner might feel tender soft/firm thickening palpable along the tibialis posterior tendon.

Also look for peroneal tendon prominence, which may indicate a peroneal spasm and an underlying tarsal coalition.

11.4 TESTS FOR ANKLE INSTABILITY

A child with a frequent giving way of the ankle or repeated ankle sprains may have chronic ankle instability. Remember to rule out a tarsal coalition in the absence of clinically demonstrable instability. The two structures requiring assessment

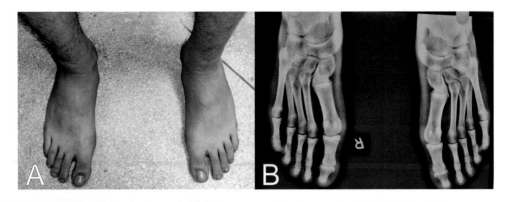

Figure 11.15 Child with bilateral accessory navicular.

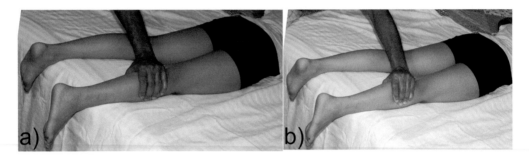

Figure 11.16 Thompson's test for testing the integrity of the tendoachilles.

are the ATFL and the CFL (calcaneao-fibular ligament). The integrity of the ATFL is assessed using the anterior drawer test, and the integrity of the CFL is assessed using the talar tilt test with the findings compared with the contralateral normal side.

11.4.1 Anterior Drawer Test

This is performed with the ankle in 10–15° of plantarflexion and is a common test in adults to assess the integrity of the anterior talofibular ligament. It is done by pulling the heel anteriorly against resistance applied by the other hand over the anterior aspect of the lower leg. If the anterior displacement of the talus is more than that of the other side and if there is the rare creation of a sulcus (skin dimple) at the attachment of the ATFL, this test is positive[14] (Figure 11.17).

11.4.2 Talar Tilt Test

With the distal tibia stabilized as described above and the ankle in neutral to slight plantarflexion,

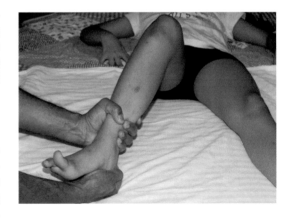

Figure 11.17 Anterior drawer test.

supination stress is applied, and the degree of laxity is compared with the other side.[14]

Note: it is important to differentiate the abnormally exaggerated valgus of the ankle from the exaggerated valgus at the subtalar joint. This is quite common in neurogenic disorders with secondary foot deformations. This is more appreciable when the patient stands weight-bearing, stressing the foot naturally with the examiner standing

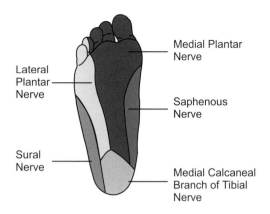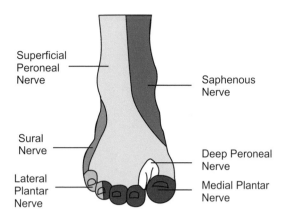

Figure 11.18 Cutaneous innervation of the foot.

behind the patient. Observe the level of the malleoli; normally, the lateral malleolus lies about a centimeter beneath the medial malleolus. If the medial malleolus is at a lower level, the valgus is from the ankle.

11.5 MOVEMENTS OF FOOT AND ANKLE

The neutral position of the foot with the ankle is a plantigrade (right-angled) position. The normal range of movements in the ankle joint is shown in Table 11.4.

Examine both the active and passive range of motion and also stress the joint to assess the integrity of the collateral ligaments. Remember that range and stability need to be compared with the other side and documented. The critical functional range required for normal gait is 15° of plantarflexion (required for normal push-off) and 15° of dorsiflexion (deceleration of heel strike phase of gait and squatting). It is important to evaluate the active and passive range of motion and to document any restriction in the movement leading to deformation. The neutral position is the plantigrade position, which is the minimum requirement for the management of many pathologies.

11.5.1 Movements of the Foot

To understand the movements of the foot, it is important to know the axis of subtalar motion. The axis of subtalar motion is oblique and passes from a posterior, plantar, lateral position to an anterior, dorsal, medial position.[15] This axis is 42° inclined from the horizontal plane and 16° inclined from the sagittal plane through the heel to space between the first and second toes.[16] The oblique axis has a longitudinal or anteroposterior component, a vertical component, and a transverse component, and the plane of motion does not correspond to any cardinal body plane. Movements in the frontal plane along a longitudinal component of the subtalar axis are referred to as inversion and eversion. Inversion is the movement where the medial border of the foot is elevated, and the lateral border gets depressed. Eversion is the opposite of inversion. Transverse plane movement occurs about the vertical component of the axis and is referred to as abduction and adduction. Abduction is an outward rotation of the foot, and inward rotation is known as adduction. Movement in the frontal plane component is about the sagittal plane and is dorsiflexion and plantarflexion. The movement of the subtalar joint occurs simultaneously in all three planes, and this resultant triplanar motion is referred to as pronation and supination. Pronation is a combination of eversion, abduction, and

Table 11.4 Movements of the Ankle

Dorsiflexion	15–30°	The anterior part of the dome of talus, which is wider, is wedged tightly between the two malleoli providing stability to the joint
Plantarflexion	30–50°	The posterior narrow part of the dome articulates with relative instability

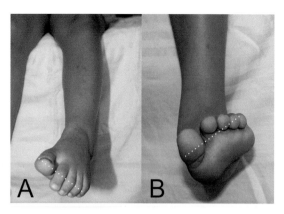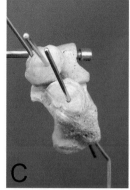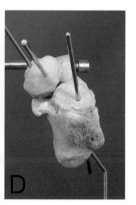

Figure 11.19 Subtalar motion. (a) Supination, (b) pronation, and (c) and (d) articulated representation of supination and pronation. Reproduced with permission from Nayagam S (2020). Equinovarus. In: Joseph B, Nayagam S, Loder R, Torde I, editors. *Paediatric Orthopaedics: A System of Decision-Making* (2nd ed., 18), Taylor & Francis.

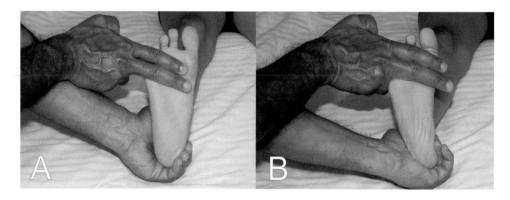

Figure 11.20 Assessment of subtalar motion. (a) Eversion. (b) Inversion.

dorsiflexion, whereas supination consists of inversion, adduction, and plantarflexion (Figure 11.19).

In the literature,[17] the terms "supination"/ "pronation" and "inversion"/"eversion" have been used interchangeably. It should be kept in mind that on an attempted elevation of the medial border, which is termed inversion/supination, plantarflexion of the subtalar joint also occurs as the talus slides beneath the calcaneus and the forefoot drifts toward the midline. The reverse occurs in eversion/pronation. It is important to constantly be reminded that the subtalar joint plantar flexes and dorsiflexes as components of the movements inversion and eversion, respectively[17](Figure 11.19).

"Varus" and "valgus" are terminologies used to describe the static position/deformation in the subtalar joint. In varus, the calcaneus angles inward with respect to the talus, and in valgus, the calcaneus angles outward with respect to the talus.

11.5.2 Assessment of Subtalar Motion

The subtalar motion assessment is done with the ankle in dorsiflexion and foot in neutral inversion/eversion (Figure 11.20). This is done keeping in view the biconical shape of the talus, which is narrower posteriorly than anteriorly. This engages the widest portion of the talar dome in the ankle mortise, which creates bony stability, and also tightens the collateral ligaments eliminating false inversion/eversion motion at that joint. The calcaneus is held in a cupped hand and is moved in the axis of the subtalar joint that is "down and in" and "up and out." The other hand is used to note the motions of the midfoot and forefoot.[17]

It should be kept in mind that some cases of rigid flatfoot may falsely show the appearance of a medial arch on heel raise. Mosca[1] mentions that the hypermobility of Chopart's joints particularly calcaneocuboid, resulting in an appearance of false flexibility of the subtalar joint in a rigid flatfoot.

11.6 DEFORMITIES PERTAINING TO FOOT AND ANKLE IN A CHILD

Remember that there are at least two segmental deformations in rotationally opposite directions from each other in all congenital and developmental deformities and most malformations of the child's foot. These rotationally opposite deformations are well appreciated in a cavovarus foot where the forefoot is pronated and the hindfoot is in varus and in flatfoot where the forefoot is in supination and the hindfoot is in valgus.[18]

The following deformations, if present, are noted as enumerated in Table 11.5.

11.6.1 Cavus

Cavus is defined as plantarflexion of the forefoot on the hindfoot with a resultant high arch. The plantarflexion may be in the medial column, lateral column, or the entire forefoot on the hindfoot.

Cavus deformity in almost all cases is the result of an underlying neuromuscular disorder, although congenital idiopathic cavus is known to exist.[19] Cavus deformation is rarely seen in isolation and can be accompanied by hindfoot varus, which is flexible/correctable or rigid. Loss of flexibility of hindfoot varus can be assessed by the Coleman block test.

11.6.1.1 COLEMAN BLOCK TEST

The need to identify the flexibility of the hindfoot during the stance phase in cavovarus deformity led to the development of the simple "cavovarus test." The patient's foot is placed on an approximately 2.5-cm (1 inch) wooden block. The foot is positioned in such a way that the heel and lateral border are placed on the block and are weight-bearing, whereas the first through third or fourth metatarsals are allowed to fall into pronation. The height of the block can be increased to avoid the first metatarsal from weight-bearing and affecting the hindfoot. The position of the hindfoot goes from varus to valgus on weight-bearing if it is flexible and is best observed from behind (Figure 11.21).[20]

The segmental deformities in a cavovarus foot are forefoot pronation, midfoot adduction, and hindfoot varus along with ankle equinus. Mosca described the modified Coleman block test to assess the hindfoot flexibility in a cavovarus foot, and it avoids the awkwardness of the Coleman

Table 11.5 Deformities of the Foot and Ankle

Deformity	Ankle Joint	Forefoot	Midfoot	Hindfoot
Equinus	Plantarflexion			
Calcaneus	Dorsiflexion			
Varus				Heel medially deviated from midline
Valgus				Heel laterally deviated from midline
Cavus			Medial longitudinal arch elevation	
Adductus		Medial deviation	Medial deviation	
Equinocavovarus	Plantarflexion	Medial deviation	Medial longitudinal arch elevation	Heel medially deviated from midline
Pes Planovalgus		Lateral deviation	Collapse of medial longitudinal arch	Heel laterally deviated from midline

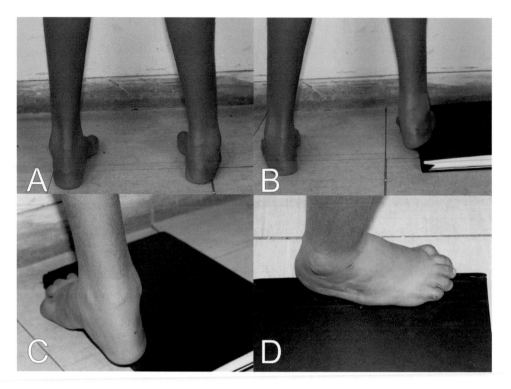

Figure 11.21 Coleman block test.

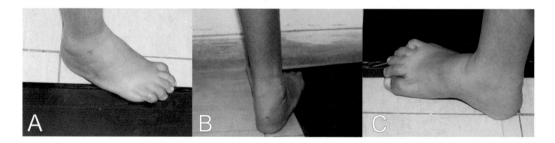

Figure 11.22 Modified Coleman block test by Mosca.

block test in which the child attempts to balance the foot on the block. Here a 2.5-cm block is placed under the lateral two or three metatarsal heads. The heel remains on the ground, and the medial metatarsal heads reach for the ground as the forefoot pronates off the block[19] (Figure 11.22).

11.6.2 Pes Planovalgus

In a flatfoot, the forefoot is in supination, the midfoot is straight or in abduction, and the hindfoot is in valgus alignment along with ankle equinus. Here the "toe standing" and "Jack toe raise test" are used to assess hindfoot flexibility.

11.6.2.1 JACK TOE RAISE TEST

This test demonstrates hindfoot/subtalar flexibility in a flexible flatfoot and is based on the principle of "windlass" action of the plantar fascia. The plantar fascia is of fixed length and is attached proximally to the plantar surface of the calcaneus and distally plantar aspect of the toes through multiple interconnections. Dorsiflex the big toe and look for the appearance of a medial arch. Dorsiflexion of the big toe pulls the plantar fascia distally under the pulley of the head of the first metatarsal. The big toe can only fully dorsiflex if the calcaneus is pulled distally toward the metatarsal heads, thereby shortening the foot, elevating the longitudinal arch, and inverting the subtalar joint [21] (Figure 11.23). Another method of assessment is asking the child to do a heel raise, which also causes the appearance of the medial arch and heel varus in a flexible planovalgus deformity.

When the foot is in supination, the articulations of the midfoot are biomechanically locked, and the foot becomes a rigid structure; this is reversed in pronation and greater mobility is allowed at the Chopart's joints. It is important to rule out hypermobile flatfoot associated with a short Achilles tendon. This condition, which is often familial, is evidenced by contracture of the gastrocnemius in association with the same clinical features as described previously. In the non-weight-bearing position, the normal arch is generally present. Contracture of the Achilles tendon is best assessed with the knee in extension and the talonavicular joint locked in inversion so that dorsiflexion is measured only at the ankle. These patients may also show evidence of hypermobility at the midtarsal joints, which allows the heel to touch the floor despite a contracted Achilles tendon.[22]

11.6.2.2 LEVER ARM DYSFUNCTION

The foot acts as an efficient lever for the generation of power during push-off, with the subtalar joint locked in inversion and the foot pointing forwards.

Lever arm dysfunction can result from the shortening of the lever arm and/or weakening of the gastrocsoleus. The lever arm is shortened when the foot is externally rotated to the sagittal plane of the knee (everted/unlocked subtalar joint or external tibial torsion).[23]

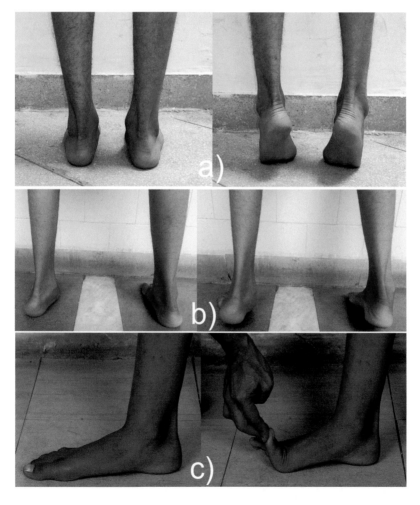

Figure 11.23 (a) Heel raise showing the appearance of the medial arch along with calcaneus swirling into varus, which is normal. (b) Rigid flatfoot on left showing absence of medial arch formation and persistent calcaneal valgus on heel raise. (c) Jack toe raise test.

11.6.3 Adductus

The "heel bisector method" (Figure 13.4e) is useful to assess the severity of metatarsus adductus. In a normal foot, the line that bisects the heel (heel bisector between the medial and lateral borders of the heel) extends to the interspace between the second and third toes.[24]

11.7.4.1 FLEXIBILITY METHOD OF ASSESSING METATARSUS ADDUCTUS

Rigid: forefoot cannot be passively abducted to create a straight lateral border.

Partly flexible: forefoot can be passively abducted to create a straight lateral border.

Flexible: forefoot can be passively abducted beyond a straight lateral border.

11.6.4 Equinus

The ankle joint should have at least 10° of dorsiflexion with the knee extended and the subtalar joint in neutral alignment.

11.6.4.1 SILFVERSKIOLD TEST

This test is used to determine the presence of a heel cord contracture and in differentiating between a gastrocnemius contracture and a tendoachilles contracture. The examiner first flexes the knee joint to relax the gastrocnemius. Maximally dorsiflex the ankle joint and record the angle between the plantar lateral border of the foot and the anterior border of the tibial shaft. Do not use the plantar medial border as the presence of supination or pronation deformity of the forefoot will give false recording and values if missed. While maintaining the subtalar joint in neutral alignment, the knee is extended to tighten the proximal end of the gastrocnemius. The ankle will lose some dorsiflexion in most cases. The inability to dorsiflex the ankle to at least 10° above neutral with the subtalar joint held in neutral alignment is abnormal. If 10° of dorsiflexion is possible with the knee flexed but not extended, it represents isolated gastrocnemius contracture. If 10° dorsiflexion is not possible regardless of the knee position (flexed/extended), then the triceps surae (gastrocnemius and soleus) are contracted (Figure 11.24).

Note: a way of ensuring the neutral alignment of the talonavicular joint is by placing the thumb on the plantar medial aspect of the talonavicular joint. If the subtalar joint is everted as in flatfoot, invert to bring it to neutral position and confirm the anatomic subtalar joint alignment with a thumb over the plantar medial aspect of the talonavicular joint. If the subtalar joint is inverted as in a cavovarus foot, evert it to bring to neutral alignment.[25]

Few authors suggest that the Silfverskiold test should be done with the foot held in inversion while assessing the foot and ankle. The inversion locks the foot and thereby eliminates instability of the hindfoot and midfoot joints.[26]

Flatfoot presents a special challenge when assessing for contracture of the heel cord. The reason is that both the ankle joint and subtalar joint dorsiflex and plantarflex. To isolate ankle joint dorsiflexion, the subtalar joint is anatomically aligned or locked using inversion to prevent subtalar dorsiflexion. The cavus foot presents a challenge to assess the heel cord contracture. Assessment of ankle equinus is done by isolating the hindfoot. The forefoot can be obscured from vision with the hand so that only the hindfoot is visualized (Figure 11.25).

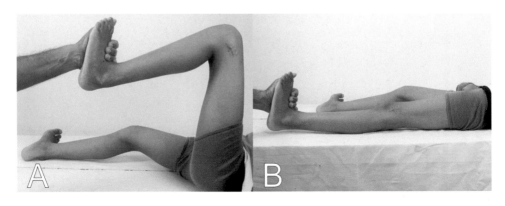

Figure 11.24 Silfverskiold test.

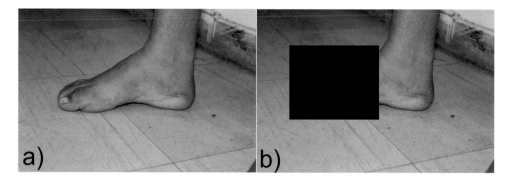

Figure 11.25 Assessment of equinus in cavus foot.

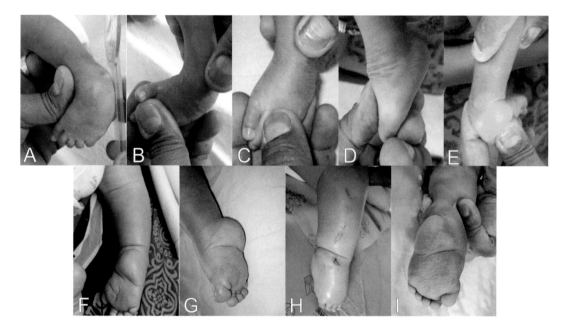

Figure 11.26 CTEV. (a) Curved lateral border. (b) Locating talar head – palpate lateral malleolus and slide your thumb down and toward dorsum (not plantar-ward) to localize talar head. (c) Derotation of calcaneopedal block around talar head. (d) Equinus appreciated from the lateral aspect. (e) Varus appreciated from the posterior aspect. (f) Adductus appreciated from the plantar aspect. (g) Complex clubfoot with short foot and extension of the big toe. (h) Swollen dorsum in complex clubfoot. (i) Transverse crease from medial to lateral aspect in a child with complex clubfoot.

11.7 NEUROLOGICAL EXAMINATION

11.7.1 Motor and Sensory Examination

Also, look for any anesthesia and paresthesia concerning the dermatomal distribution (Figure 11.18).

Assess muscle balance by asking the child to dorsiflex the foot or by stimulating the plantar aspect of the sole. Normally the tibialis anterior and the peroneus tertius are balanced, and the plane of the metatarsal heads is perpendicular to the tibial shaft. The plane of the metatarsal heads is supinated in relation to the tibial shaft in a child with corrected, flexible clubfoot due to the relative overpull of the normal tibialis anterior against the weak peroneus tertius and longus. The intrinsic muscles of the foot can be examined by evaluating the interossei and the lumbricals. A child with a neurogenic talipes equinovarus may not have the reactive dorsiflexion of the toe on stimulation of the sole, and this is known as a drop toe sign.

The axis of foot is formed by the second metatarsal, and the dorsal interossei are responsible for fanning out of the webs and the plantar interossei are responsible for closing the webs. They can be tested by placing a card between the toes and asking the patient to resist pull by closing the web. The lumbricals along with the interossei are responsible for flexion of the metatarsophalangeal joints and extension at the interphalangeal joints.

The examination should include regional lymph node examination in relevant pathologies and evaluation of other joints of the lower limb.

REFERENCES

1. Mosca VS. *Principles and management of pediatric foot and ankle deformities and malformations.* Baltimore, MD: Lippincott Williams & Wilkins, 2014 May 6. p. 1.
2. Andersen KS. *Clinical orthopaedic diagnosis*, 2nd ed. S. Pandey, A.K. Pandey, 2000;501 pp., New Delhi: Jaypee Brothers Medical Publishers Ltd. *Int Orthop.* 2000;24(4):238–238.
3. Mosca VS. *Principles and management of pediatric foot and ankle deformities and malformations.* Philadelphia, PA: Wolters Kluwer/ Lippincott Williams & Wilkins, 2014. p. 12.
4. Mosca VS. *Principles and management of pediatric foot and ankle deformities and malformations.* Philadelphia, PA: Wolters Kluwer/ Lippincott Williams & Wilkins, 2014. p. 25.
5. Mickle KJ, Steele JR, Munro BJ. The feet of overweight and obese young children: Are they flat or fat? *Obesity (Silver Spring).* 2006;14:1949–1953.
6. Nemeth B. The diagnosis and management of common childhood orthopedic disorders. *Curr Probl Pediatr Adolesc Health Care.* 2011;41:2–28.
7. Herrera-Soto JA. Pediatric foot and ankle disorders. *Curr Opin Orthop.* 2004;15:417–422.
8. Johnson KA. Tibialis posterior tendon rupture. *Clin Orthop Rel Res.* 1983;177:140–147.
9. Devas MB. Stress fractures in children. *J Bone Joint Surg Br Vol.* 1963;45(3):528–541.
10. Kasparek M, Schneider W. Surgical treatment of Morton's neuroma: Clinical results after open excision. *Int Orthop.* 2013;37(9):1857–1861.
11. Vijayalakshmi S, Raghunath G, Shenoy V. Anatomical study of Dorsalis pedis artery and its clinical correlations. *J Clin Diag Res.* 2011;5:287–290.
12. Akdogan M, Atilla HA, Barca F. Pediatric Achilles tendon laceration: A case report and systematic review of literature. *MOJ Sports Med.* 2018;2(5):153–156.
13. Thompson TC. A test for rupture of the tendo achillis. *Acta Orthop Scand.* 1962;32:461–465.
14. Gruskay J, Brusalis CM, Heath MR, Fabricant PD. Pediatric and adolescent ankle instability: Diagnosis and treatment options. *Curr Opin Pediatr.* 2019;31:69–78.
15. Rockar PA. The subtalar joint: Anatomy and joint motion. *J Orthop Sports Phys Ther* 1995;21:361–372.
16. Manter IT: Movements of the subtalar and transverse tarsal joints. *Anat Rec* 1941;80:397–410.
17. Mosca VS. *Principles and management of pediatric foot and ankle deformities and malformations.* Philadelphia, PA: Wolters Kluwer/ Lippincott Williams & Wilkins, 2014. p. 10.
18. Mosca VS. *Principles and management of pediatric foot and ankle deformities and malformations.* Philadelphia, PA: Wolters Kluwer/ Lippincott Williams & Wilkins, 2014. p. 6.
19. Mosca VS. *Principles and management of pediatric foot and ankle deformities and malformations.* Philadelphia, PA: Wolters Kluwer/ Lippincott Williams & Wilkins, 2014. p. 19.
20. Coleman SS, Chesnut WJ. A simple test for hindfoot flexibility in the cavovarus foot. *Clin Orthop Relat Res.* 1977; 123:60–62.
21. Mosca VS. *Principles and management of pediatric foot and ankle deformities and malformations.* Philadelphia, PA: Wolters Kluwer/ Lippincott Williams & Wilkins, 2014. p. 23.
22. Weinstein SL, Buckwalter JA, editors. *Turek's orthopaedics: Principles and their application.* Philadelphia, PA: Lippincott Williams & Wilkins, 2005. p. 639.
23. Mosca VS. *Principles and management of pediatric foot and ankle deformities and malformations.* Philadelphia, PA: Wolters Kluwer/ Lippincott Williams & Wilkins, 2014. pp. 10–11.
24. Mosca VS. *Principles and management of pediatric foot and ankle deformities and malformations.* Philadelphia, PA: Wolters Kluwer/ Lippincott Williams & Wilkins, 2014. pp. 94–96.
25. Mosca VS. *Principles and management of pediatric foot and ankle deformities and malformations.* Philadelphia, PA: Wolters Kluwer/ Lippincott Williams & Wilkins, 2014. pp. 26.
26. Robb JE, Brunner R. *Orthopaedic management of cerebral palsy. Children's orthopaedics and fractures 2010.* London: Springer, 2010. pp. 307–325.

12

Evaluation of the Spine in a Child

ASHISH DAGAR, SARVDEEP SINGH DHATT, DEEPAK NERADI,
AND VIJAY G GONI

This chapter on pediatric spine examination starts with information on the relevant basic anatomy of the spine and then goes on to an elaborate discussion on relevant points in history-taking. This chapter discusses the examination of the spine in the pediatric age group with a special focus on pathologies specific to the pediatric age group. All important points regarding inspection, palpation, movements, special tests, deformity evaluation, and neurological examination have been covered in detail.

12.1 BASIC ANATOMY OF THE SPINE

There are 33 vertebral bodies in the spine – 7 cervical, 12 thoracic, 5 lumbar, 5 sacral, and 4 coccygeal. All vertebral bodies (except C1–C2) are separated from each other by a fibrocartilaginous intervertebral disc. The spinal cord lies in the spinal canal and ends at the lower border of L1 or the upper border of L2. At birth, the cord ends at L3 level but recedes to adult level by the age of 2 months. In the region of the D12 and L1 vertebrae, an expanded portion of the spinal cord coexists with emerging nerve roots (conus medullaris). Below L1, only the lumbosacral roots exist, forming the cauda equina. The spinal cord is segmented into 31 segments, each segment giving out a pair of nerves that supply a definite set of muscles (myotome) and area of skin (dermatome). There are 8 cervical, 12 thoracic, 5 lumbar, 5 sacral, and 1 coccygeal segment. The association of the spinal segments with the vertebral levels is given in Table 12.1.

12.2 BASICS OF PEDIATRIC SPINE EXAMINATION

12.2.1 History

The onset, duration, and progression of presenting complaints should be documented in chronological order. Symptoms should be described pertaining to their location, severity, quantity, quality, duration, frequency, associated symptoms, relieving and aggravating factors, and relation to physical activity.

Table 12.1 Association of Spinal Segments with Vertebral Level

Vertebral Level	Spinal Segments
Cervical	+1
T1–T6	+2
T7–T9	+3
T10	L1 and L2 segments
T11	L3 and L4 segments
T12	L5 segments
L1	Sacral segments

12.2.2 Age

A differential diagnosis of certain pathologies can be made depending on age. In children, the spectrum of disease is quite different from adults. Growth-related disturbances, such as deformities of the spine and spondylolisthesis,[1] are common in children. Spina bifida can be diagnosed in a newborn. Back pain in a child younger than 4 years is usually caused by either an infection or a malignancy. Children in the first decade of life commonly present with discitis and osteomyelitis and primary orthopedic neoplasms. Patients older than 10 years are most likely to have back pain secondary to trauma, spondylolysis, disc herniations, or apophyseal fractures. Scheuermann's kyphosis manifests in adolescence. Inflammatory arthritis, like ankylosing spondylitis and juvenile rheumatoid arthritis, commonly present in the adolescent age group.[2]

12.2.3 Pain

Pain should be described in terms of site, onset, nature of pain, radiation, aggravating factors, and relieving factors. Insidious onset pain is usually a feature of developmental conditions like Scheuermann's kyphosis and benign neoplasms. On and off pain associated with sports and relieved by rest is seen in spondylolysis. Sharp shooting pain aggravated by coughing, sneezing, defecation, or Valsalva maneuver is a feature of a prolapsed disc. Continuous throbbing pain is seen in acute infective lesions. Dull aching pain with girdle pain and night cries are present in Pott's spine. Night pain may also be seen in primary tumors/tumor-like conditions, e.g., osteoid osteoma. Inflammatory arthropathies are associated with morning stiffness.

12.2.3.1 AXIAL VERSUS RADICULAR PAIN

On the one hand, axial pain is a marker of ligamentous, osseous, muscular, joint, and annular pathologies. Radicular pain, on the other hand, is usually caused by irritation of neurological tissue due to compression because of an etiology like disc fragment, canal stenosis, and foraminal stenosis. Patients with nerve root symptoms usually present with paresthesia, hyperalgesia, tingling, numbness, and burning pain. Patients with cervical radiculopathy usually obtain relief on abduction of the ipsilateral shoulder, while a patient with shoulder pathology usually has painful abduction of the shoulder. The pelvic cause of low back pain must be considered in differential diagnosis, particularly sacroiliitis. Pathology in retroperitoneal structures like the kidney, ureter, pancreas, etc. can present as back pain.

12.2.3.2 CONSTITUTIONAL SYMPTOMS

Fever in a child with acute onset back pain points to an infectious or neoplastic etiology. Ask for a history of malaise, anorexia, and evening rise of temperature. A rash or abnormal bruising with back pain can be the presenting complaint in a child with leukemia.

12.2.4 Birth History

Birth history includes antenatal, natal, and neonatal history. The mother should be clearly asked about any previous miscarriage, history of any fever during the antenatal period, any drug intake (if present, then determine the type of drug, its frequency, and duration), substance abuse, alcohol intake, smoking, etc. Ask about the type of delivery, vaginal or cesarean. If cesarean, then ask if there was an indication for operative intervention. Elicit further history regarding the newborn: did the newborn cry after birth? What was the weight of the baby at birth? Was it a premature birth? Was intensive care required at that time? Was there any abnormality/deformity of the spine noted at the time of birth?

12.2.5 Past Medical History

History of infections and disease of the immune system should be sought. Congenital or genetic diseases, such as Marfan syndrome and Down syndrome, have a predisposition for spinal anomalies.

12.2.6 Family History

Certain spinal pathologies have a familial inheritance. A history of congenital spinal deformities such as scoliosis, kyphosis, meningocele, etc. should be sought after. A family history of inflammatory diseases such as rheumatoid, ankylosing spondylitis, and inflammatory bowel disease can predispose a child to spinal problems.

12.2.7 Psychosocial History

A child with chronic pain not collaborating with radiological findings and disability out of proportion to that expected can be a result of child abuse or a personality disorder. A child psychologist must be consulted if such a history is suspected.

12.2.8 Development History

Developmental history is important as it tells us about the mental and physical growth pattern of the patient. Ask about all motor and social milestone achievements within the timeframe.

12.2.9 Tanner's Stages of Development

The Tanner stages[3,4] of maturation are based on breast size in girls, genital size in boys, and pubic hair stages for both girls and boys. The onset of menstruation is also an important milestone in the physical maturation of girls and can also guide in the possible progression of spinal deformities.

12.3 EXAMINATION OF SPINE

12.3.1 Inspection

Inspection starts as soon as the patient enters the room and should be done from the front, side, and back. Notice the patient's attitude, gait, how he/she carries their head, whether he/she requires support with the hands to the neck or head to avoid pain. A child with a painful inflammatory lesion in the spine will walk with caution to avoid any jerks with the trunk held stiff and a broad base formed by the lower limbs. He/she may stand with his/her hands kept on the knees to bypass weight transmission across the dorsolumbar spine. A child with paraparesis will modify his/her gait according to the type of paresis. In spastic paresis, the child may walk with scissoring (adductor spasm) or circumduction gait with the loss of normal rhythmic movements of the gait cycle. A patient with flaccid paresis may walk with assistance to clear ground. A high-stepping gait will be present in case of weakness of ankle dorsiflexion. Observe fine movements of the hands, such as unbuttoning of the shirt while the patient gets ready for examination.

Inspection should include all regions of the back, neck, triangles of the neck, supraclavicular fossa, axilla, arms, chest, abdomen, gluteal region, thigh, and legs. Look for stigmata of spinal dysraphism such as hair patches, puckering of the skin, dimples, or sinuses. Notice any café au lait spots and neurofibromas. Swellings should be described in terms of site, size, shape, number, margins, skin changes, pulsations, and signs of inflammation

such as redness and erythema. Scars and sinuses should also be described in terms of site, size, number, edges, margins, floor, base, type of discharge, surrounding skin changes such as pigmentation and associated signs of inflammation such as redness and erythema. Comment on the central furrow. Obliteration of the central furrow can be due to wasting of the paraspinal muscles or a minimal kyphotic deformity. A prominent central furrow may be seen in paraspinal muscle spasm. The pectus carinatum (prominent sternum) and pectus excavatum (sunken or funnel chest) should be noted.

Check for the position of the head on shoulders, short or webbed neck, low hairline, level of shoulders, position of scapulae, symmetry of the trunk, and symmetry of the pelvis. With the patient standing in his/her normal posture with the hip and knees in neutral position, notice any abnormal deviations of the spine in the sagittal and coronal planes. Also take note of the position and orientation of the pelvis in the sagittal and coronal planes as abnormal curvatures of the spine in both the coronal and sagittal plane can be secondary to pathologies of the hip and pelvis. Coronal plane curves compensate for adduction/abduction deformities, and sagittal plane curves compensate for fixed flexion deformities of the spine (e.g., exaggerated lumbar lordosis in flexion deformity of the hip and scoliosis in adduction/abduction deformities of the hip).

Abnormal deviation of the trunk to one side (list) can also be due to a painful herniated disc. List usually causes truncal shift due to the uniplanar sideway tilt of the spine. If a herniated disc is present at the shoulder of the exiting nerve root (lateral to the exiting nerve root), the list will be toward the opposite side to prevent pain. In an axillary presentation of a herniated disc, the list will be toward the side of prolapse (Figure 12.1).

12.3.2 Palpation

Look for temperature differences using the back of the hand. Compare symmetrical areas on both sides of the body.

The level of tenderness should be noted (Table 12.2). Different methods are described for eliciting tenderness.

1. Holdsworth test: It is a method of eliciting tenderness in which a fingertip is run over the spinous process of the spine.

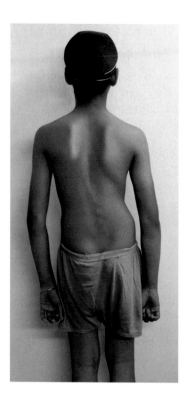

Figure 12.1 Direction of list in a herniated disc.

2. Direct method: Direct pressure over the spinous process of a vertebra elicits pain. It is positive in advanced anterior diseases or posterior element disease.

3. Rotatory tenderness: Spinous processes of two consecutive vertebrae are rotated in opposite directions by applying laterally directed forces in the opposite direction; anterior element diseases are usually painful in this technique.

4. Thrust tenderness: The spine is thrust with a fist. It is positive in mild anterior element involvement or when a pathological process is in its early phase.

Table 12.2 Bony Landmarks Correlating with Vertebral Levels

Vertebral Level	Landmark
C7	First prominent spinous process as we come down from the occiput
D3	Spine of the scapula
D7	Inferior angle of the scapula
D12	Last rib
L4	Highest point of the iliac crest
S2	Posterior superior iliac spine (PSIS)

Confirm findings of inspection as the site, size, number, shape, consistency, margins, and mobility of any swelling palpated. Bony palpation should include palpation of the hyoid bone, thyroid cartilage, cricoid cartilage, carotid tubercle on the C6 transverse process, manubrium sterni, clavicle, acromion, mastoid process, occiput, spinous processes, facet joints, scapula, ribs, costovertebral junction, iliac crest, posterior superior iliac spine (PSIS), and coccyx. Palpating each spinous process, notice any tenderness, malalignment, and gap or step. A step may be palpable in cases of spondylolisthesis and fracture dislocations. The absence of or a defect in any spinous process may be a sign of spina bifida. Facets can be palpated lateral to the spinous processes.

Soft tissue palpation includes palpation of the paraspinal muscles. Palpate the sternocleidomastoid for consistency in cases of torticollis. This muscle can be made prominent by asking the child to look to the contralateral side and then bend the neck against resistance to the ipsilateral side. Palpation of the trapezius starts from the occiput and follow its muscle laterally toward the acromion and then move downwards along the muscle span. A spasm of the paraspinal muscles can be demonstrated by the *Kibler test*. The movement of pinched skin along the axis of the paraspinal muscles is restricted in the presence of spasm.

Whiplash injury can present with tenderness at the insertion of ligaments. The superior nuchal ligament is a continuation of the supraspinatus ligament in the cervical spine extending from T1 to the occiput in the midline. Tenderness of the nuchal ligament is seen in whiplash injury.

Palpation of the supraclavicular fossa, axilla, triangles of the neck, chest, abdomen, iliac fossa, groin, hip, and thigh should be part of the lumbosacral spine examination. Any swelling should be looked for in the loin, iliac fossae, pettit's triangle, groin, and medial aspect of the thigh and, if present, should raise the suspicion of a cold abscess.

12.4 MOVEMENTS

12.4.1 Cervical Spine

Flexion/extension: at the zero starting point, the neck is aligned with the trunk as observed in the sagittal profile. The trunk should be stabilized, and the range of movement measured in degrees with a goniometer, as shown in Figure 12.2. Normally, the child is able to touch chin to chest on flexion and is able to see the roof on extension.[5]

Lateral bending: at the zero starting point, the nose is vertical and perpendicular to the shoulders. Now the child is asked to do a lateral bending movement of the neck with the trunk kept stable. The angle between the vertical line and mid-axis of the face is the range of movement (Figure 12.3). Normally, a child should be able to touch the ear to the ipsilateral shoulder.

Rotation: the zero starting point is the same as for lateral bending, but the examiner should observe from above while the child sits on a stool. The child is now asked to rotate his/her neck, keeping the trunk stable. The angle between the vertical line and mid-axis of the face is the range of movement of rotation (Figure 12.4). Normally a child can touch the chin to the shoulder when rotating the head.

12.4.2 Thoracolumbar Spine

Movements in the thoracolumbar spine are a combination of individual movement of individual motion segments of the spine. A goniometer and inclinometer are usually used for clinical assessment.[6-8]

12.4.2.1 FLEXION

Always rule out non-spinal causes of decreased flexion at the lumbar spine as tight hamstrings or hip flexion restriction. The zero starting point is a neutral anatomical position with the patient standing straight with the feet shoulder-width apart, hip and knee extended, trunk aligned to the lower limbs, and arms by the side. The patient is now asked to bend forward and touch the ground with the fingertips keeping the hip and knee extended.

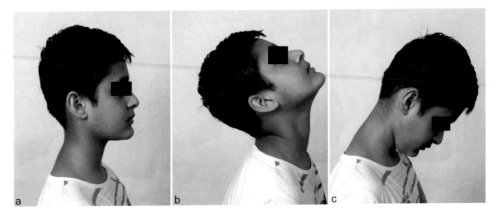

Figure 12.2 Cervical spine flexion and extension measurement from zero starting point.

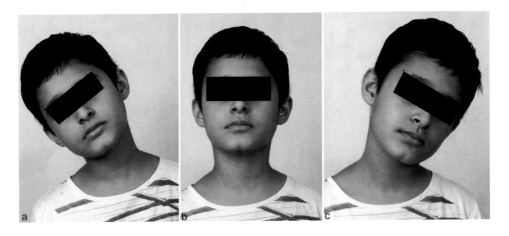

Figure 12.3 Cervical spine lateral bending measurement from zero starting point.

In this position, flexion can be quantified in a couple of ways:

- The inclinometer is a more accurate method[8]: it requires two inclinometers, one at the sacrum and the other at D12. Subtracting the sacral reading from the dorsal readings will give the lumbar spine range of motion.
- By measuring the finger to floor distance: this is a simple but not reliable method. A normal individual can reach up to 7 cm from the ground (Figure 12.5).
- Goniometer: it can also be used to measure the angle between the mid-truncal lines in zero position and the flexion position (Figure 12.5).

12.4.3 Ott Test

This test is used to quantify movements of the dorsal spine. The C7 vertebra is marked. Another point is marked at the midline, 30 cm distal to C7. Now, ask the patient to flex forward as described above. An increase in distance between the two marked points denotes dorsal spine flexion. The normal value is 3 cm or more.

12.4.4 Schober's Test

With the patient standing, a point is marked midway between the two PSISs, which is the level of S2. A second point is marked 10 cm above this point. Now the child is asked to bend forwards, keeping the knees straight. The distance between the

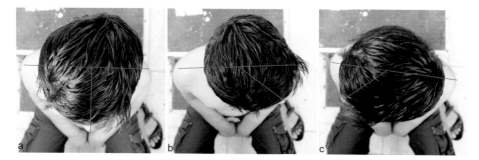

Figure 12.4 Cervical spine rotation measurement from zero starting point.

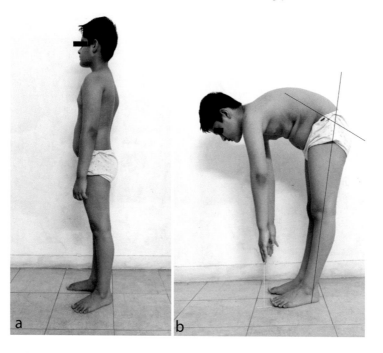

Figure 12.5 Thoracolumbar spine flexion measurement by finger to floor distance measurement.

two points is measured again in this position. An increase in distance between the two points over 10 cm denotes movement occurring at the lumbar spine.[9] It should not be less than 5 cm.

12.4.5 Modified Schober's Test

For a detailed description, refer to Chapter 9.

12.4.5.1 EXTENSION

The zero starting position is the same as for flexion testing. The patient is now asked to extend the trunk over the pelvis, keeping the hips and knees straight. The range of movement can be measured as in flexion either by a goniometer or two inclinometers (Figure 12.6). The normal range of active extension is 25–40°.

12.4.5.2 LATERAL BENDING

The zero starting point is the same as for lateral bending, except the examiner observes from behind. The patient is now asked to bend laterally, keeping the feet on the ground, the hips and knees straight, and the pelvis stable. The degree of movement can be measured by finger floor distance or by goniometer (Figure 12.7). The normal range of active lateral bending is 20–40°.

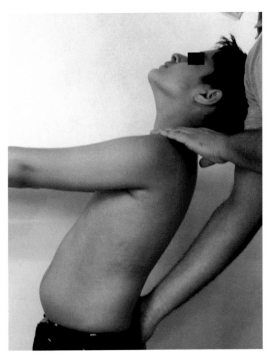

Figure 12.6 Thoracolumbar spine extension measurement.

12.4.5.3 ROTATION

Rotation mostly takes place at the dorsal spine as the facet orientation of the lumbar spine in the sagittal plane prevents rotation. With the patient sitting and the examiner observing from above, the child is instructed to rotate the trunk to one side, keeping the pelvis stable. Measure the movement of the shoulders using a goniometer. Normal rotation is around 45° on each side (Figure 12.8).

12.5 THORACIC EXPANSION TEST

The child is asked to inhale maximally, and the chest circumference is measured using measuring tape at the level of the fourth intercostal space. A normal person is able to expand his/her chest by 5 cm or more. Expansion of 3 cm or less is indicative of ankylosing spondylitis.

12.6 SPECIAL TESTS

12.6.1 Foramina Compression Test (Modified Spurling's Maneuver)

With the child seated on a stool, stand behind and place a hand on the patient's head. Rotate the head to the side of radiculopathy and then side bend and extend the neck simultaneously. A positive test is indicated by the appearance of symptoms of radiculopathy (Figure 12.9).

12.6.2 Lhermitte's Test

Flexion of the neck forwards causes a sensation of tingling, shooting pain, or weakness in the arms or legs. It is seen in anterior compressive lesions and is a sign of compressive myelopathy.

12.6.3 Adson's Test

Palpate the radial pulse on the wrist with the patient sitting. Now abduct, extend, and externally rotate the arm while still palpating the radial pulse. At this point, ask the child to take a deep breath and hold it and rotate the head toward the test side. A positive test is indicated by the weakening of the pulse or loss of pulse. It denotes compression of the subclavian artery due to any pathology such as a cervical rib or scalenus anticus syndrome (Figure 12.10).

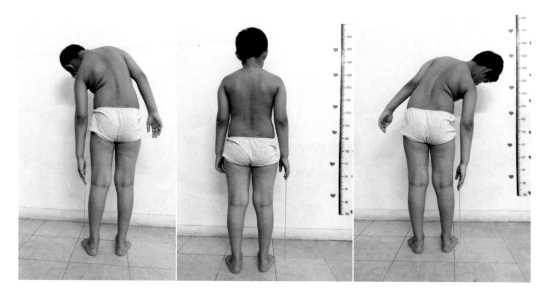

Figure 12.7 Thoracolumbar spine lateral bending measurement by finger to floor distance measurement.

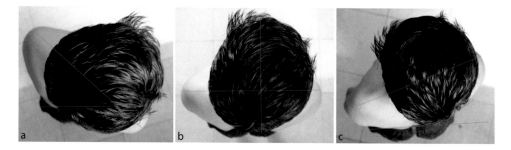

Figure 12.8 Thoracolumbar spine rotation assessment.

12.6.4 Passive Straight Leg Raise (PSLR)/Lasègue's Test

Ask the patient to lie relaxed in a supine position. Hold the patient's leg at the ankle and start raising it passively, keeping the patient's knee extended. Stop at a point where the patient winces with pain radiating down his/her leg. PSLR is significant if pain occurs below 40–60° of leg raise (Figure 12.11).

12.6.5 Braggard's Test

Do a PSLR test and stop when it becomes positive. At this point, lower the leg gradually until the pain subsides. Keeping the leg in this position, dorsiflex the foot. If symptoms are reproduced, the test is said to be positive.

12.6.6 Bowstring Test

Do a PSLR test and stop when it becomes positive. At this point, flex the knee joint, which will relieve pain. Now, using your hand, firmly press in the popliteal fossa. If symptoms are reproduced, the test is said to be positive.

12.6.7 Crossed SLR

A crossed SLR is the occurrence of symptoms in the involved leg on doing the PSLR of the normal leg. It is positive in cases of a central disc bulge.

12.6.8 Slump Test

With the patient sitting on the edge of the table and legs hanging, the involved leg is gradually

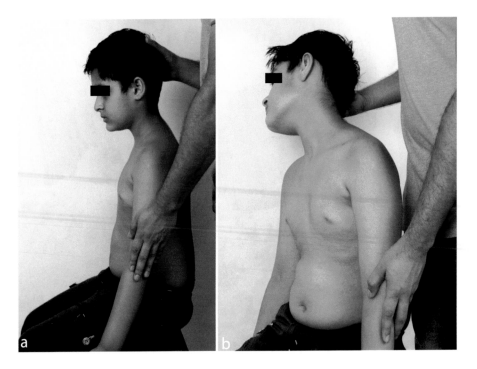

Figure 12.9 Modified Spurling's maneuver.

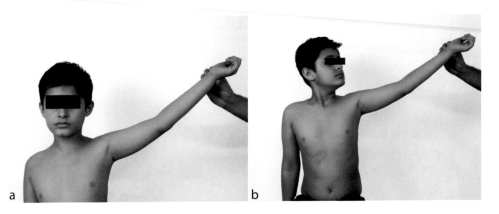

Figure 12.10 Adson's test.

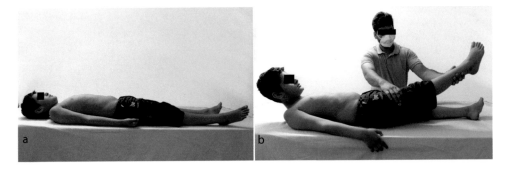

Figure 12.11 Passive straight leg raising test.

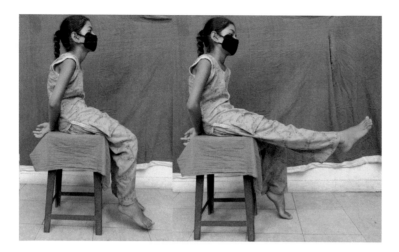

Figure 12.12 Slump test.

extended at the knee. A patient with a herniated disc will lean backward for support due to the radiation of pain down the leg (Figure 12.12).

12.6.9 Femoral Nerve Stretch Test/ Reverse Straight Leg Raise Test

The patient lies prone on the examination table. Now the knee is passively flexed, followed by passive hip extension (Figure 12.13). The test is said to be positive if anterior thigh pain is reproduced. A positive test is found in higher (L2–L3, L3–L4) disc herniations.

12.7 DEFORMITY EVALUATION

12.7.1 Kyphosis

Normal curvature of the dorsal spine is that of kyphosis of around 40°. An abnormal increase over the normal value of kyphosis, either segmental or global, constitutes deformity. A *knuckle* is kyphosis caused by the involvement of a single vertebra appreciated as prominence of one spinous process on palpation. A knuckle can easily be missed on inspection or can present as a subtle loss of central furrow on inspection. *Angular* kyphosis is the involvement of two or three vertebrae. *Round* kyphosis is the involvement of more than three vertebrae. Round kyphosis can be postural or pathological, such as Scheuermann's kyphosis (Figure 12.14). To differentiate between the two, ask the patient to bend forward, keeping the knees in neutral position. If deformity disappears or reduces, it is postural. However, if the deformity

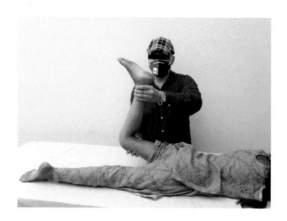

Figure 12.13 Femoral nerve stretch test/reverse straight leg raise test.

becomes more prominent, it is Scheuermann's kyphosis. Flexibility of the curve can be assessed by making the patient do an extension of the spine in prone position. If deformity reduces with extension, a curve is flexible.

12.7.2 Scoliosis

In a normal individual, a pendulum held at the C7 spinous process should pass through the natal cleft. Any deviation from the midline denotes a truncal shift and should be measured in centimeters. Any curve of the spine in the coronal plane should be described in terms of the level of curve and direction of convexity. A coronal curve in the thoracic spine can be compensatory to primary curves in the cervical spine, lumbar spine, or a pelvic obliquity. A secondary curve due to pelvic obliquity

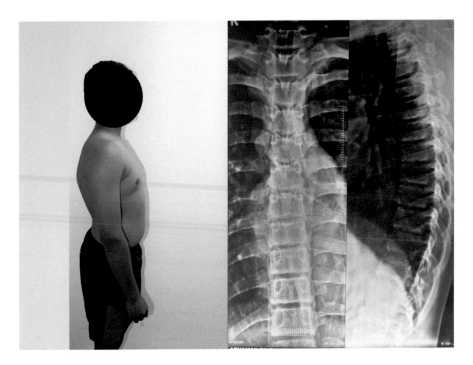

Figure 12.14 Scheuermann's kyphosis.

and fixed deformity of the hip can be identified by making the patient sit. In the sitting position, the pelvis will balance, and the curve disappears.

12.7.2.1 THE ADAM'S FORWARD BENDING TEST

Adam's forward bending test can be used to distinguish between a fixed (primary) and flexible (secondary) curve. Over a period of time, secondary curves can become fixed and rigid. Ask the patient to bend forwards with the legs shoulder-width apart and knees straight. In this position, a flexible curve disappears or reduces in size while a primary curve becomes prominent (Figure 12.15).

A scoliometer can also be used in this position to measure rib hump. Rib hump becomes more prominent in a flexed position. Rib hump is seen on the side of convexity of a spinal curve, but anterior rib hump is prominent on the side of concavity of the spinal curve.

- Shoulder asymmetry: This can be measured by measuring the angle between the line passing through both the coracoid processes and a horizontal reference line.
- Limb length and pelvic obliquity: Limb length discrepancy can give rise to spinal deformity.

Correction of limb length should be included in the management plan. Pelvic obliquity arising out of internal pelvic pathologies or hip joint pathologies should be considered in the final management plan.

12.7.3 Flexibility of Curve

- Three-point bending test: With the shoulders and pelvis stabilized, an attempt is made to correct the deformity at the apex by pushing it.
- Unweighting of the curve: The child is lifted off the ground with the examiner's hands in the axilla (Figure 12.16).

12.8 EXAMINATION OF SACROILIAC JOINTS

Pelvic distraction test: Pain on distraction of the pelvis by applying outward force on the bilateral anterior superior iliac spine (ASIS) simultaneously.

Patrick's four-part sign/FABER test: Refer to Chapter 9.

Gaenslen's test: Refer to the chapter on examination of the hip joint.

Gillie's test: The patient lies prone on the examination table, and the normal side of the pelvis is

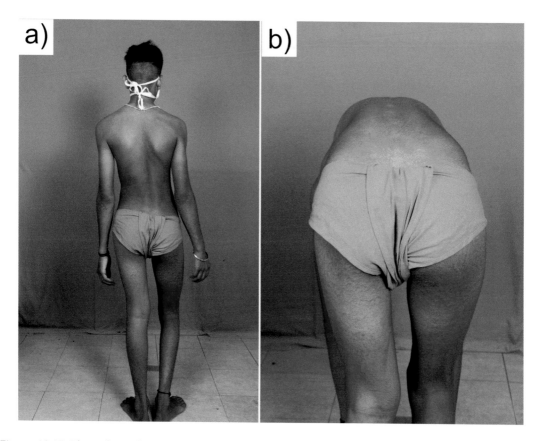

Figure 12.15 The Adam's forward bending test: obliteration of nonstructural scoliosis by forward bending test. (a) Nonstructural scoliosis lumbar spine with convexity to right. (b) Obliteration of scoliotic curve on forward bending.

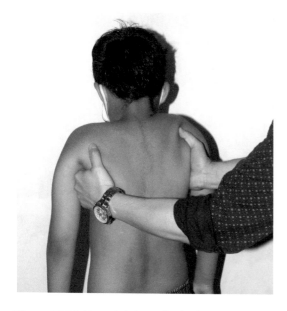

Figure 12.16 Unweighting of spinal curve.

stabilized by the examiner's hand by pressing upon it. Now the involved hemipelvis is lifted off the table by holding the leg at the ankle, with the knee extended and hip extended (Figure 12.17). Pain on this maneuver implies sacroiliac joint pathology.

12.9 ADDITIONAL ORTHOPEDIC EXAMINATION

Always make a point to examine the pelvis, hip, shoulder girdle, distal vascular status, and per rectal examination as part of the spine exam. The coccyx can be palpable through a rectal examination.

12.10 NEUROLOGICAL EXAMINATION

The aim of the neurological examination is to ascertain the level and type of pathological process. Neurological examination includes the examination

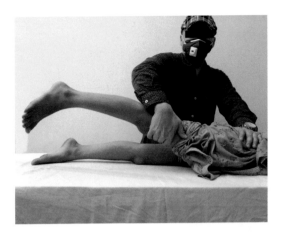

Figure 12.17 Gillie's test.

of the cranial nerves, higher mental function, motor system, sensory system, autonomic system, and cerebellar function. In addition to these usual heads of neurological examination, developmental reflexes should be checked for in a neonate.

12.11 MOTOR EXAMINATION

12.11.1 Bulk

The focal atrophy of muscle usually denotes a neurological disease. Fasciculations, along with muscular atrophy, is usually seen in lower motor neuron type of lesions. On palpation, wasted muscles are soft and flabby. In longstanding pathology, fibrosis may cause the muscle to become inelastic and hard-cord-like on palpation. Wasting is quantified by limb circumference measurement. The circumference is measured at the site of the maximum bulk of muscle in the normal limb. This point is measured from a fixed nearby bony landmark, and then the circumference is measured at a similar point in the contralateral limb.

12.11.2 Tone

Tone is defined as the inherent capacity of muscle to resist passive stretching. It is a function of the reflex arc controlled by the reticulospinal pathways in the spine. Tone is reduced in lower motor neuron type lesions, while increased tone is present in upper motor neuron type lesions. An increase in tone can be clasp-knife rigidity (lesions of corticospinal tracts), cogwheel rigidity (extrapyramidal diseases), and lead-pipe rigidity (extrapyramidal diseases).

In clasp-knife rigidity, there is initial resistance to movement, which increases on increasing the speed of passive movement followed by sudden giveaway. In cogwheel rigidity, the tone keeps on increasing and decreasing alternatively during the range of motion of a joint. In lead-pipe rigidity, there is uniform resistance to passive movement throughout the range of motion of a joint.

Tone can be assessed by:

- Passive rolling of limbs with palms and feeling for resistance offered.
- Passive flexion and extension of joints of the limb and feeling for resistance offered.
- Sudden lifting of the limb off the examining table by placing a hand below the lower aspect of the thigh. In the case of hypertonia, the heel will remain in the air as the knee gets flexed. However, in cases of hypotonia, the heel will drag along, touching the examining table as the knee gets flexed.

12.11.3 Muscle Strength

Grading muscle strength in a pediatric patient can be a herculean task. The basic idea can be derived from observation of the spontaneous activities of the infant or child. The Moro reflex is also said to be of value in assessing muscle strength in an infant.[10] The examiner should also try to determine the cause of weakness – myogenic or neurogenic. Systemic or generalized causes, such as electrolyte imbalance, myasthenia gravis, myopathies, and polyneuropathies, should be considered. The most commonly used muscle grading system is the Medical Research Council (MRC) scale, as shown in Table 12.3. The individual muscles tested are also shown in Table 12.4.

Table 12.3 Medical Research Council Scale

Grade	Description
0	No muscular contraction detected
1	Trace of contraction barely detectable
2	Active movement with gravity eliminated
3	Active movement against gravity
4	Active movement against gravity and some resistance
5	Active movement against full resistance

Source: Used with the permission of the Medical Research Council.

Table 12.4 Spinal Segments, Related Nerves, and Associated Muscles to Be Tested

Level	Motor Testing	Muscles Tested	Reflex
C4	Resisted bilateral scapular elevation	Trapezius: cranial nerve (CN) XI Levator scapulae: C3, C4	
C5	Shoulder abduction Elbow flexion (C5, C6)	Deltoid: axillary nerve C5 Supraspinatus: suprascapular nerve C5, C6 Brachialis: musculocutaneous nerve C5, C6 Biceps: musculocutaneous nerve C5, C6	Biceps reflex
C6	Wrist extension	Extensor carpi radialis longus: radial nerve C5, C6 Extensor carpi radialis brevis: radial nerve C5, C6 Extensor carpi ulnaris: radial nerve C6	Brachioradialis reflex
C7	Elbow extension Wrist flexion	Triceps: radial nerve C7 Flexor carpi radialis: median nerve C7 Flexor carpi ulnaris: ulnar nerve C8	Triceps reflex
C8	Finger flexion	Flexor digitorum profundus: ulnar nerve and anterior interosseous branch of median nerve C8, T1 Flexor digitorum superficialis: median nerve C7, C8, T1	
T1	Little finger adduction Finger abduction	Palmar interossei: ulnar nerve C8, T1 Dorsal interossei: ulnar nerve C8, T1 Abductor digiti minimi: ulnar nerve C8, T1	
L1, L2	Hip flexion	Iliopsoas	
L2, L3	Hip adduction	Adductor brevis, adductor longus, adductor magnus – obturator nerve	
L3, L4	Knee extension	Quadriceps – femoral nerve	Patellar tendon reflex
L4	Ankle dorsiflexion Standing on heels	Tibialis anterior	
L5	Big toe extension	Extensor hallucis longus – deep peroneal nerve	
L5	Hip abduction	Gluteus medius – superior gluteal nerve (L5)	
S1	Plantarflexion Hip extension	Peroneus longus and peroneus brevis, gastrocnemius–gastrocsoleus complex – superficial peroneal nerve Gluteus maximus – inferior gluteal nerve (S1)	Ankle reflex
S2, S3, and S4	Intrinsic muscles of the feet, anal sphincter, and bladder function		

12.11.4 Bevor's Sign

Instruct the patient to do a sit-up and hold the position. In a normal person, the umbilicus remains symmetrical in a central position of the abdomen. Asymmetric movement of the umbilicus denotes a positive Bevor's sign. If it moves upwards, the lesion is below T10. If it moves downwards, the lesion is above T10.

The American Spinal Injury Association (ASIA) impairment scale (Figure 12.18) is frequently used

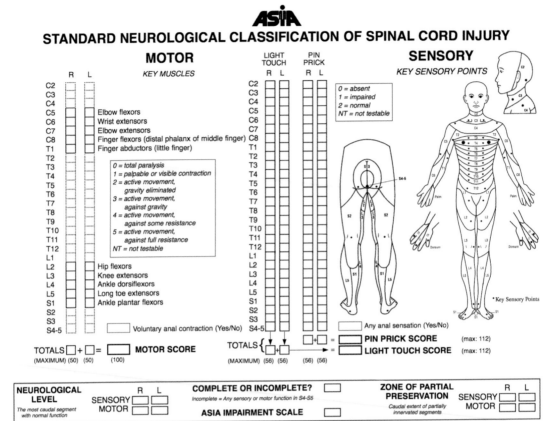

Figure 12.18 ASIA score chart. (Marino RJ. Introduction. In *Reference Manual for the International Standards for Neurological Classification of Spinal Cord Injury.* Chicago, IL: American Spinal Injury Association; 2003:1–6.).

in traumatic spine cases to describe the type of neurological deficit.

- A (complete): No motor or sensory function is preserved in the sacral segments S4–S5.
- B (incomplete): Sensory but not motor function is preserved below the neurologic level of injury and extends through the sacral segments S4–S5.
- C (incomplete): Motor function is preserved below the neurologic level of injury, and the majority of key muscles below that level have a muscle grade less than three.
- D (incomplete): Motor function is preserved below the neurologic level of injury, and a majority of key muscles below the neurologic level have a muscle grade greater than or equal to three.

- E (normal): Motor and sensory function are normal.

12.12 REFLEXES

12.12.1 Deep Tendon Reflexes

Deep tendon reflexes (DTR) are monosynaptic stretch reflexes; check the integrity of the reflex arc consisting of the afferent pathway, efferent pathway, and anterior horn cells in the spinal cord. DTR are graded according to the Reflex Grading Classification System.

- Grade 0: No reflex.
- Grade 1: Slight response.
- Grade 2: Normal reflex.
- Grade 3: Hyperactive.
- Grade 4: Hyperactive with clonus.

Hyperactive deep tendon reflexes and clonus indicate an upper motor neuron lesion, while absent reflex suggests a lower motor neuron type of lesion.

12.12.2 Biceps Reflex (C5, C6)

The patient is instructed to sit or stand with the forearm flexed and relaxed at an angle of 90° with exposed biceps and muscle belly. The patient's forearm rests over the examiner's forearm. Grasp the patient's elbow with your hand, placing your thumb over the biceps tendon (Figure 12.19). Strike your thumb over the tendon with the reflex hammer, watching for a contraction of the biceps muscle.

12.12.3 Triceps Reflex (C7)

The triceps reflex appears after 6 months of age. A sudden tap is given to the triceps tendon near the olecranon process with the elbow placed in flexion (Figure 12.20). Look for a contraction of the triceps muscle.

12.12.4 Supinator Reflex/ Brachioradialis Reflex (C6)

With the elbow flexed and forearm in pronation, a sudden gentle tap is given just proximal to the radial styloid (Figure 12.21). Look for contraction of the brachioradialis muscle.

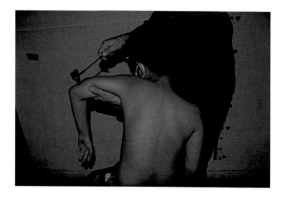

Figure 12.20 Triceps reflex.

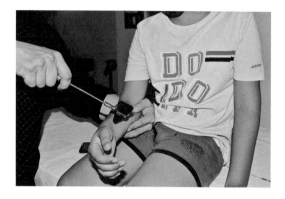

Figure 12.21 Supinator reflex/brachioradialis reflex.

12.12.5 Crossed Radial Reflexes

A crossed reflex is positive when both biceps' and a wrist extensor reflex are elicited simultaneously on percussing the biceps tendon with a hammer. It is a sign of an upper motor neuron lesion.

12.15.5.1 INVERTED RADIAL REFLEX

Inverted radial reflex is positive when both wrist extension and finger flexion response are elicited when eliciting the brachioradialis reflex. It is a sign of upper motor neuron lesion.

12.12.6 Knee Reflex (L3–L4)

With the knee flexed and supported by one forearm, a sudden tap is given to the quadriceps tendon just below the patella (Figure 12.22). Look for contraction of the quadriceps muscle, which should be kept exposed for examination.

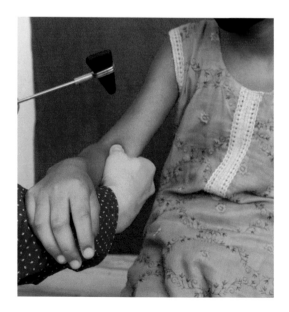

Figure 12.19 Biceps reflex.

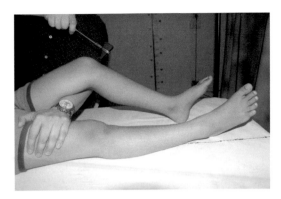

Figure 12.22 Knee reflex.

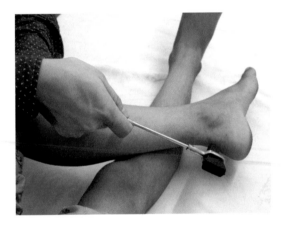

Figure 12.23 Ankle reflex.

12.12.7 Ankle Reflex (S1)

The patient lies supine on the table. The limb is positioned so as to keep the heel of the limb to be tested on the contralateral shin. Now, with the ankle gently dorsiflexed, a sudden tap is given to the Achilles tendon with the fingertips or hammer (Figure 12.23). This should elicit contraction of the gastrocnemius muscle or plantar-directed jerk of the ankle joint.

12.12.8 Clonus

The clonus is present in cases of exaggerated DTR where a single stimulus causes repetitive contraction of the muscle.

- Ankle clonus: With the hip and knee flexed to 90°, a sudden but gentle dorsiflexion of the ankle is carried out. If present, there will be alternating contraction and relaxation of the

gastrocnemius and soleus. Sustained clonus (more than six beats) is a sign of an upper motor neuron lesion.[11]
- Patellar clonus: With the patient supine and knee extended, a sudden distally directed push is given to the patella.

12.12.9 Peripheral Reflexes/ Superficial Reflexes

Peripheral and superficial reflexes are polysynaptic reflexes.

12.12.9.1 BABINSKI'S REFLEX/PLANTAR REFLEX

With a bluntly pointed object, the patient's foot is stroked along the lateral aspect of the sole starting from the heel and continuing along the lateral aspect reaching up to but not touching the base of the big toe. Normally, there is plantarflexion of the toes. In an abnormal reflex, there is an extension of the big toe with extension and fanning out of all other toes. An abnormal reflex indicates an upper motor neuron lesion. In children, Babinski's reflex can normally be present for up to 2 years of age. Various named methods of eliciting plantar reflex are:

- Oppenheim's sign: To perform the Oppenheim's test, run a thumb pressing down along the crest of the tibia.
- Gordon's reflex: Squeeze the patient's calf.
- Chaddock reflex: Scratch the skin along the region of the lateral malleolus.

12.12.9.2 HOFFMANN'S REFLEX

This reflex is elicited by tapping or flicking the patient's middle finger. Normally, there is no response. In an abnormal reflex, there will be flexion of the index finger or thumb. It is usually positive in upper motor neuron lesions.

12.12.9.3 CREMASTERIC REFLEX

In a normal response, gentle stroking of the inner portion of the thigh in the distal to proximal direction will cause symmetric contraction of the scrotum in a male child. Absence or an asymmetric response indicates an upper motor neuron lesion.

12.12.9.4 ABDOMINAL REFLEX

In a normal response, gentle stroking of the abdomen in all four quadrants from lateral to the medial direction toward the umbilicus will cause contraction of the rectus abdominis muscle and the umbilicus migrates toward the quadrant being stroked. Absence or an asymmetric response indicates an upper motor neuron lesion.

12.12.9.5 BULBOCAVERNOSUS REFLEX (S2, S3, S4)

The patient lies on their side with hips and knees flexed. Now, insert a gloved and lubricated finger into the rectum, and with the other hand, squeeze the glans penis or clitoris. In a normal response, the gloved finger in the rectum should feel the contraction of the anal sphincter.

12.12.9.6 ANOCUTANEOUS REFLEX (S3, S4, S5)

The patient lies on their side with hips and knees flexed. Now, stimulate the skin around the anal orifice and watch for contraction of the anal sphincter.

12.12.10 Coordination of Movements

The coordination of movements exam assesses the function of the posterior column of the spinal cord and cerebellum. Coordination is assessed by rapid alternating hand and foot movements and finger-to-nose test.[12]

12.12.10.1 STATIC ROMBERG'S TEST

Make the child stand with their arms at 90° of flexion, hands outstretched, and palms facing upwards. Now, ask the child to close his/her eyes. If he/she loses balance or the arms go above parallel, the test is positive and is indicative of myelopathy or cerebellar dysfunction.

12.12.10.2 DYNAMIC ROMBERG'S TEST

Ask the child to do a heel-to-toe walk in a straight line. The difficulty in doing this task denotes a positive test.

12.13 SENSORY EXAMINATION

The dermatomal distribution of the body is given in Table 12.5, Table 12.6, and Figure 12.24.

All dermatomes should be checked for various sensory modalities carried by different pathways of the spine. The patient should be asked to close their eyes, and the symmetrical parts of the body should

Table 12.5 Dermatomes of the Upper Limb

Level	Sensory Testing
C1	No sensory supply
C2–C4	Back of skull and neck
C5	Lateral aspect of the upper arm
C6	Lateral aspect of forearm, thumb, and index finger
C7	Middle finger
C8	Ulnar side of the distal forearm, the ring finger, and the little finger
T1	Medial aspect of the arm

Table 12.6 Dermatomes of the Lower Limb

Level	Sensory Testing
L1	Groin
L2	Lateral groin and anterior aspect of the thigh
L3	Anteromedial aspect of the thigh to the malleoli
L4	Anterolateral aspect of the thigh and leg to the medial aspect of the big toe
L5	Lateral aspect of the foot
S1	Posterior aspect of the thigh and lower leg, lateral aspect of the foot, lateral aspect of the fifth toe
S2	Posterior aspect of the thigh and lower leg
S3	Medial aspect of the thigh, perianal region
S4	Perineum, perianal region
S5	Perianal region (innermost around anus)

be compared. In cases of bilateral symmetrical sensory involvement, the examiner should start testing from the area of sensory loss and proceed gradually toward the normal dermatomes.

Pain sensation: This is tested with the back or head of a pin. Take care to test pain and not pressure. The pinhead should be firmly pushed onto the skin without breaching the skin.

Light touch: This is tested with a wisp of cotton.

Deep/crude touch: This is tested by giving a firm touch with the hands.

Temperature: A test tube containing water at a temperature of 110°F (hot) and 45°F (cold) should be used. Alternatively, an alcohol swab, ice cube,

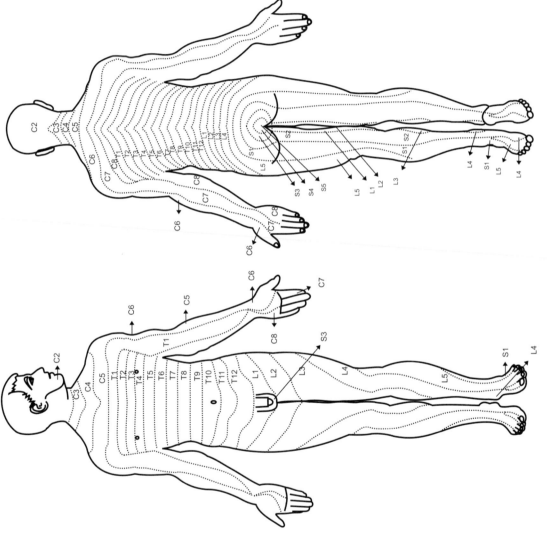

Figure 12.24 Dermatomal distribution in the body.

Table 12.7 Two-Point Discrimination

Fingertip	2 mm
Palm	10 mm
Forehead	20 mm
Back of hand	25 mm
Back	40 mm

steel handle of a reflex hammer (in winter) can be used for cold testing.

Two-point discrimination: This should be tested with a fine calibratable instrument such as a mathematical divider. The two ends of a divider are gradually brought closer until the child perceives them as a single stimulus. Different regions of the body have different thresholds for minimum distance appreciable as two different points (Table 12.7).

Vibration: A tuning fork of 256 Hz is used to test this. The tuning fork must be placed on the subcutaneous bones such as the medial malleolus, lateral malleolus, proximal tibia, tibial tuberosity, greater trochanter of the femur, anterior superior iliac spine, styloid process of the radius and ulna, olecranon, lateral epicondyle of the humerus, acromion process, and mastoid process.

Proprioception: This is checked by positioning a patient's joint at an extreme range of motion and asking the patient for the position of the joint.

Stereognosis: This is analyzed by asking the patient to identify common things of daily use such as a coin, pen, etc. just by palpating the things for size and feel.

12.14 AUTONOMIC NERVOUS SYSTEM

Autonomic nervous system dysfunction is represented by anhidrosis, vasomotor instability, trophic skin changes, impaired temperature control, erectile dysfunction, and bladder and bowel dysfunction. Spinal segments S2, S3, and S4 innervate the bladder and bowel (Table 12.8). The bladder and bowel can be examined by checking for sensations in the S2, S3, and S4 dermatome, anal tone, voluntary anal contraction, anal wink, and bulbocavernosus reflex.

To test the voluntary contraction of the external anal sphincter, instruct the patient to lie on his/her side and bring the hips and knees into flexion.

Table 12.8 Difference between UMN Type and LMN Type of Urinary Bladder Involvement – Developmental Reflexes

	UMN Bladder	LMN Bladder
Bladder volume	Normal to decreased	Increased
Detrusor	Overactive	Hypoactive
Pressure	High	Low
Incontinence	Urge	Overflow
Symptoms	Urgency Frequency Leaking of urine	Dribbling of urine

Abbreviations: UMN – upper motor neuron, LMN – lower motor neuron

Instruct the patient to relax and then insert a gloved and lubricated finger into the rectum. Now, ask the patient to contract the anal sphincter and feel for a change in sphincter tone.

The time of appearance and disappearance of these infantile reflexes is of utmost importance as a guide to normal neurological development and associated impairment, if any. The infantile reflexes are described in Chapter 13.

REFERENCES

1. Micheli LJ, Wood R. Back pain in young athletes: Significant differences from adults in causes and patterns. *Arch Pediatr Adolesc Med.* 1995;149:15–18.
2. Hosalkar H, Dormans J. Back pain in children requires extensive workup. *Biomechanics* 2003;10:51–58.
3. Tanner J. Growth and endocrinology of the adolescent. In: Gardner L, editor. *Endocrine and genetic diseases of childhood.* Philadelphia: WB Saunders, 1975.
4. Tanner JM. *Growth at adolescence.* New York: Blackwell Scientific, 1982.
5. Hoppenfield S. *Physical examination of the spine and extremities.* New York: Appleton-Century-Crofts, 1976.
6. Gill K, Krag MH, Johnson GB, et al. Repeatability of four clinical methods for assessment of lumbar spinal motion. *Spine* 1988;13:50.
7. Macrae IF, Wright V. Measurement of back movement. *Ann Rheum Dis.* 1969;28:584.
8. Salisbury PJ, Porter RW. Measurement of lumbar sagittal mobility: A comparison of methods. *Spine.* 1987;12:190.
9. Solomon J, Nadler SF, Press J. Physical examination: Of the lumbar spine. In Malanga G, Nadler SF, editors. *Musculoskeletal physical examination:*

An evidence-based approach. Philadelphia: Hanley & Belfus; 2006. pp. 189–226.

10. Johnson EW. Examination for muscle weakness in infants and small children. *JAMA.* 1958;168:1306.

11. Swaiman KF. Neurologic examination after the newborn period until 2 years of age. In: Swaiman KF, editor. *Pediatric neurology: Principles and practice*, Vol 1. St. Louis: CV Mosby, 1993. p. 43.

12. Bates B. *A guide to physical examination and history taking*, 5th ed. Philadelphia: JB Lippincott, 1991.

13

Examination of a Child with Cerebral Palsy

NIRMAL RAJ GOPINATHAN

In this chapter we will be going through the clinical examination of a child with neuromuscular disorder focusing on cerebral palsy (CP). Emphasis will be placed on detailed lower limb examination; upper limb involvement is also touched upon. The main aim of this chapter is to have a detailed overview of the outpatient clinical evaluation, which can be of help in formulating the management plan for these patients.

13.1 DEFINITION OF CP

Before learning how to examine a child with CP, it is imperative to know the definition of CP.

> CP describes a group of permanent disorders of the development of movement and posture, causing activity limitations that are attributed to non-progressive

disturbances that occurred in the developing fetal or infant brain. The motor disorders of CP are often accompanied by disturbances of sensation, perception, cognition, communication and behavior, epilepsy, and by secondary musculoskeletal problems.[1]

The movement disorder is clinically an upper motor neuron syndrome, and the examiner must look for the positive and negative signs enumerated in Table 13.1.

13.2 HISTORY-TAKING

The diagnostic matrix of cerebral palsy includes detailed history-taking, detailed evaluation, and supportive investigations; it is important to have a multidisciplinary approach.

The history-taking includes a detailed evaluation of prenatal, natal, and postnatal events with specific importance given to illness encountered or medications taken during pregnancy, duration of pregnancy/prematurity, multiple pregnancies, birth weight, any difficulties encountered during labor, signs of birth asphyxia, or any early neonatal illness requiring ventilatory assistance or hospitalization.

Developmental milestones and the presence of any primitive reflex beyond the timeline helps us to assess the selective motor control to an extent; this must be carefully evaluated according to the child's age (Table 13.2). It will also be of help in prognosticating the outcome for the given child.

Also, ask for and observe other clues like preferential use of a limb or early handedness/dragging a limb while crawling or scooting/abnormal positioning like keeping the upper limb flexed at the elbow while running, etc. which may suggest hemiparetic CP. Passing the child an object like a toy or a pen may reveal the child is selectively using one extremity. Also ask for other things like neonatal intensive care admission, seizures, strabismus, frequent choking, dysphagia, dribbling of saliva, delayed speech, and poor eyesight, which may indicate the possibility of neurological insult in the perinatal period.

Table 13.2 Common Motor Milestones and Time of Achievement[2]

Motor Milestone	Time of Establishment[a]
Head control	3–6 months
Sitting	6–9 months
Crawling	9 months
Standing and cruising[b]	10–12 months
Walking	12–18 months

[a] Adjustment for prematurity should be made – subtract the number of weeks of prematurity from the child's actual age in weeks.
[b] Walking by holding hands/objects.

13.3 INFANTILE REFLEXES

The newborn possesses some infantile reflex mechanisms that usually disappear by 3–6 months of age when the motor cortex matures. In CP, these reflexes might be retained and aid in diagnosing the disorder (Table 13.3).

13.4 ASSESSMENT OF AMBULATORY POTENTIAL

The timing and attainment of developmental milestones can be of help in predicting the child's ability to walk.

Negative prognosticators:

• Not able to sit by 2 years of age.
• Presence of two or more infantile reflexes beyond 12–15 months of age.
• No head control by 20 months of age.

Table 13.1 Movement Disorders in CP

Positive Signs	Negative Signs
Abnormal phenomena because of absent inhibition from cortical circuits	Failure of formation of proper sensorimotor control mechanisms
Spasticity	Weakness
Dyskinesia	Poor coordination of movements
Hyperreflexia	Poor balance and walking ability
Retained developmental reactions	
Secondary musculoskeletal malformations	

Table 13.3 Infantile Reflexes and Their Time of Appearance/Disappearance

Reflex	Time	How to Elicit?	Positive Response
Startle or Moro	Disappears by 3–6 months of age	It is elicited in supine position with slight elevation by suddenly letting the infant's head drop back into extension	Results in abrupt extension of legs and arms
		A sudden loud noise in an older child	Results in extension and lurching from the wheelchair
Parachute	Present from 5 months of age	Hold the child prone in the air and lower him/her quickly headfirst toward the examination table	Child will reach out with both arms to protect itself
			A CP child will not do that, and a hemiplegic child will use only one extremity
Tonic neck reflex	Disappears in infancy	Turn the supine infant's head to one side	Arm and leg extend on ipsilateral side while the contralateral arm and leg flexes

Table 13.4 Topographical Classification of CP[3]

Monoplegia	Involves one limb
Paraplegia	Involves legs only
Hemiplegia	One half of the body affected
Triplegia	Involves three extremities
Quadriplegia/Tetraplegia	Involves all four extremities
	Patients with significant involvement of lower limbs are usually spastic
	Patients with significant involvement of the upper limbs are usually those with dyskinetic CP, including athetoid CP
Diplegia	Paralysis involving like parts on both sides of the body; bilateral paralysis

The ability to walk plateaus by 7 years of age, and if a child is non-ambulatory by 7 years of age, it is unlikely that the child will ever attain ambulatory potential.[2]

13.5 PHYSICAL EXAMINATION

13.5.1 Classification

There are many classification systems available depending upon the topography, neurological involvement, functional impairment, etc. But we will be restricting our discussion to topography and the commonly presenting spastic CP. It is important to classify the child according to the topographical involvement[3] (Table 13.4) and the respective Gross Motor Function Classification System (GMFCS) classification[4] (classify per age, i.e., up to 2 years, 2–4 years, 4–6 years, 6–12 years, and 12–18 years) as that will help us in the

documentation, management, as well as prognostication of these children. Tabulating the GMFCS for individual age groups is beyond the scope of this book, but in general, the GMFCS for a child of ambulatory age is given in Table 13.5.

Diplegia refers to the involvement of symmetrical parts of the body, and quadriplegia refers to the involvement of all four limbs, but not essentially symmetrical.

13.5.2 Gait

The examination starts with observation of the child's ability to ambulate independently or with the help of an assistive device if the child can do so. A detailed description of gait evaluation is given in Chapter 3. It should also be kept in mind that physical examination often gives a clue to the static pathophysiology and should be correlated with a dynamic assessment like gait analysis for effective

Table 13.5 GMFCS Classification

GMFCS Level	Ambulatory (Motor) Ability
I	Walks without any restrictions; limitations in more advanced gross motor activities
II	Does not require assistive devices for walking; limitations in outdoor and community walking
III	Uses assistive devices for walking; limitations in outdoor and community walking
IV	Limited self-mobility; children are transported or use powered mobility in outdoors and community
V	Severely limited self-mobility even with assistive technology; needs manual wheelchair for transport

interpretation. A note is also made upon the balance, equilibrium, and standing posture of the child.

Apart from gait evaluation, the physical examination evaluates the following:

- Power and selective motor control of individual muscle groups.
- Muscle tone and muscle tendon reflexes.
- Presence of joint contractures.
- Skeletal deformations including torsional and lever arm abnormalities.

13.5.3 Power/Strength

Although children with cerebral palsy are weak, strength assessment is essential to document the child's current motor capabilities and to plan for management according to the available group of muscles that can be recruited for a selective or coordinated function. We use the Medical Research Council (MRC) grading[5] (Table 13.6), which is a five-point scale; it is a quick and reliable way to assess power.

13.5.4 Selective Motor Control

One of the hallmarks of CP is impairment of selective motor control, which affects the functional motor capabilities of the child, including ambulatory capacity and potential. It is graded in the following manner: grade 0, no ability, grade 1, partial ability, and grade 2, complete ability in terms of isolating movement and demonstrating maximum voluntary contraction in the absence of overflow movement in the appropriate time. For example, it is essential to differentiate the strength and selective control of a given group of muscles, as a child

Table 13.6 Royal Medical Research Council of Great Britain Strength Grading Scale

Grade	Strength
0	No contraction
1	Flicker or trace of contraction
2	Active movement, with gravity eliminated
3	Active movement against gravity
4	Active movement against gravity and resistance
4−	Slight resistance
4	Moderate resistance
4+	Strong resistance
5	Normal power

Source: Used with the permission of the Medical Research Council.

may have 3/5 strength in the tibialis anterior but may not be able to selectively dorsiflex the ankle when asked and may demonstrate a mass hip and knee flexion in response, which will be grade 0 with respect to selective motor control. This is again important in terms of expectations following management and prognostication (Figure 13.1). It is important to rule out established contractures in the assessed joint so that the joint has an adequate range of motion possible for performing the act.

13.5.5 Tone Assessment

Tone is resistance felt to a passive stretch in a relaxed state of muscle activity and is best demonstrated by passive movement about a joint. The child is assessed in a relaxed state and can be examined in the parent's lap. It may be increased in the form of spasticity, dystonia, or rigidity. The

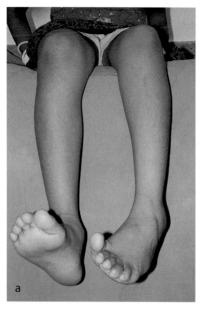
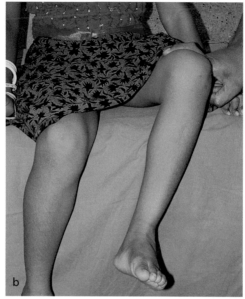

Figure 13.1 Absence of selective motor control. (a) Attempted ankle dorsiflexion possible only on the right side in this child with left hemiplegic CP. (b) The left ankle dorsiflexes on hip flexion against resistance indicating preserved power. Reproduced with permission from Joseph B (2020). General principles of management of upper motor neuron paralysis. In Joseph B, Nayagam S, Loder R, Torde I, editors. *Paediatric Orthopaedics: A System of Decision-Making* (2nd ed., 456), Taylor & Francis.

criteria described by Sanger et al.[6] to assess hypertonia can be followed:

- Palpate the muscle to be examined to assess whether there is muscle contracture at rest.
- Define the available passive range of motion by moving the limb gently.
- Now move the limb at different speeds through the available range to look for catch, i.e., sudden resistance offered to the passive range and further possible slow stretch.
- Now the patient is asked to move the same joint on the other side and look for an alteration in resistance to movement or involuntary movement on the side being examined, which may indicate the presence of dystonia.

13.5.5.1 SPASTICITY

Spasticity is defined as "velocity dependent resistance of muscle to passive stretching."[7] Spasticity increases with speed, and resistance is felt as a catch. It is assessed by passively moving the extremity through the range of motion to stretch the individual muscle groups, and Ashworth has described a five-point ordinal scale to grade the resistance felt. This scale was modified by Richard

W. Bohannon and Melissa B. Smith,[7] is widely used, and is given in Table 13.7.

13.5.5.2 TARDIEU SCALE

The other method of assessing spasticity is to use the *Tardieu scale*. The Tardieu scale is considered to be more sensitive and specific with respect to other scales. It measures spasticity with the help of two parameters, namely spasticity grade Y and spasticity angle X, with respect to three stretch velocities, V1, V2, and V3.

Grading is done with the muscle to be tested at rest. It should be kept in mind that other joints must be kept in a constant position, including the neck, throughout the test and also in between tests.

The velocity of the stretch is quantified as follows:

V1: As slow as possible (minimizing stretch reflex).
V2: Limb segment allowed to fall under gravity.
V3: As fast as possible, faster than the natural drop of a limb with gravity.

V1 is used to assess the passive range of motion, whereas V2 and V3 are used to assess spasticity.

Table 13.7 Modified Ashworth Scale for Grading Spasticity

Grade	Description
0	Muscle tone not increased
1	Slight increase in muscle tone, felt as a catch and release or as minimal resistance at the terminal arc of motion when the affected part(s) is moved into flexion or extension
1+	Slight increase in muscle tone, felt as a catch, followed by minimal resistance throughout the remaining (less than half) range of motion (ROM)
2	Muscle tone is increased more markedly through most of the ROM, but affected part(s) can be easily moved
3	Considerable increase in muscle tone making passive movement difficult
4	Affected part(s) kept rigid in flexion or extension

13.5.5.2.1 Spasticity Grade (Y)

0: No resistance during passive movement.

1: Slight resistance all along the course of the passive movement, with no definite catch at a precise angle.

2: Clear catch at a particular angle, interrupting the passive movement, followed by release.

3: Fatigable clonus (<10 seconds when maintaining pressure) occurring at a particular angle.

4: Infatigable clonus (>10 seconds when maintaining pressure) occurring at a particular angle.

13.5.5.2.2 Spasticity Angle (X)

Spasticity angle X is the difference between the angles of arrest at slow speed and catch-release/clonus at fast speed.

The evaluation involves two stretch maneuvers of the comfortably resting limb, one slow (V1) and one at the maximum speed possible for the examiner (V3). V1 measures the passive range of motion, and the examiner makes a note of any movement arrest due to discomfort or mechanical resistance. The difference (Xv1 – Xv3) is the spasticity angle (X), which indicates the velocity-dependent stretch

reflex. The larger this difference, the more spastic the muscle. V2 is only feasible for extensors of the knee, wrist, and flexors of the elbow.[8]

Note: it should be kept in mind that the angles are measured with respect to the muscle tested and not according to the anatomic principles so that 0° represents the position of minimal stretch on the muscle. For example, when the plantar flexors of the ankle are assessed, the angle 0° corresponds to the full plantarflexion position at the ankle.

13.5.5.2.3 Modified Tardieu Scale

To keep it simple, with the modified Tardieu scale (MTS), the examiner measures two joint angles, namely R1 and R2. R1 is the "angle of catch/resistance," which is elicited after a rapid velocity stretch, and R2 is the angle measured after a passive joint range of motion elicited after a slow velocity stretch to the maximum extent of exertion. The difference between these two measurements indicates the dynamic component of spasticity, i.e., R2–R1. If there is not much difference between R2 and R1, then it indicates static contractures that have been established in the affected muscle[9] (Figure 13.2).

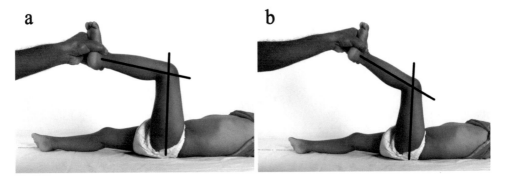

a   b

Figure 13.2 R1 and R2 of spasticity assessment. (a) R1, (b) R2 indicating hamstring spasticity.

13.5.5.3 DYSTONIA

These are a group of involuntary movements from sustained or intermittent muscle contractions. They result in twisting repetitive movements, abnormal postures, or sometimes both. In a case of dystonia, there is an increase in muscle activity while at rest, and there is a tendency to go back to a fixed posture. Also, there is an increase in resistance with the movement of the opposite limb and changes with alteration of behavior or posture. It is also important to diagnose children with mixed tone (both spasticity and dystonia) as the management protocol differs in these children, and the results are less predictable. Make a note of the presence or absence of dystonia.

13.5.6 Muscle Tendon Reflexes

CP, being an upper motor neuron disorder, results in an exaggeration of deep tendon reflexes. Repetitive tapping or sudden passive stretch results in the elicitation of clonus. The reflexes will be asymmetric in hemiparetic children. The deep tendon reflexes are graded, as given in Table 13.8.

13.5.7 Joint Contractures

The static examination of muscle length provides details about the evolution of spasticity into contracture. It is important to differentiate these two as the management differs and is more invasive for managing an established contracture. Contracture, unlike spasticity, is not velocity dependent, and the fixed-length phenomenon of the muscle tendon unit should be examined slowly. It is also important to differentiate contracted biarticular and monoarticular muscles (for example, the Silfverskiold test is used to identify isolated gastrocnemius contracture versus gastrocsoleus contracture). A detailed evaluation will be elaborated under individual joint examination.

Table 13.8 Grading of Deep Tendon Reflexes[10]

Grade	Response
0	Absence of response – abnormal
1+	Slight response
2+	Brisk response – normal
3+	Very brisk response
4+	Clonus – abnormal

13.5.8 Evaluation of Skeletal Deformation: Torsional Anomalies of Femur and Tibia

13.5.8.1 LEVER ARM DISEASE

Lever arm disease is defined as "deviation in gait resulting from malalignment of the musculotendinous forces because of skeletal anatomic abnormalities in rotation" (Figure 13.3).

13.5.8.2 FEMORAL ANTEVERSION

In a child with cerebral palsy, the normal reduction in femoral neck anteversion during growth may be affected due to abnormalities in muscle balance. The method of quantifying femoral neck version is described in Chapter 9 and the values at different age groups are described in Chapter 2.

It is of the utmost importance to keep in mind while assessing femoral rotation that pelvic rotation may be present, and it may confound the

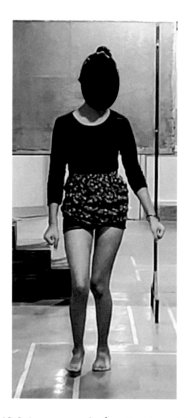

Figure 13.3 Lever arm dysfunction in a child with CP (left hip appears adducted due to flexion deformity and exaggerated femoral anteversion leading to internal rotation).

clinical picture. This is commonly seen in patients with spastic hemiplegia in whom the hemipelvis on the affected side retracts and is externally rotated, which partially masks the increase in femoral anteversion.

13.5.8.3 TIBIAL TORSION

13.5.8.3.1 Thigh-Foot Angle Method

To measure the tibial torsion, the thigh-foot angle can be used provided that midfoot and hindfoot

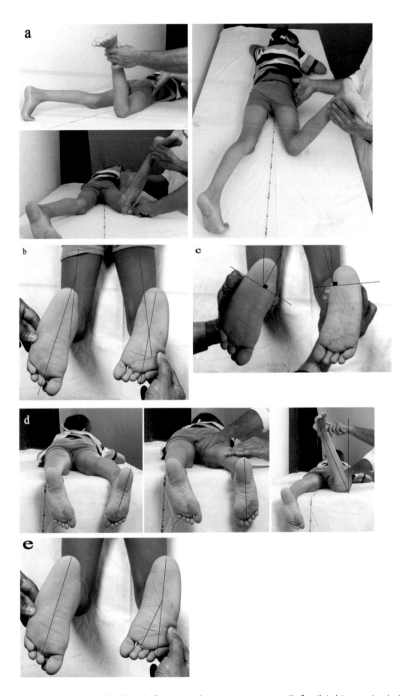

Figure 13.4 (a) Craig's method. (b) Thigh-foot angle measurement (left tibial intorsion). (c) Bimalleolar axis method (right tibial intorsion). (d) Second toe method. (e) Heel bisector method.

mobility is preserved to adequately align the foot with the talus.[11] In children with foot deformation, this measurement may not be feasible or accurate. The patient is placed prone, and both knees are flexed to 90° with the ankle in neutral position and the sole kept parallel to the floor. The angle subtended between the longitudinal axis of the thigh and the longitudinal axis of the foot marks the thigh-foot angle and is normally positive, implying external rotation of about 10–15°. If the value is less than 10–15° or on the negative side, it implies internal rotation (Figure 13.4).

13.5.8.3.2 Transmalleolar Axis Method

In patients with CP spasm, the tibialis anterior and tibialis posterior lead to varus foot deformation and an inward foot deviation that, in turn, leads to false thigh-foot angle values. In such cases and in children with rigid foot deformation, the bimalleolar axis/transmalleolar axis method can be utilized as the foot deformity, if any, will not interfere with the torsional assessment in this method.

The difficulty in this method is correctly aligning the knee joint and accurately identifying the bimalleolar axis. With the patient prone and knees flexed to 90°, the angle between the longitudinal axis of the thigh and a line perpendicular to the axis that connects the most prominent points of both malleoli is measured. Under normal circumstances, the lateral malleolus must be 25° posterior to the medial malleolus, which is the normal value range attained by about 8 years of age (Figure 13.4).

13.5.8.3.3 Second Toe Test

The patient is placed prone with the knees in extension. Now the lower extremity is rotated internally or externally until the second toe points directly down at the floor. Now, without altering the thigh rotation, the knee is flexed to 90°. The angle between the line perpendicular to the floor and the shank's longitudinal axis gives the value of tibial torsion, internal or external (Figure 13.4).

13.6 INDIVIDUAL JOINT ASSESSMENT IN A CHILD WITH CEREBRAL PALSY

13.6.1 Examination of Foot

13.6.1.1 EQUINUS DEFORMITY

It is important to have knowledge of normal dorsiflexion possible in a child. It is around 20–25° of

dorsiflexion at 3 years of age, which diminishes to 10° by 15 years of age. Equinus can be either due to contracture of the gastrocsoleus, which is fixed plantarflexion deformity or may be dynamic due to overactivity of the gastrocsoleus during gait where the foot can be brought to neutral position or even dorsiflexion on persistent, passive, gentle stretch. The examiner should keep in mind other etiologies of toe-walking like idiopathic toe-walking with isolated congenital short Achilles tendon, muscular dystrophies, spina bifida, arthrogryposis, etc. Children with muscular dystrophy may have a history of delayed walking and/or positive Gower's sign apart from abnormal laboratory values of creatinine phosphokinase.

The examiner performs a Silfverskiold test to differentiate isolated gastrocnemius contracture from gastrocsoleus or Achilles tendon contracture. Remember that during the stance phase, the greatest degree of dorsiflexion at the ankle is required just before heel lift with the knee in maximal extension. When this normal dorsiflexion at the ankle is not possible, various compensatory mechanisms come into play to facilitate normal-looking ambulation. Various compensations to mask equinus deformity are given in Table 13.9 and are to be looked for (Figure 13.5).

Patients with longstanding equinus may develop hindfoot valgus, hallux valgus, and midfoot break with the talar head prominent in the longitudinal arch (plantar aspect) with the development of painful callosities.

13.6.1.2 EQUINOVARUS

When the invertors of the foot (tibialis posterior and tibialis anterior) are strong and overactive in comparison to the evertors (peroneals), the patient develops a varus in addition to the equinus deformity (more common in spastic hemiplegics). The patient might develop painful calluses on the lateral border over the fifth metatarsal, where he/she bears weight while walking. Also, the child may demonstrate an internal foot progression angle due to the inversion foot deformation (Figure 13.6).

13.6.1.3 PES EQUINOVALGUS

In children with spastic diplegia and quadriplegia, bilateral pes equinovalgus is also common. Here the child presents with deformity and painful calluses/blisters in the plantar aspect due to prominence of the talar head in the arch of the foot. The child may also have a painful hallux valgus, which

Table 13.9 Compensatory Mechanisms in Knee Associated with Equinus Foot Deformation (see Figure 13.5)

Compensation	Biomechanical Cause
Genu recurvatum	Due to tightness of the gastrocsoleus, the tibia is unable to move forward over the plantigrade foot in midstance with resultant backward thrust
Forward leaning, pelvic rotation, hip flexion, knee hyperextension, and external rotation of leg	To balance the center of gravity/ground reaction force facilitating gait
Pronation of subtalar joint[12]	This leads to unlocking of the midfoot resulting in abduction and dorsiflexion at the subtalar joint[a]

[a] Equinus might get masked in a hypermobile flatfoot, which has exaggerated midtarsal mobility and subtalar abduction and dorsiflexion.

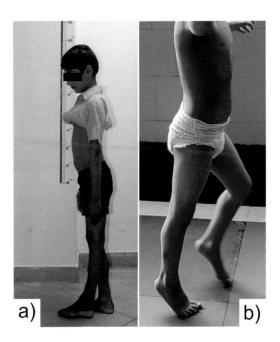

Figure 13.5 Compensations for equinus deformation. (a) Recurvatum at knee, anterior tilting of pelvis with flexion at hip. (b) Toe-walker.

develops in response to the longstanding everted position (Figure 13.6).

The examiner must be aware of the fact that valgus deformity masks equinus and the triceps surae does not feel tight on initial examination. The examiner must bring the hindfoot to neutral position before passively dorsiflexing the ankle. These children might not demonstrate equinus while standing due to the hypermobile midfoot that maintains the plantigrade position even in the presence of hindfoot equinus with the talar head in significant plantarflexion (midfoot break). It is also

important to remember that the pes valgus may be accompanied by ankle valgus.

13.6.1.4 HALLUX VALGUS

The patient's first toe may lie beneath the second, the head of the first metatarsal gets uncovered as the toe deviates laterally, and the child may develop a painful bunion (uncovered metatarsal head). There may be a concomitant external tibial torsion that pushes the toe laterally due to weight-bearing by the everted forefoot (Figure 13.6).

Also look for dorsal bunion (prominence/uncovering of first metatarsal head dorsally) that may be the result of soft tissue balancing procedures.

13.6.2 Examination of Knee Joint

The hamstrings are affected (either spastic or contracted) in patients with cerebral palsy.

Reasons for crouch knee (excessive knee flexion in stance phase):

- Hamstring spasticity/contracture.
- Quadriceps weakness.
- Gastrocsoleus weakness.

Clinically, hamstring tightness is measured by measuring the popliteal angle. The hip joint is flexed to 90° during the assessment to passively stretch the hamstrings, which are extensors of the hip joint.

13.6.2.1 POPLITEAL ANGLE TEST

The popliteal angle (PA) measurement test is used very commonly for the assessment of hamstring

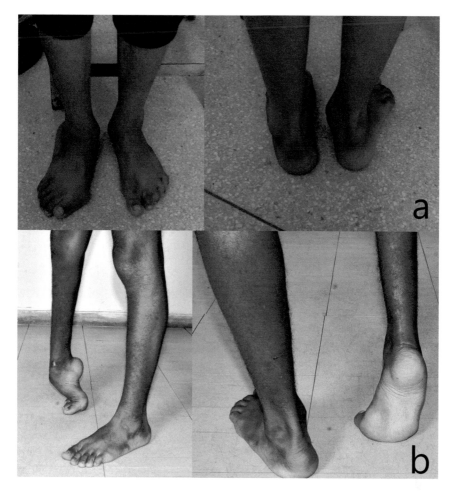

Figure 13.6 Foot deformation in CP. (a) Planovalgus with hallux valgus on right side. (b) equinus.

contracture in patients with cerebral palsy. Here the child lies supine, and the examiner flexes the hip joint to 90° while the contralateral hip is in neutral position and the limb is extended at the knee. The examiner gradually extends the knee with hip flexed at 90°. When the examiner feels a substantial resistance to knee extension, the acute angle formed between the long axis of the femur and tibia is measured. The modified PA test is the bilateral popliteal angle (PAB) test.[13] Here, after assessment of the PA in the standard way and maintaining the position of the limb, the examiner flexes the child's contralateral hip to align the anterior superior iliac spine (ASIS) and posterior superior iliac spine (PSIS) vertically. The value (acute angle between the femur and long axis of the tibia) changes now and is noted, and the difference between the two measurements is defined as the hamstring shift, which indicates the amount of hip

flexion contracture in CP patients. The value of the PA tends to increase with age and normally is less than 30–40° in adolescent children. The values in CP children tend to be between 37° and 66° (mean being 51.9°).

The PAB was an attempt to eliminate the ambiguity in measuring the PA by aligning the pelvis in a way to simulate the upright posture adapted while walking. The PA is considered to reflect functional hamstring muscle contractures, whereas the PAB reflects the true hamstring contracture. In the PAB test, there is posterior tilting of the pelvis due to the relaxation of the hip flexors on the opposite limb. This leads to a distal shift of the shortened hamstrings on the ipsilateral limb leading to a smaller PA compared to the standard measurement technique (Figure 13.7). A hamstring shift more than 20° denotes excessive anterior pelvic tilt due to tight hip flexors or weak hip extensors.

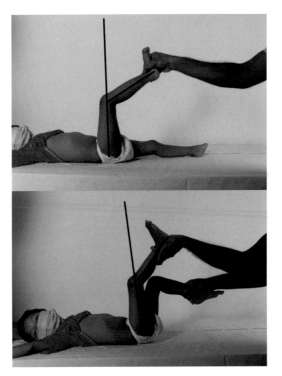

Figure 13.7 Popliteal angle test. (a) Unilateral popliteal angle. (b) Bilateral popliteal angle test.

The normal values of the popliteal angle may differ from the mean reported in the literature, which is 26° in children of 4 years and more. When it crosses 50°, it is considered abnormal. The straight leg raise angle is also reduced in patients with tight hamstrings. When the hamstrings are significantly tight, hip flexion gets constrained. It is very important to identify and address concomitant hip flexion contractures as the correction of hamstring tightness without managing hip flexion contractures leads to an exaggeration of hip flexion deformity and an increase in the anterior pelvic tilt during gait (hamstrings being extensors of the hip).

It is important to differentiate capsular contracture of the knee joint from hamstring contracture in a child with cerebral palsy. In capsular contracture, the position of the hip will not alter the knee extension, and in hamstring contracture, the knee extension will improve with hip extension/ankle plantarflexion and reduces with hip flexion to 90°.

13.6.2.2 RECTUS

The examiner must also assess rectus tightness. Rectus also crosses two joints, namely the hip and knee, and it acts as a flexor of the hip at the initial swing and an extensor of the knee. Normally, the knee flexes up to 60° in early swing. This knee flexion might get restricted in rectus tightness, which leads to difficulty in clearing the foot during the swing phase.

Clinical methods of assessing rectus femoris tightness:

- The Duncan–Ely test: The patient is positioned prone with knees kept in extension. The knee joint is passively flexed on the side of examination by the examiner. Normally, there is no motion of the hip or pelvis while the knee flexes completely. In patients with rectus femoris contracture, complete passive knee flexion results in involuntary flexion at the hip, elevating the buttocks off the examination table (Figure 13.8). The disadvantage of this test is that it is not specific for rectus femoris in patients with hip flexion contracture secondary to iliopsoas tightness.
- Rectus grab: The patient is positioned supine, and the knee is rapidly flexed. If the examiner feels resistance to flexion, then the test is

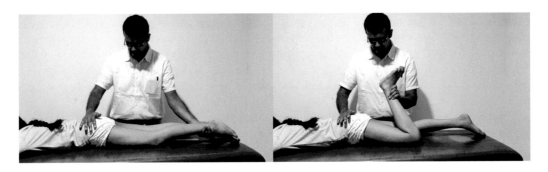

Figure 13.8 Duncan–Ely test.

positive, and the rectus is spastic. The positive grab along with increased popliteal angle is an indication for distal hamstring lengthening with simultaneous rectus femoris transfer.

13.6.3 Examination of Hip Joint

13.6.3.1 HIP FLEXION CONTRACTURE

Hip flexion contractures are commonly seen in patients with spastic diplegia or quadriplegia. It is very important to stabilize and control the pelvis while assessing for contractures around the hip joint. Hip flexion contracture is assessed by the Thomas test for unilateral involvement and by Staheli's prone test for bilateral involvement.

13.6.3.2 ADDUCTION CONTRACTURE

Patients with adductor spasticity have a narrow base of gait with resultant scissoring. It is important to identify the adduction contracture with concomitant flexion contracture, which may predispose subluxation/dislocation of the hip joint. Apart from adductors, the other two muscles involved here are the gracilis and the pectineus. On examination, there is an inability to abduct the hips both in flexion and extension. Differentiating contractures of biarticular and monoarticular muscles is important to plan management. For example, assessment of hip abduction with knee flexion tests the adductor longus, brevis, and magnus, eliminating the gracilis, whereas examination of hip abduction with knee extension includes the gracilis, and if abduction increases with the knees

flexed than extended, it implies that the gracilis is contracted (Phelps test) (Figure 13.9).

It is important to differentiate true adduction from pseudo-adduction deformities. In pseudo-adduction, there is increased femoral anteversion along with crouch at the knee resulting in the appearance of scissoring. But the examiner will be able to appreciate the internal rotation while examining the gait by observing the patella. In children with hip subluxation or dislocation, loss of range of motion is the first clue. These children usually have a flexion contracture at the hip joint, and the abduction is limited to less than 30°. They also have increased internal rotation and reduced external rotation. When there is frank dislocation, the child will have a positive Galeazzi sign on the involved side.

13.6.3.3 ILIOTIBIAL TRACT

13.6.3.3.1 Ober's Test

The child is positioned in lateral decubitus position with the side to be assessed facing up. The patient's knee joint is flexed 90°. The hip joint is then abducted about 40° and extended to its limit. Maintaining knee flexion and hip extension and with pelvis stabilized, the limb is gradually adducted toward the examination table. In a normal child, the hip must be able to adduct past the midline of the body. The inability to do this indicates the contracture of the iliotibial tract (Figure 13.10).

Another way of doing the test where both sides can be compared is by doing it in prone position on a flat surface. The examiner stands on the side opposite the side being tested and places the hip

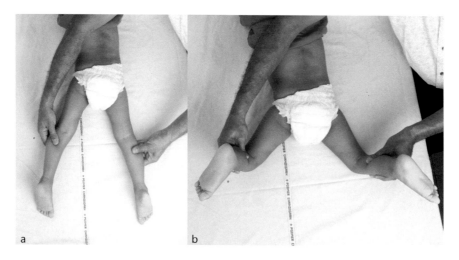

Figure 13.9 Phelps test. (a) Abduction in knee extension. (b) Abduction in knee flexion.

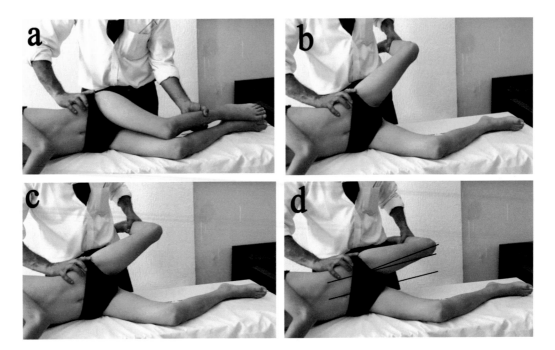

Figure 13.10 Ober's test. (a) In lateral decubitus position, (b) abduction, (c) extension in abduction, and (d) inability to reach midline confirms iliotibial tract contracture.

to be tested in maximum abduction at the hip, holding the lower leg near the ankle. The examiner ensures that the pelvis is flattened without any flexion at the hip by using the other hand. Now the examiner tries to adduct the limb with the knee in 90° flexion, and the angle between the vertical axis of the body and the thigh quantifies the residual abduction beyond which adduction is not possible.[14]

13.7 EVALUATION OF UPPER LIMB INVOLVEMENT IN CEREBRAL PALSY

The child's upper limb involvement must also be noted and documented in detail.[15,16] The spasticity needs to be quantified and the joint position/attitude/active and passive range of motion and presence of any contracture are noted. For example, the shoulder might have an adduction or internal rotation contracture, the elbow might be flexed and pronated, and the wrist might be flexed and deviated. All these are to be documented in detail and it is essential to do a functional assessment. There are many scoring methods for functional assessment but a description of all of them is beyond the scope of this book. The clinician must be aware of the Manual Ability Classification System (MACS) (Table 13.10) to categorize upper limb involvement and functional ability.

Thumb deformation in cerebral palsy is another important part to be examined and is the result of an imbalance between the extrinsic and intrinsic muscles acting across the joints, namely the carpometacarpal (CMC), metacarpophalangeal (MCP), and interphalangeal (IP) joints. Thumb involvement can significantly impair upper limb function in every way and can impede overall care, including hygiene. We will see a few points regarding the clinical examination of thumb deformity in a child with cerebral palsy.

Table 13.10 Manual Ability Classification System (www.macs.nu/)

Level	Activity Description
I	Handles objects easily
II	Handles objects with reduced quality and speed
III	Handles object with difficulty requiring modification
IV	Handles objects only in adapted situations
V	Does not handle objects

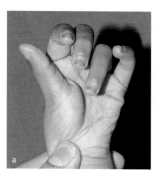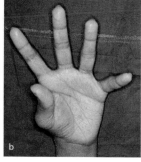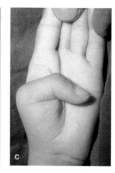

Figure 13.11 Thumb deformity in CP. (a) Type 1. (b) Type 2. (c) Type 3. Reproduced with permission from Joseph B (2020). The spastic thumb. In Joseph B, Nayagam S, Loder R, Torde I, editors. *Paediatric Orthopaedics: A System of Decision-Making* (2nd ed., 500), Taylor & Francis.

Table 13.11 Classification of Thumb Involvement in Cerebral Palsy

Type of Deformation	Position of Thumb	Deforming Forces	Paretic Muscles	Remarks on the Deformity
Type 1	Metacarpal adduction, flexion at MCP joint, and extension at IP joints	Adductor pollicis, first dorsal interosseous and flexor pollicis brevis	Abductor pollicis longus, extensor pollicis longus and brevis	Flexion at MCP joint and extension of IP joint implies an *intrinsic deformity*
Type 2	Flexion at MCP and IP joints. Metacarpal adduction is less marked	Flexor pollicis longus	Extensor pollicis longus	It is an *extrinsic deformity*. Extension of wrist accentuates the deformity
Type 3	Metacarpal is in adducted position. MCP and IP joints are flexed, giving a true *"thumb in palm"* appearance	Flexor pollicis longus, adductor pollicis, first dorsal interosseous, and flexor pollicis brevis are all involved	Abductor pollicis longus, extensor pollicis longus and brevis	It is a combined spasticity of intrinsic and extrinsic muscles and deformity

The classification of the thumb in palm deformity by House et al.[17] is given in Table 13.11 and is useful in classifying as well as identifying the deforming forces.

The examiner asks the child to make a fist with the thumb in the lateral pinch position (Figure 13.11) and makes a note of the things given in Table 13.11.

REFERENCES

1. Rosenbaum P, Paneth N, Leviton A, Goldstein M, Bax M, Damiano D, et al. A report: The definition and classification of cerebral palsy April 2006. *Dev Med Child Neurol Suppl.* 2007;109:8–14.

2. Karol LA. Disorders of the brain. In. Herring JA, editor. *Tachdjian's pediatric orthopaedics: From the Texas Scottish Rite hospital for children*, 5th ed. Philadelphia: Elsevier Saunders; 2014. pp. e3–e97.

3. Minear WL. A classification of cerebral palsy. *Pediatrics.* 1956;18:841–852.

4. Palisano R, Rosenbaum P, Walter S, Russell D, Wood E, Galuppi B. Development and reliability of a system to classify gross motor function in children with cerebral palsy. *Dev Med Child Neurol.* 1997;39:214–223.

5. Aids to the Examination of the Peripheral Nervous System. *Medical research council memorandum, no. 45, superseding war memorandum no. 7, 1.* London: Her Majesty's Stationery Office, 1976.

6. Sanger TD, Delgado MR, Gaebler-Spira D, Hallett M, Mink JW; Task Force on Childhood Motor Disorders. Classification and definition of disorders causing hypertonia in childhood. *Pediatrics.* 2003;111:e89–97.

7. Bohannon RW, Smith MB. Interrater reliability of a modified Ashworth scale of muscle spasticity. *Phys Ther.* 1987;67:206–207.

8. Gracies J-M, Burke K, Clegg NJ, Browne R, Rushing C, Fehlings D, et al. Reliability of the Tardieu scale for assessing spasticity in children with cerebral palsy. *Arch Phys Med Rehabil.* 2010;91:421–428.

9. Boyd R, Graham H. Objective measurement of clinical findings in the use of botulinum toxin type A for the management of children with cerebral palsy. *Eur J Neurol.* 1999;6:S23–35.

10. Walker HK. Deep Tendon reflexes. In: Walker HK, Hall WD, Hurst JW, editors. *Clinical methods: The history, physical, and laboratory examinations,* 3rd ed. Boston: Butterworths; 1990. Chapter 72. www.ncbi.nlm.nih.gov/books/NBK396/

11. Lee SH, Chung CY, Park MS, Choi IH, Cho T-J. Tibial torsion in cerebral palsy, validity and reliability of measurement. *Clin Orthop Relat Res.* 2009;467:2098–2104.

12. Gourdine-Shaw MC, Lamm BM, Herzenberg JE, Bhave A. Equinus deformity in the pediatric patient: Causes, evaluation, and management. *Clin Podiatr Med Surg.* 2010;27:25–42.

13. Manikowska F, Chen BP, Jóźwiak M, Lebiedowska MK. The popliteal angle tests in patients with cerebral palsy. *J PediatrOrthop B.* 2019;28:332–336.

14. Gautam VK, Anand S. A new test for estimating iliotibial band contracture. *J Bone Joint Surg [Br].* 1998;80:474–475.

15. Leafblad ND, Van Heest AE. Management of spastic wrist and hand in cerebral palsy. *J Hand Surg Am.* 2015;40:1035–1040.

16. Tonkin MA, Hatrick NC, Eckersley JR, Couzens G. Surgery for cerebral palsy part 3: Classification and operative procedures for thumb deformity. *J Hand Surg Br.* 2001;26:465–470.

17. House JH, Gwathmey FW, Fidler MO. A dynamic approach to the thumb-in-palm deformity in cerebral palsy. Evaluation and results in fifty-six patients. *J Bone Joint Surg [Am].* 1981;63(2):216–225.

14

Peripheral Nerve Examination in a Child

ANIL AGARWAL

14.1 INTRODUCTION

In a younger child, symptoms are most often reported by parents/relatives. As such, it is imperative that a close relative responsible for the child's care be present at the time of examination. As is necessary for every pediatric examination, the child must be made comfortable before any interaction. The part to be examined is appropriately exposed, and adequate illumination is ensured. A clinician must be ready with all devices/tools required for completion of the examination. Sometimes, a child may need a distractor (in the form of a toy, music, light, etc.) to ensure his/her participation. In neonates and infants, skillful observation of the child's activities with methodical posturing may be the only way to assess active muscle power and range of movements.

14.2 HISTORY

Peripheral nerves have good soft tissue coverage providing protection, except for selected areas. Examples of such selected areas are the ulnar nerve curving behind the medial epicondyle of the humerus and

195

the common peroneal nerve winding around the posterolateral aspect of the fibular neck; at these points, the nerves are superficial and they are more prone to trauma. It is necessary to elicit all relevant history, the chief being trauma. The trauma could have been a fracture/dislocation (e.g., supracondylar humerus fracture, fracture midshaft humerus, fracture dislocation elbow, fracture medial epicondyle humerus, etc.), incisional cut (e.g., with broken glass/bangle, agricultural injuries, iatrogenic injuries, etc.) or penetrating injuries (e.g., foreign body, stab, etc.). It is important to keep in mind that the manifestation of nerve injury may be far distant from the apparent site of trauma. The trauma can as well have a late presentation when the original injury might be altogether forgotten or not remembered (e.g., tardy ulnar nerve palsy in deformities secondary to the lateral condyle fracture of the humerus, entrapment of a nerve in evolving callus, etc.). Partially recovered nerve lesions may also present with a similar history. Another common cause of nerve lesions in children is intramuscular injections close to nerves, although the problem is less common in upper limbs. The noxious nature of medicine injected, if any (e.g., chemotherapy), should be documented. A history of massage or tight bandaging is sometimes forthcoming in cases of ischemic contracture. The child may report secondary trophic changes, especially in involved digits due to sensory loss. A history of critical illness and the morbid condition of the child may be relevant in common peroneal nerve lesions (recent history of significant weight loss may as well lead to the loss of subcutaneous fat and compression of the common peroneal nerve at the fibular head).

There are certain conditions where the onset of peripheral nerve lesions may be insidious. A growing osteochondroma, enlarging tumor, or a progressive limb deformity can progressively stretch the regional nerves resulting in symptoms. In many cases, primary infection (tuberculosis, leprosy) or subsequent fibrosis has insulted the nerves.

Brachial plexus lesions form an altogether different category of nerve lesion. In such lesions, the mode of delivery/labor characteristics (prolonged labor, breech presentation), any recovery since birth, age of the child at presentation, dominance of upper limb, etc. have an important bearing on the nature of the treatment. When eliciting the history, it is essential to inquire whether the symptoms are improving, static, or progressive and the exact duration elapsed since the primary insult to plan for further management. Nonetheless, a note of any previous treatments/interventions/surgeries performed/splint usage is also required.

14.3 GENERAL EXAMINATION

Although many times findings in peripheral nerve involvement are confined to the involved limb, one must exclude systemic conditions leading to nerve palsy like Hansen's disease, multiple osteochondromas, and neurofibromatosis, etc. The examiner must be able to identify café au lait spots in neurofibromatosis or hypopigmented patches in Hansen's disease. In conditions like multiple osteochondromatosis, the metaphyseal long ends will have expansions all over the body. In Klumpke's type of brachial plexus lesion, the neonate may present with Horner's syndrome. The examiner should also keep in mind that there are conditions like scurvy, hemophilia, and acute infection/trauma that may present as pseudoparalysis.

14.4 LOCAL EXAMINATION

14.4.1 Inspection

Remember that a peripheral nerve can be motor, sensory, or a mixed nerve, and presentation depends upon the composition of motor and sensory fibers. For example, the anterior interosseous nerve, which is a branch of the median nerve, and the posterior interosseous nerve (a branch of the radial nerve) are purely motor. Motor deficits produce certain characteristics, attitude, and deformity of the concerned limb, which can pinpoint the nerve involved and the site of the lesion. A wrist drop in the radial nerve (Figure 14.1), foot drop in the common peroneal nerve (Figure 14.2), claw hand in ulnar (Figure 14.3a) or combined ulnar median nerve lesions, pointing index, and Benediction hand of the median nerve (Figure 14.3b) fall under this category. The policeman tip hand deformity (Figure 14.4) is indicative of brachial plexus injury.

In longstanding lesions, the denervated muscles undergo atrophy, and the change can be readily appreciated when compared to the opposite side (Figure 14.3a). The skin supplied by the peripheral nerve may show trophic changes or vasomotor disturbances due to the involvement of accompanying sympathetic supply. The skin may be dry, smooth, and glossy. The vasomotor changes may manifest in the form of pallor, cyanosis, excessive sweating, and even ulcers. Also, do not miss healed scars in the vicinity of the nerve that might give a clue to the nerve and the level of injury.

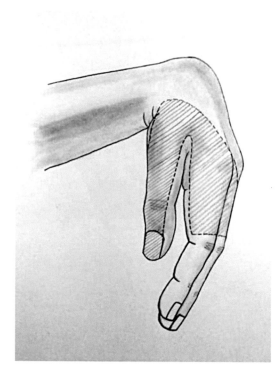

Figure 14.1 Wrist drop due to radial nerve lesions in the radial groove of the humerus. There is motor paralysis of all the extensors of the elbow, wrist, metacarpophalangeal joints, and all joints of the thumb. The child may demonstrate active extension of the interphalangeal joints of other digits if the knuckle is stabilized. This is due to the preserved action of the interossei innervated by the ulnar nerve. The shaded area demonstrates the accompanying area of sensory loss.

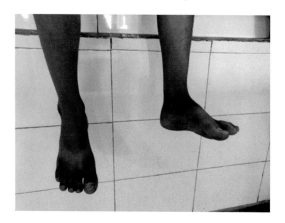

Figure 14.2 Foot drop due to common peroneal nerve paralysis near the fibular head in the right lower limb. There is motor paralysis of the dorsi-flexors and evertors of the foot. There is foot slap when the patient walks.

14.4.2 Palpation

The denervated region may have a colder feel/excessive sweating. The wasted muscles become soft and flabby. If there are any telltale signs like a scar, the same should be carefully palpated as it may be a possible site for nerve entrapment.

14.4.3 Muscle Power

A clinician should be well aware of the nerve anatomy, the origin of its branches supplying various muscles, cross innervations, and double supply. Thus, to test whether a particular nerve is injured or not, the key muscle that is exclusively innervated by that particular nerve is preferably tested. This forms the basis of many clinical signs.

14.4.4 Radial Nerve

The nerve receives supply from C5–C8 and T1. Its branches and their approximate origin are depicted in Figure 14.5. The following muscles are tested for this nerve.

14.4.4.1 BRACHIORADIALIS

It is an important muscle as it is supplied before the nerve divides into the superficial and deep branch at the level of the lateral epicondyle. By testing this muscle, one can assess the level of the radial nerve injury. Test the muscle by instructing the patient to flex the elbow further from 90° in forearm neutral pronation and supination against resistance (Figure 14.6).

14.4.4.2 EXTENSOR MUSCLES OF WRIST JOINT

The extensor carpi radialis longus is supplied by the radial nerve before it crosses the elbow joint. All other extensor muscles of the wrist are supplied by the posterior interosseous nerve (deep branch of the radial nerve). The patient is asked to extend the wrist against resistance (forearm in pronation) with the elbow flexed (Figure 14.7).

The muscles that contribute to wrist extension but are tested as a group are:

Extensor carpi radialis longus (ECRL).
Extensor carpi radialis brevis (ECRB).
Extensor digitorum (ED).
Extensor digiti minimi (EDM).
Extensor carpi ulnaris (ECU).
Extensor indicis (EI).

(a) (b)

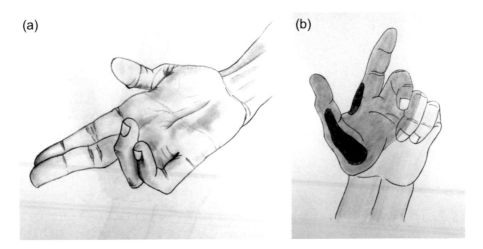

Figure 14.3 (a) Mild degree of clawing due to ulnar nerve lesions at the elbow. A paralysis of all inter-ossei and medial two lumbricals supplied by the nerve results in hyperextension of the metacarpo-phalangeal joints and flexion of the proximal and distal interphalangeal joints of the medial two digits. A characteristic flattening of the hypothenar eminence and depressions in interdigital space due to atrophy of the interossei accompanies this nerve lesion. The claw hand, due to combined lesions of the ulnar and median nerve, is more severe as the remaining first and second lumbricals are also para-lyzed. The combined lesions commonly occur in the elbow region and are also seen in Klumpke's type of brachial plexus lesion (C8, T1). There is an extended wrist, hyperextended metacarpophalangeal joints, accompanied by flexion of interphalangeal joints. (b) When a patient with median nerve injury at the elbow tries to make a fist, the index finger stands out prominently due to paralysis of the lateral half of the flexor digitorum profundus resulting in a pointing index deformity. There is a loss of flexion at the metacarpophalangeal and interphalangeal joints in the second and third digits resulting in Benediction hand ("preacher's hand"). The muscles of the thenar eminence are paralyzed and gradu-ally wasted (dark shaded area in figure). The thumb apparently comes to lie in the same plane as the other metacarpal bones. This is called "simian" or "ape-like thumb." The light shaded area represents the accompanying sensory loss.

Extensor pollicis longus (EPL).
Extensor pollicis brevis (EPB).
Abductor pollicis longus (APL).

Extensor digitorum: This muscle is responsible for the extension of the metacarpophalangeal joints. To test this muscle, the patient is instructed to extend the knuckles against resistance with the interphalangeal joints relaxed (Figure 14.8). A cau-tion here is that the interossei innervated by the ulnar nerve can extend the interphalangeal joint of the digits and can be used by the child to show the apparent extension of the fingers.

14.4.5 Median Nerve

The nerve receives supply from C5–C8 and T1. Its branches and their approximate origin are given in Figure 14.9. The following are tested for this nerve.

14.4.5.1 FLEXOR POLLICIS LONGUS

The proximal phalanx is first stabilized by the examiner. The patient is then asked to flex the interphalangeal joint of the thumb against resis-tance (Figure 14.10).

14.4.5.2 FLEXOR DIGITORUM SUPERFICIALIS AND LATERAL HALF OF PROFUNDUS

This is also known as the Ochsner's clasping test. The index finger stands proud as a pointing index if the patient is instructed to clasp the hands. This happens because of the inability to flex the finger (Figure 14.11).

14.4.5.3 ABDUCTOR POLLICIS BREVIS

The pen test is performed to identify the power of the abductor pollicis brevis. Instruct the patient to keep his/her hand flat on the table and touch the

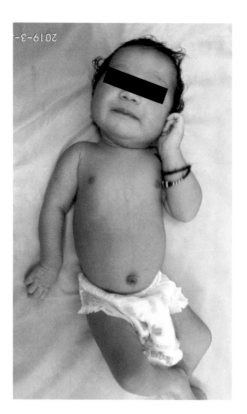

Figure 14.4 The policeman tip hand deformity is characteristic of upper brachial plexus lesion (Erb's palsy), mainly involving C5 and C6. The abductors and lateral rotators of the shoulder (deltoid, supraspinatus, infraspinatus, and teres minor) and the flexors and supinators of the elbow (biceps, brachialis, brachioradialis, and supinator) are paralyzed. In this nerve lesion, the affected arm assumes the posture of internal rotation. The forearm is extended at the elbow and fully pronated.

The Peripheral nervous system: Anatomy and function

- Triceps, long head
- Triceps, lateral head
- Triceps, medial head
- Radial nerve
- Brachioradialis
- Extensor carpi Radialis longus
- Posterior interosseous nerve (deep branch)
- Extensor carpi Radialis brevis
- Supinator
- Extensor carpi ulnaris
- Extensor digitorum
- Extensor digiti minimi
- Abductor pollicis longus
- Extensor pollicis longus
- Extensor pollicis brevis
- Extensor indicis
- Superficial radial nerve

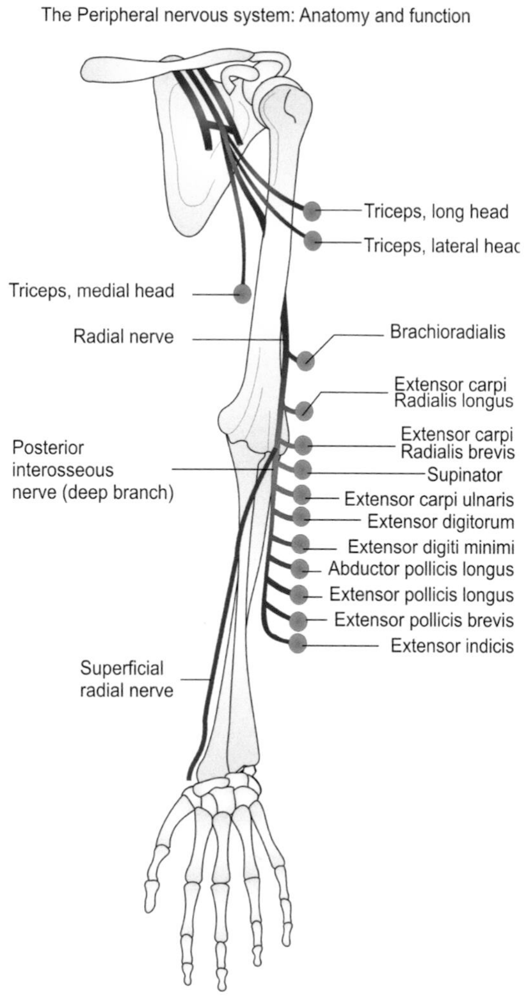

Figure 14.5 The radial nerve and its branches at various levels.

pen with his/her thumb, which is kept at a slightly higher level than the palm in a plane perpendicular to it. The inability to perform indicates loss of abduction of the thumb, a function of the median nerve (Figure 14.12).

14.4.5.4 OPPONENS POLLICIS

To test this muscle, the patient moves the thumb across the palm in an attempt to touch other fingertips. In the case of muscle paralysis, the patient is unable to perform this action properly (Figure 14.13). Be cautious of a trick movement the patient might show utilizing the adduction movement of the thumb carried out by the adductor pollicis, which is innervated by the ulnar nerve.

14.4.6 Ulnar Nerve

The nerve receives supply from C8 and T1. Its branches and their approximate origin are given in Figure 14.14. The following muscles are tested for this nerve.

14.4.6.1 FLEXOR CARPI ULNARIS

In the case of ulnar nerve lesions, when the patient tries to flex the wrist joint against resistance, the hand tends to deviate toward the radial side.

14.4.6.2 INTEROSSEI

The patient is asked to abduct his/her fingers against resistance to test the dorsal interossei (Figure 14.15).

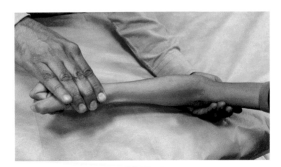

Figure 14.6 Testing the strength of the brachioradialis muscle in mid prone position of the forearm.

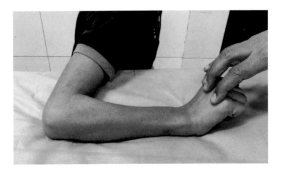

Figure 14.7 Testing of the extensor muscles of the wrist as a group. The examiner should exert counter-pressure against the second and third metacarpals.

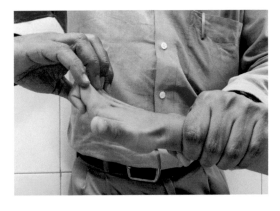

Figure 14.8 Testing the strength of the extensor digitorum.

Card test: To test the palmar interossei, the patient is asked to hold a card by adducting two fingers. The examiner tries to pull the card out of the fingers (Figure 14.16).

The examiner stabilizes the proximal phalanx, and the patient extends the middle and distal interphalangeal joints against resistance to test the interossei and lumbricals (Figure 14.17).

14.4.6.3 FIRST DORSAL INTEROSSEI AND ADDUCTOR POLLICIS

The patient is asked to grasp a book between the two thumbs (Figure 14.18). In the case of intact nerve function, the thumb remains extended due to the action of the first palmar interossei and adductor pollicis. In the case of nerve lesion, with these muscles paralyzed, the patient now attempts to hold the book by flexing the thumb interphalangeal joint with the help of the flexor pollicis longus. The flexor pollicis longus is innervated by the median nerve and is still functional. This is also known as Froment's sign. A similar test can be performed by asking the patient to hold a card against an extended thumb and other fingers.

14.4.7 Common Peroneal Nerve

It should be remembered that the peroneal division of the sciatic nerve is the more superficial and smaller component than the tibial division, and hence it is more prone to injury.

The superficial peroneal nerve supplies motor innervation to the peroneus longus and brevis. It has sensory innervation for the lower lateral part of the leg and dorsum of the foot. The deep peroneal nerve travels with the anterior tibial artery. The deep peroneal nerve supplies the tibialis anterior, extensor hallucis longus, extensor digitorum longus, and the peroneus tertius. It terminates as a sensory branch in the first dorsal web space. The clinical findings in individual nerve involvement are listed in Table 14.1.

14.4.7.1 PRESENTATION

The patient may give a history of catching toes during ambulation along with numbness. Two things can be noticed in the gait, one being the ipsilateral knee lifting higher than normal during swing to avoid dragging toes on the ground and the other being slapping of the forefoot on the ground following heel strike due to weakness in the ankle/toe dorsiflexors. The tibial nerve is examined by instructing the patient to invert the dorsiflexed foot against resistance (normally, inversion is weak in a plantar flexed foot).

The involvement of both tibial and peroneal components of the sciatic nerve will result in additional

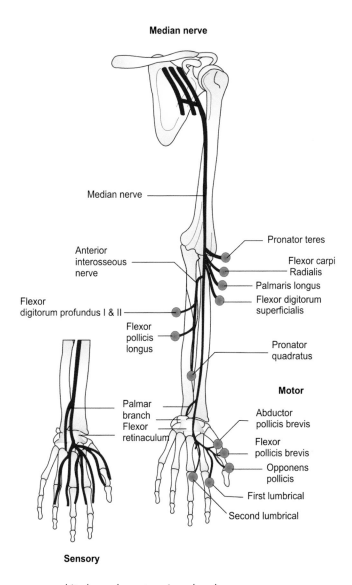

Median nerve

Median nerve

Pronator teres

Flexor carpi
Radialis

Anterior
interosseous
nerve

Palmaris longus

Flexor digitorum
superficialis

Flexor
digitorum profundus I & II

Flexor
pollicis
longus

Pronator
quadratus

Motor

Palmar
branch

Abductor
pollicis brevis

Flexor
retinaculum

Flexor
pollicis brevis

Opponens
pollicis

First lumbrical

Second lumbrical

Sensory

Figure 14.9 Median nerve and its branches at various levels.

weakening of knee flexion, ankle plantarflexion, and toe flexion, along with weakness of muscles of the anterolateral compartments of the leg.

14.4.8 Combined and Mixed Nerve Lesions

Combined and mixed nerve lesions can occur in brachial plexus lesions and ischemic contractures. Sometimes partial recovered nerve lesions present with such a picture. In upper brachial plexus palsy (Erb's palsy) involving the C5 and C6 nerve roots, the affected muscles will be the deltoid, biceps, brachialis, and brachioradialis. Sensory deficit may not be minimal and restricted to the area over the deltoid muscle and on the radial (lateral) side of the arm and hand. Lower brachial plexus palsy (Klumpke's palsy) involves lesions of the C8 and T1 nerve roots and will have an effect on the long flexors of the fingers, intrinsic muscles of the hand, and sometimes the wrist flexors. The triceps brachii is usually spared. The child may have concomitant Horner syndrome. Sensory deficit is present on the ulnar side of the forearm, hand, and fingers. Muscle and nerve involvement in ischemic contractures can be variable depending upon the severity of the condition.

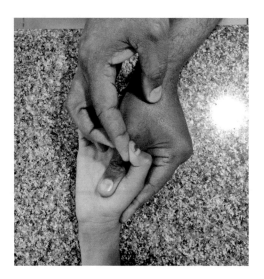

Figure 14.10 Testing the strength of the flexor pollicis longus at the thumb interphalangeal joint.

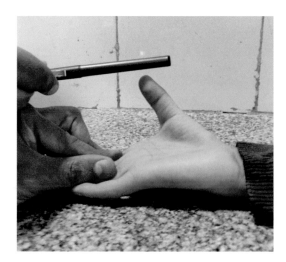

Figure 14.12 Pen test for strength of abductor pollicis brevis.

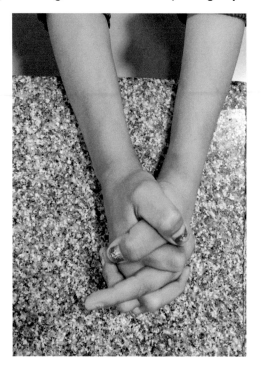

Figure 14.11 Ochsner's clasping test. Note the pointing index deformity of the index finger.

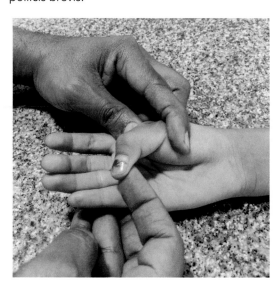

Figure 14.13 Test for strength of opponens pollicis.

14.4.9 Sensations and Reflexes

Sensation testing in a younger patient may be an uphill task as it involves both the child's mental ability and cooperation. The different forms of sensation that can be tested are pain, temperature, tactile sensation (namely, light touch, pressure, and two-point discrimination), stereognosis, position localization, and vibration. A sensory stimulus is applied first to an area of impaired sensation and then gradually moved to the normal regions. Each peripheral nerve has a distinct pattern of sensory loss (Figure 14.19; Chapter 11). The main portion of hand supplied by the radial nerve is its dorsal aspect on the lateral aspect, excluding the digits. The median nerve supplies the palmar and distal dorsal aspects of the lateral three-and-a-half digits and the lateral palm. The ulnar nerve supplies the palmar and dorsal aspects of the medial one-and-a-half digits and medial palm.

Ulnar nerve

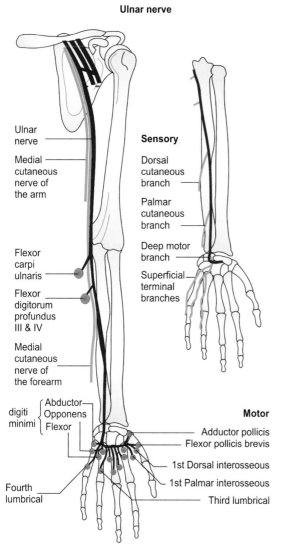

Ulnar nerve

Medial cutaneous nerve of the arm

Sensory

Dorsal cutaneous branch

Palmar cutaneous branch

Deep motor branch

Superficial terminal branches

Flexor carpi ulnaris

Flexor digitorum profundus III & IV

Medial cutaneous nerve of the forearm

digiti minimi { Abductor Opponens Flexor

Motor

Adductor pollicis
Flexor pollicis brevis
1st Dorsal interosseous
1st Palmar interosseous
Third lumbrical

Fourth lumbrical

Figure 14.14 Ulnar nerve and its branches at various levels.

The corresponding reflexes will also be diminished or abolished.

14.4.10 Nerve Course and Tinel's Sign/Formication Sign

An appraisal of complete nerve course is essential in any peripheral nerve injury because it can indicate the approximate site of insult. The nerve may be found thickened in nerve tumors and leprosy. An important palpatory sign is Tinel's sign. It refers to a tingling/creeping sensation experienced by the patient and is produced by slight percussion of

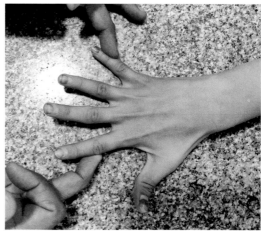

Figure 14.15 Test for strength of dorsal interossei.

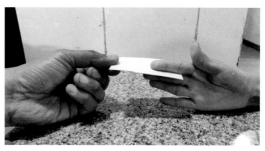

Figure 14.16 The card test to demonstrate strength in the palmar interossei.

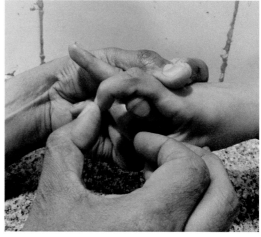

Figure 14.17 Test for strength of the interossei and lumbricals. The examiner steadies the proximal phalanx.

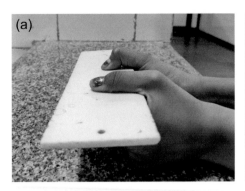
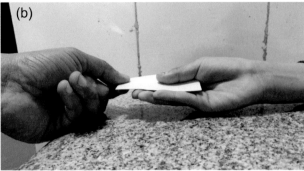

Figure 14.18 (a) Froment's sign: first palmar interossei and adductor pollicis are paralyzed on the right side. (b) Alternate method to show the strength of the first palmar interossei and adductor pollicis.

a nerve trunk following a nerve injury. The sign is elicitable after about 4–6 weeks following a peripheral nerve injury and is described as perceiving mild electric current/pins and needles/hyperesthesia referred to the cutaneous distribution of the nerve. It should be kept in mind that the tingling of regeneration of touch fibers is barely perceived in the area of percussion and radiates only into the cutaneous distribution of the specific nerve.

The examiner percusses distal to proximal along the nerve route to elicit this test. The sequential recording of Tinel's sign can corroborate with nerve regeneration. If the sign remains fixed in one

Table 14.1 Clinical Findings in Peroneal Nerve Palsy

	Deep Peroneal Nerve	Superficial Peroneal Nerve
Muscle weakness	Foot/toe dorsiflexion	Foot eversion
Decreased or abnormal sensation	Dorsal aspect of the first web space of the foot	Lower portion of the lateral aspect leg and dorsum of the foot

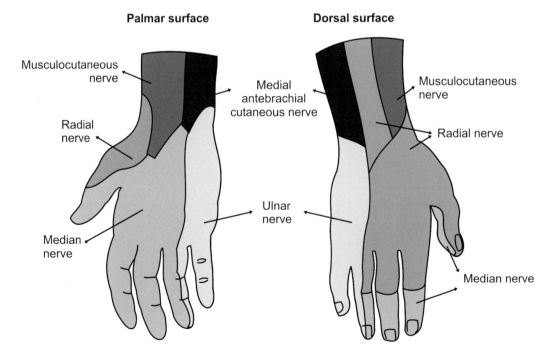

Figure 14.19 The various sensory zones of the peripheral nerves in the hand.

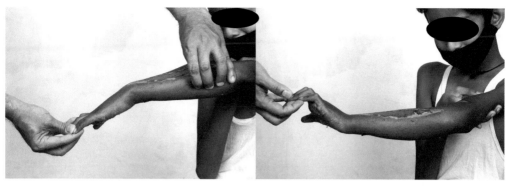

Figure 14.20 Fixed-length phenomenon seen in Volkmann's ischemic contracture (VIC) (Volkmann's sign).

spot for several consecutive weeks or even months, there may be an obstacle, and they may be grouped together, forming a neuroma. If the location of the sign moves progressively in a distal direction, this is a favorable sign. The sign can be elicited by gentle tapping with the eraser on the end of a pencil to avoid widespread mechanical stimulus over the involved nerve trunk or branches of the nerve distal to the site of injury or tapping over the belly of the muscle innervated by the nerve. A genuine Tinel's sign is never considered painful and is due to the growth of touch fibers. If there is pain on tapping, this is not Tinel's sign but evidence of neuroma or a neuroma-like sign.

Tinel's sign cannot be elicited in patients with a nerve-root lesion proximal to the dorsal root ganglion because the sensitive touch fibers that are healing are proximal to the ganglion under these circumstances.

14.4.11 Movements of Joints and Deformities

A distinction needs to be made between active and passive range of movements. Following paralysis of a muscle, the passive range of motion of a joint may still be preserved, but the active movement will be impaired. With longstanding nerve lesions or ischemic contractures, the muscle fibers and soft tissue undergo fibrosis resulting in fixed deformities across the joints (e.g., equinus contracture following common peroneal nerve palsy). The deformities may also develop due to unopposed action of the active group of muscles, wasting of paralyzed muscles, skin contractures, dislocation of joints, etc.

In Volkmann's ischemic contracture, the nerves sustain a two-fold insult. The ischemia can affect both muscle and nerves directly. Secondarily, the nerves may get compressed by the cicatricial contracture of the degenerating muscles and skin. The deformity spectrum can vary from flexion contracture of two or three fingers to complete involvement of all flexor group muscles and partial involvement of extensor muscles. A clinical sign sometimes observed in a less severe variety of ischemic contracture, is acquired contracture of the digits due to fibrosis of the muscles of the flexor compartment of the forearm. A tenodesis effect can be demonstrated, i.e., the contracted fingers can be extended by flexing the wrist, but if the wrist is extended, the clawing of the affected fingers become more marked. This is also known as *fixed-length phenomenon* of the long flexors/Volkmann's sign (Figure 14.20).

BIBLIOGRAPHY

1. Immerman I, Price AE, Alfonso I. Lower extremity nerve trauma. *Bull Hosp Jt Dis.* 2014;72:43–52.
2. Poage C, Roth C, Scott B. Peroneal nerve palsy: Evaluation and management. *J Am Acad Orthop Surg.* 2016;24:1–10.
3. Grant GA, Goodkin R, Kliot M. Evaluation and surgical management of peripheral nerve problems. *Neurosurgery.* 1999;44:825–839.
4. Chaudhry S, Ipaktchi KR, Ignatiuk A. Updates on and controversies related to management of radial nerve injuries. *J Am Acad Orthop Surg.* 2019;27:e280–e284.
5. Costales JR, Socolovsky M, Sánchez Lázaro JA, Álvarez García R. Peripheral nerve injuries in the pediatric population: A review of the literature. Part I: Traumatic nerve injuries. *Childs Nerv Syst.* 2019;35:29–35.
6. Costales JR, Socolovsky M, Sánchez Lázaro JA, Costales DR. Peripheral nerve injuries in the pediatric population: A review of the literature. Part II: Entrapment neuropathies. *Childs Nerv Syst.* 2019;35:37–45.

Evaluation of Swelling/Tumor in a Child

MANISH PRUTHI AND NIRMAL RAJ GOPINATHAN

15.1 INTRODUCTION

Any enlargement or protuberance of body tissue is usually called a swelling. In a child, the causes of swelling could be grouped under congenital, traumatic, infective/inflammatory, and neoplastic.

Evaluation of a swelling in a child requires good history and clinical examination before we proceed for imaging studies. This chapter is written, keeping various differential diagnoses in mind so that by the end of the clinical evaluation, we are able to narrow down to a few diagnoses. Every heading in the history or examination will be described in a way to help the clinician accept or refute a differential. Wherever possible, a case scenario/clinical pictures are added to better understand the importance of a relevant point.

15.2 HISTORY

History is imperative in the evaluation of a child with swelling as it allows the clinician to narrow the differentials and reach a correct diagnosis. In this chapter, only salient points in the history pertaining to the swelling are highlighted.

As far as history-taking in the swelling goes, it can be grouped under two categories:

- About the swelling itself.
- About the associated symptoms.

15.2.1 History of Swelling

15.2.1.1 ONSET

This is one of the very important questions that a clinician should ask the child or parents. If a swelling has appeared immediately after a trauma, we know it can be a hematoma or a fracture. Usually, inflammatory swellings have a rapid onset; neoplastic swellings will have a slower onset but could have a rapid onset in certain aggressive tumors like Ewing's sarcoma. A swelling appearing weeks to months after trauma could be myositis ossificans.

Also, it should be kept in mind that most patients with malignant bone tumors will also have a history of some trauma, which at times may be misleading (Figure 15.1).

15.2.1.2 DURATION

As a rule, the longer the duration, the more slow-growing the swelling is and the more chances of it being less aggressive. However, we should not presume a swelling to be benign or malignant just on the basis of duration. There are certain malignant soft tissue tumors like synovial sarcoma that can have a history of years.

15.2.1.3 PROGRESSION

This point in the history gives a valuable insight into the type of swelling we are dealing with. A very rapid progression (in days) is usually seen in inflammatory swellings; malignant swellings usually show fast progression, which is most often a

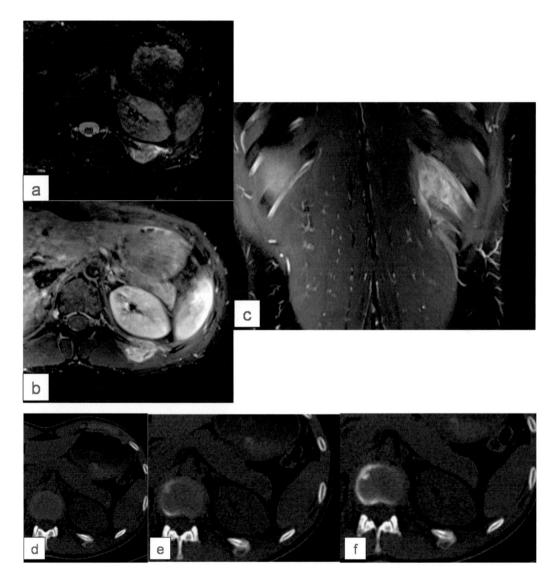

Figure 15.1 Eighteen-year-old male with history of a fall 4 months back. MRI was reported as suspected mesenchymal neoplasm arising from the left 12th rib. (a) and (b) axial MRI pictures showing lesion arising from the left 12th rib. (c) Coronal film showing the extent of the lesion. (d), (e), (f) Axial CT films showing a lesion abutting the 12th rib with peripheral ossification and central lucency, classical of myositis ossificans.

doubling of size in less than 6 months if untreated. Benign tumors usually do not grow or grow at a slow pace over years or sometimes decades.

15.2.1.4 NUMBER

Swellings can be multiple, which is often seen in certain hereditary/congenital syndromes like neurofibromatosis type 1, hereditary multiple exostosis, enchondromatosis (Figure 15.2) (including Ollier's disease and Maffucci syndrome), and familial multiple lipomatosis.

15.2.2 History of Associated Symptoms

15.2.2.1 PAIN

Pain is the most common associated symptom, and most times, it precedes swelling. As clinicians, we should always try to elucidate the site of pain, its onset, type or the nature of pain, and any diurnal variation. It will usually precede swelling in cases of inflammatory swellings or in cases of malignant bone tumors.

15.2.2.2 CONSTITUTIONAL SYMPTOMS

Like fever, weight loss and loss of appetite are classically seen in chronic infections or malignancies. Often, the constitutional symptoms are absent in chronic limb infections like pyogenic or tubercular osteomyelitis or certain slow-growing malignant tumors like synovial sarcoma in a child. So, the absence of these symptoms should not lead a clinician to refute these diagnoses. Acute inflammatory swellings often present with high-grade fever.

15.2.2.3 LOSS OF FUNCTION

A swelling close to a nerve or a joint can impair function; similarly, a large swelling in the muscles can restrict function (Figure 15.3). Sometimes a child can present with pseudoparalysis; most often, it is caused by osteomyelitis or septic arthritis in the child, and it can also be associated with local fullness or swelling.

By the end of the history, a clinician should be able to classify the swelling into the above-mentioned groups (congenital/traumatic/neoplastic or inflammatory) and further proceed with the examination keeping differentials of each type in mind.

15.3 EXAMINATION

Clinical examination has two components: general physical examination (GPE) and local examination of the involved region.

15.3.1 GPE

The aim of GPE is to find out systemic signs, if any, associated with the swelling. This could pertain to a syndromic association (café au lait spots of neurofibromatosis/polyostotic fibrous dysplasia or hemangiomas of Maffucci syndrome) or to a side effect of abnormal tissue growth in the body (pallor, cachexia, lymph nodal enlargements, etc.) or identify any underlying chronic ailment.

Standard GPE signs that need to be seen are vital examination (temperature, pulse, respiratory rate, and blood pressure), pallor, nutrition, and appearance and status of lymph nodes, etc.

The local examination of a child with swelling starts from an inspection.

15.3.2 Local Examination of Swelling

Before focusing our attention on the swelling per se, we should first see the attitude of the limb. This will tell us about the position of comfort and involvement of nerves/muscles/joints.

15.3.2.1 INSPECTION

- *Shape*: Most of the neoplastic swellings will be round to oblong in shape; however, most of the inflammatory swellings will be diffuse and not well defined.
- *Size*: The size per se does not help us to differentiate between benign versus malignant swellings, but it is important to document the size as it helps in identifying further change and the rapidity of growth. In inspection, we can roughly identify the size in the mediolateral, anteroposterior, and superior-inferior dimensions; this finding has to be confirmed in the palpation.
- *Surface*: Can appear smooth, lobulated, or bosselated. Osteochondromas usually have a lobulated surface.
- *Margins*: Inflammatory swellings are diffuse with ill-defined margins. Benign tumors have

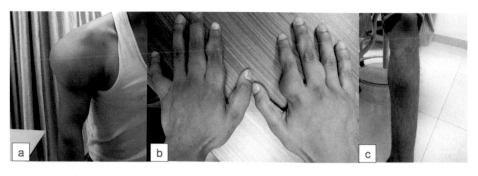

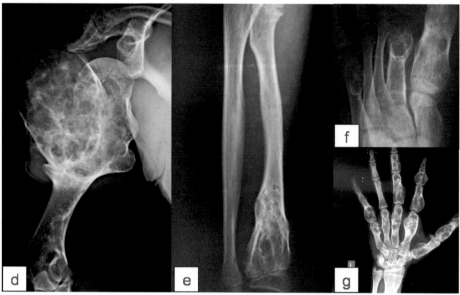

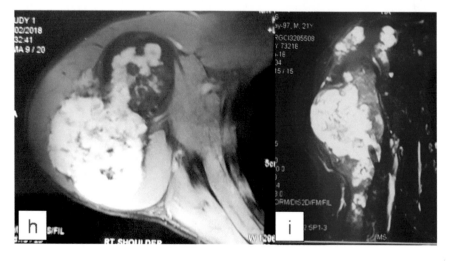

Figure 15.2 Seventeen-year-old male patient with multiple bony swellings all around the body. (a) Right shoulder, (b) bilateral fingers, (c) left leg, (d) radiographs showing multiple enchondromatosis involving the humerus, (e) radius, (f) foot, (g) hand, (h) and (i) MRI film of the right proximal humerus enchondroma showing a large extra-osseous mass suspicious of chondrosarcomatous transformation.

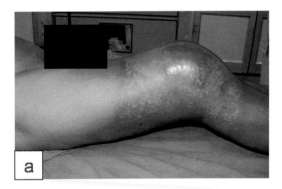

Figure 15.3 Clinical picture of a large tumor around the knee, causing fixed flexion deformity due to tumor invasion of the surrounding muscles.

well-defined margins; margins of malignant bone/soft tissue tumors can be well/ill-defined.

- *Color*: The color of swelling usually is not that important but is diagnostic in certain tumors like malignant melanoma, which is classically a pigmented lesion; however, it is usually not seen in a child. A common pigmented lesion in a child is usually a pigmented nevus or a hemangioma. Inflammatory swellings like cellulitis are expected to appear red in color.
- *Pulsation*: It is very difficult and rare to appreciate pulsations on inspection. Pulsations can be seen in swellings arising directly from arteries like aneurysms.
- *Number*: Usually primary malignant bone/soft tissue tumors present as solitary swelling. Multiple swellings in the same limb or all limbs can be part of congenital/hereditary syndromes (e.g., neurofibromatosis, enchondromatosis, hereditary multiple exostosis, and lipomatosis) or sometimes part of a regional metastasis of a malignant tumor situated distally (e.g., epithelioid/clear cell sarcomas, which are unlikely to occur in children).

15.3.2.2 PALPATION

The aim of palpation is to confirm the inspected findings and to add additional information on swelling so as to narrow our differentials.

- *Temperature*: Checking the temperature first in palpation cannot be overemphasized. A local rise in temperature is a feature of all acute inflammatory swellings but is also sometimes seen in chronic infections and certain neoplastic swellings like osteosarcoma and Ewing's sarcoma.
- *Tenderness*: It is difficult to examine a tender swelling in a child. Eliciting tenderness in a child first requires calming the child and gaining his/her confidence before jumping to palpate the swelling and eliciting this sign. It is important for the examiner to pursue with the utmost care and gentleness without multiple attempts as this may increase the child's apprehension.
- *Size*: We can measure the size of the swelling exactly with a measuring tape. This helps in future comparison if we plan to observe the swelling. Size is measured and documented in two perpendicular dimensions.
- *Margins*: The margins of swelling are palpated with the tip of the finger. The margins or edges could be well defined or indistinct. Sometimes, one of the margins could be well defined, and the other could be indistinct. Usually, all benign swellings and chronic infections have a well-defined margin, while acute inflammatory swellings having indistinct margins. Margins in malignant tumors could be well- to ill-defined depending upon the rate of growth.
- *Surface*: The surface of the swelling could be smooth or bosselated. A bosselated surface can be seen in certain benign bone tumors like osteochondroma and giant cell tumors, etc.
- *Consistency*: It is important to know how the swelling feels on pressure, whether it is cystic or solid and if solid, whether it is soft, firm, or hard. The best way to differentiate a cystic swelling from a soft one is by examining the margin. The margin of a soft swelling will slip away from the palpating finger while that of a cystic swelling will yield on pressure (slip sign). Another way to differentiate between the two is to do a fluctuation/translucency, described below.

Cystic swelling in a child could be a ganglion cyst, while a soft swelling could be a lipoma. A firm swelling in a child could be a benign neurofibroma. It is important to mention here that most of the malignant or aggressive bone/soft tissue tumors are firm in consistency and not hard (e.g., fibromatosis,

Ewing's sarcoma, osteosarcoma, or any other soft tissue sarcomas). Hard swellings are usually bony and are most commonly a benign bone tumor like osteochondroma or an enchondroma. Often, a swelling can show a variegated consistency, being firm to soft in different regions; this can happen due to spontaneous tumor necrosis in malignant bone tumors.

- *Fixity to skin*: Fixity to the skin usually happens due to dermal infiltration and can be seen in superficial soft tissue sarcomas. It is an important sign as it helps the clinician in planning the treatment (how much skin needs to be removed in case of malignant tumors). If a child presents with a recurrent swelling at the same place, it is important to document the fixity of the previous scar to the swelling.
- *Fixity to underlying structures*: This sign gives us some idea about the depth of swelling and the tissues involved. A subcutaneous swelling usually is mobile in all planes, and the overlying skin remains freely mobile even if we contract the underlying muscle. A swelling arising from the deep fascia is less mobile than a subcutaneous swelling but remains free on muscle contraction. The mobility of a swelling arising from the muscles will reduce in the longitudinal plane but will remain in the transverse plane after muscle contraction. Bony swellings are fixed. With advances in imaging techniques like MRI, tissue involvement and infiltration are visualized clearly.
- *Fluctuation*: This sign is only seen in cystic swellings. It is the fluid movement in the swelling that is captured with another finger/s. We need to press the swelling at one end; the other finger placed on the other end of swelling will be passively lifted due to an increase in the pressure. For a very mobile swelling, this test requires stabilization of the swelling by another finger/thumb.
- *Translucency*: This test identifies the transmission of light through the swelling and is positive only in swellings with clear fluids like lymph/water, etc. Darkness is required for this test, otherwise, a roll of black paper can be used. The examiner will pass light through the swelling by placing a torchlight on one side of the swelling and will see if the light is transmitted to the other side of the swelling using

the rolled paper (one end of the rolled paper is placed against the swelling opposite to the light source and the other end of the rolled paper is used as an eye piece).

- *Pulsations*: A pulsatile swelling can directly arise from an artery (aneurysm) or is located very close to a major artery (transmitted pulsations).
- *Compressibility*: Some swellings like hemangiomas are compressible, meaning they disappear on compression and slowly reappear after. This is different from yielding on pressure as the swelling disappears rather than redistributing itself as in yielding. Sometimes a Baker's cyst in a child can also disappear on compression, only to reappear slowly; this happens due to redistribution of fluid into the joint.
- *Distal neurovascular status*: This should be examined and documented properly. Signs of venous compression, and examination of motor and sensory nerves should be done meticulously.

15.3.2.3 MOVEMENTS

- *Neighboring joints*: Movements of the nearby joints should be documented, if feasible. Sometimes, in cases of severe pain (from a fracture or large swelling), the child will not cooperate with testing this. It is important to compare the movement of the ipsilateral side with the other, as sometimes the movement loss is subtle.
- *Distal joints*: A swelling sometimes involves or originates from the major motor nerves of the limb; this could lead to paralysis distally.

15.3.2.4 MEASUREMENTS

Limb measurements should be done as long duration swellings/disuse/neurological impairment can lead to muscle wasting. The measurements are done bilaterally in the middle of the extremities at a symmetrical distance from fixed bony points.

15.4 DRAINING LYMPH NODES

Regional lymphadenopathy can be seen in inflammatory/neoplastic swellings. Although regional lymphadenopathy is uncommon with primary bone tumors, it could be a part of multisystem disease like Langerhans cell histiocytosis (LCH). Many high-grade soft tissue sarcomas of children can metastasize to regional lymph nodes (rhabdomyosarcoma, synovial sarcoma, angiosarcoma, clear cell sarcoma, epithelioid sarcomas). The chances of lymph node metastasis in these tumors could be between 10% and 25%. Any enlarged lymph nodes in the draining region in a setting of a high-grade sarcoma should be evaluated with further imaging.

16

Evaluation of a Child with Short Stature

NIRMAL RAJ GOPINATHAN, ANUPRIYA KAUR, AND CHAKSHU CHAUDHRY

A child of short stature (SS) brought to the outpatient clinic raises many questions with no definite answers. The attending orthopedician must be well versed in identifying a child with short stature and must be capable of categorizing it accordingly for further evaluation. The process of evaluating a child with suspicion of short stature is multidisciplinary again and involves a pediatrician, endocrinologist, geneticist, etc. The reduction in height has wider implications with respect to the child's psychological development, self-confidence, peer pressure, and performance apart from being an indicator of an underlying organic disorder and needs to be attended to with diligence. The following questions are to be answered while evaluating a child with short stature.

16.1 IS THE CHILD REALLY SHORT?

16.1.1 One-Time Measurement

By definition, a child is labeled as short stature if the child's height falls below the third percentile/two standard deviations or more short of the average height on the gender and population specific growth charts. The clinician must be using a recommended gender specific growth chart like the one shown in Figure 16.1.[1,2]

16.1.2 Serial Monitoring

Although outpatient examination offers only one index opportunity to assess the child, serial measurements can be of more help. It is beyond doubt that a single point measurement of height is not as accurate as *poor growth velocity* to assess growth disturbance.[2] A growth rate of <4.5 cm/year in children between 2 and 12 years of age is not normal and calls for evaluation.[2]

Growth velocity is calculated by the given formula:

Growth velocity (cm / year)

$$= \frac{(T_2 - T_1) \times 12}{[\text{Number of months in between } T_1 \text{ and } T_2]}$$

T1: Height recorded earlier
T2: Height recorded later

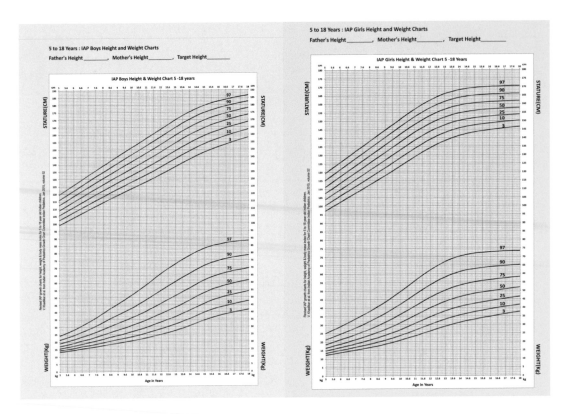

Figure 16.1 Growth chart.

The expected growth velocity at different ages is depicted in Table 16.1.

16.2 MEASUREMENTS

16.2.1 Measuring Length/Height

The evaluation of a child with SS starts with detailed and accurate anthropometric measurements. Height measurement starts with the removal of footwear and head accessories. The child is made stand upright against the wall or a firm structure like a vertical stadiometer with the child's heels, buttocks, thoracic spine, and occiput touching the vertical measure (Figure 16.2). The child is instructed to look straight ahead to avoid head tilt, which can be assured by bringing the lower margin of the eye socket and external auditory meatus at the same level.

Alternatively, a steel tape placed on the head with the horizontal surface placed perpendicular to the vertical surface (wall) can be used. For length measurement of a small child, an infantometer, which is a horizontal board with a head plate that is fixed and a mobile footplate, can be used. The child needs to be held by at least two people, knees kept straight, and feet held against the footplate (Figure 16.3).

16.2.2 Measurement of Body Proportions

Once it is known that the child is short, it is important to know whether the growth is as

Table 16.1 Linear Growth Velocity According to Age[2]

Age	Growth Velocity
0–3 months	3.5 cm/month
3–6 months	2 cm/month
6–9 months	1.5 cm/month
9–12 months	1.3 cm/month
1–2 years	10–11 mm/month; 12 cm/year
2–3 years	8 cm/year
3–4 years	7 cm/year
4–9 years	5–6 cm/year

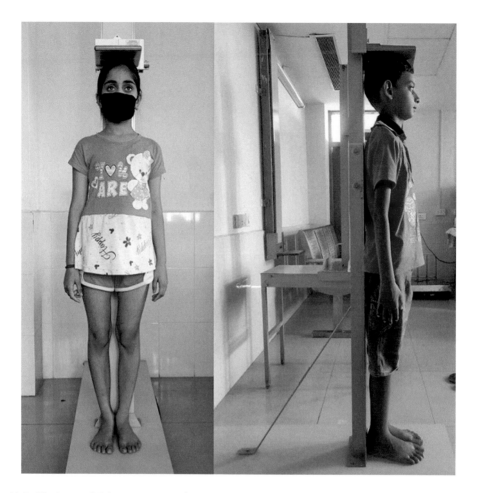

Figure 16.2 Placing a child against a stadiometer.

proportionate as it should be. To facilitate this, it is important to individualize the upper segment and lower segment measurements. The upper segment (US) can be measured by measuring the height of the child made to sit on the stadiometer (Figure 16.4). Otherwise, the lower segment (LS) is measured with the child erect and feet kept 4 cm apart to facilitate the measurement. The distance from the upper border of the pubic symphysis to the floor is measured, and this comprises the LS. The US is obtained by subtracting the LS from the total height. The US/LS ratio is obtained by dividing the US by the LS value.

The proportionate short-statured child might have an underlying treatable medical cause, which needs to be evaluated. Disproportionate short stature can be divided into those characterized mainly by the shortened trunk or shortened limbs (short limb/short trunk dwarfism) (Figure 16.5). Table 16.2 depicts the US:LS ratio per age.[2, 3]

16.2.3 Arm Span – Height Difference

Arm span is measured by making the child stand against a vertical surface with both the arms abducted 90° at the shoulder and elbows fully extended (Figure 16.6). The distance between the tips of the middle fingers of both the hands are marked and measured to get the arm span. Arm span measurement has proven to be a good complementary measure for understanding body proportions. It is shorter than height in conditions where long bone growth is primarily affected like achondroplasia.[3] Engelbach documented an average arm span – height difference of –3.0 cm and –3.5 cm in boys and girls at age 4 years, with values

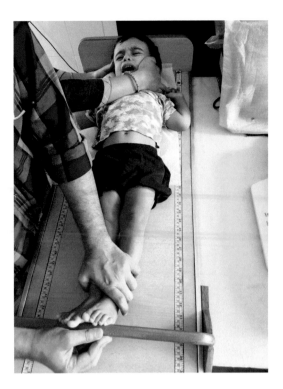

Figure 16.3 Measuring length with an infantometer.

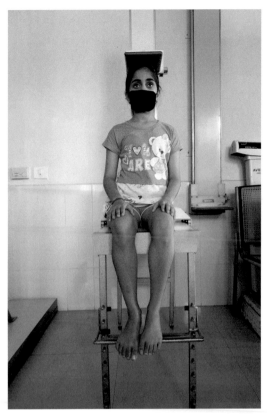

Figure 16.4 Upper segment measurement.

approaching zero at 9 years in boys and 12 years in girls.[2,4] In general, arm span reaches the value of height at approximately 8 years of age.[5]

16.3 GROWTH POTENTIAL

Genetic and environmental factors largely influence a child's growth potential. A child born to parents who are short is expected to be short. On the basis of this concept, the mid-parental height (MPH) is used to detect familial short stature (FSS). MPH[2] gives a reasonable assessment of genetic growth potential and is calculated by using the following formulas:

$$MPH\ boys = \left\{ \begin{array}{l} Father's\ height\ (cm) \\ + \left(Mother's\ height\ (cm) + 13 \right) \end{array} \right\} / 2$$

$$MPH\ girls = \left\{ \begin{array}{l} \left(Father's\ height\ (cms) - 13 \right) \\ + \left(Mother's\ height\ (cms) \right) \end{array} \right\} / 2$$

The obtained value is plotted on the gender specific growth chart (18/20 years). The height curve of the child is then extrapolated up to adult height (i.e., 18/20 years). The projected height at 18/20 years should fall within ±10 cm of MPH for boys, and for girls ± 8.5 cm of MPH. If it falls within this range, the short stature is probably an FSS. But if the child's height falls below the MPH percentiles in the chart, even when the height is above the third centile or two standard deviations, the child needs to be investigated. Pathological SS should be considered when the difference between the projected height and the MPH is more than 8 cm (Figure 16.7).

16.4 HISTORY AND PHYSICAL EXAMINATION

This part of the evaluation starts from the time the patient steps into the clinic, even before assessing whether the child is short or not and is of great importance. For the convenience of the reader, it is described here. Apart from anthropometry, history-taking and physical examination should

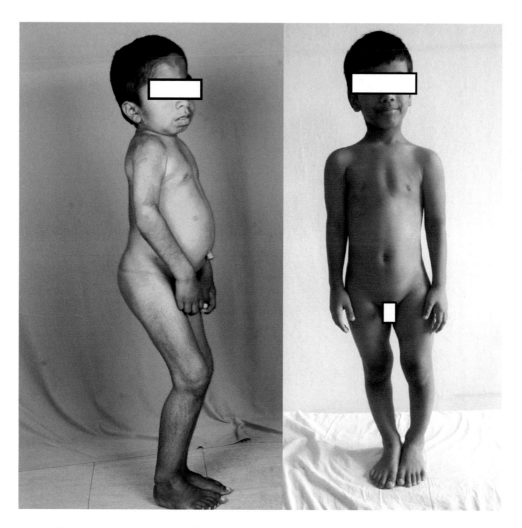

Figure 16.5 Short trunk/short limb children.

Table 16.2 Upper Segment Lower Segment Ratio per Age

Age	US:LS ratio
Birth	1.7:1
3 years	1.3:1
7 years	1.1:1
10 years	0.9:1

be elaborately done to find out telltale features of inherited/sporadic syndromes and endocrine and metabolic disorders if any. For example, even long duration drug intake (chronic steroid use, anticonvulsants, and drugs used for attention deficit hyperactivity disorder) can result in short stature and should be kept in mind while eliciting history. Special importance should be given to examination

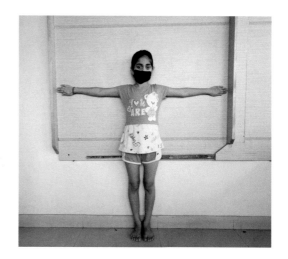

Figure 16.6 Arm span measurement.

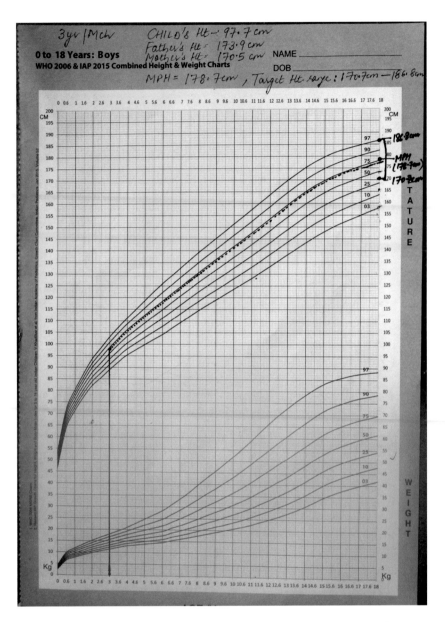

Figure 16.7 MPH calculation and charting: father's height 173.9 cm, mother's height 170.5 cm, child's present height 97.7 cm. MPH calculated is 178.7 cm, with a target height range of 170.7 cm to 186.8 cm. The child's projected height falls within the target range, as shown in the chart.

of the craniofacial region and physical examination for a wide variety of abnormalities with short stature, a few of which are given in Table 16.3 and Table 16.4.

Apart from craniofacial characteristics, there are other findings that are not to be missed (Tables 16.3 and 16.4). For example, diastrophic dysplasia is characterized by a markedly abducted thumb ("hitchhiker's thumb"). Ellis–van Creveld syndrome is characterized by exceptionally

well-formed polydactyly. One of the hallmarks in achondroplasia is a trident hand where there is relative abduction of the index and middle finger one way and the ring and little finger the other way (Figure 16.10). Coccygeal tail is seen in metatropic dysplasia apart from an inguinal hernia. Although the workup of skeletal dysplasia comprises clinical, radiographic, and genetic workup, careful physical examination can help us proceed in a focused way toward further workup.

Table 16.3 Characteristic Craniofacial Findings in Skeletal Dysplasia with Short Stature

Finding	Associated Syndrome/Disorder
Calcification or generalized thickening of ears	Diastrophic dwarfism
Clouding of cornea (Figure 16.8)	Mucopolysaccharidoses
Midfacial hypoplasia	Achondroplasia
Nasal depression	Achondroplasia
Broadening of nasal region	Mucopolysaccharidoses
Abnormalities of the teeth and gums	Ellis–van Creveld syndrome/Osteogenesis imperfecta
Cleft palate	Diastrophic dysplasia and numerous other skeletal dysplasias

Table 16.4 Characteristic Clinical Features of Skeletal Dysplasias Associated with Short Stature

Skeletal Dysplasia	Clinical Features	Remarks
Achondroplasia	Severe short stature with rhizomelic short limbs, trident hands, large head, depressed nasal bridge	Condition is identifiable at birth
Hypochondroplasia	Mild short stature, muscular appearance, rhizomelic shortening of limbs, bowed legs, mild lumbar lordosis	
Pseudo achondroplasia	Shortening of limbs similar to achondroplasia but with normal skull and face, hypermobility of joints except elbow, genu varus or valgum, small broad hands	Onset 2 years or later, at risk of osteoarthrosis of hips or knees, waddling gait
Osteogenesis imperfecta type III	Multiple fractures throughout life, bowed and short limbs, blue sclera, often wheelchair-bound (Figure 16.9)	Identifiable at birth
Osteogenesis imperfecta type I and IV	Recurrent pathologic fractures, hearing loss, dentinogenesis imperfecta	Identifiable later in life
Spondyloepiphyseal dysplasia tarda	Short stature with short trunk	Pain in hips, knees, back
Multiple epiphyseal dysplasia	Mild short stature	Pain or arthritis in hips, knees, ankles, waddling gait
Metaphyseal dysplasia (multiple types)	Bowing of legs, short stature with short limbs	
Progressive pseudo rheumatoid arthropathy of childhood (PPRAC)	Enlargement of interphalangeal joints of hands, progressive restricted mobility of all joints, absence of signs of inflammation	Onset of arthropathy usually between ages 3 and 6 years
Larsen syndrome (multiple congenital dislocations)	Dysmorphism, cleft palate, hyperextensible joints, scoliosis/kyphosis	At risk for spinal cord compression
Cleidocranial dysplasia	Box-shaped head with large fontanelles, droopy shoulders, dental anomaly	
Chondrodysplasia punctata	Flat face, depressed nasal bridge, short limbs, joint contractures	

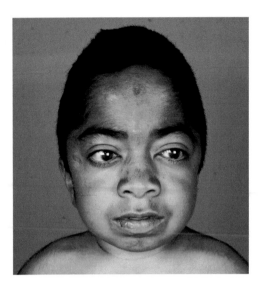

Figure 16.8 Corneal clouding in a child with mucopolysaccharidosis.

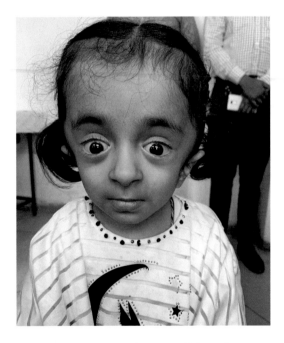

Figure 16.9 Triangular facies and blue sclera in a child with osteogenesis imperfecta.

16.5 CORRELATION OF CLINICAL FINDINGS

16.5.1 Skeletal Age

Bone age (BA) estimation is an important part of the workup of a child with SS. Routinely, left hand

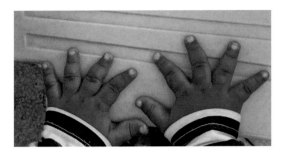

Figure 16.10 Achondroplasia with trident hand (relative abduction of the index and long finger one way and ring and small finger the other way).

and wrist radiograph is taken, and bone maturity is assessed. One way of assessing BA is by comparison of the radiograph with standard radiographs from the Greulich–Pyle atlas.[6] Another method is by scoring individual bones of the hand and wrist, described as Tanner–Whitehouse method.[7–9] When BA is less than 2 standard deviations (SD) or <2 years of chronological age, it is labeled as delayed (Table 16.5).

16.5.2 Height Age

Height age (HA) is the age at which the child's present height is at the 50th percentile on the growth chart.

Constitutional short stature (CSS) is a delay in attaining normal growth/expected growth potential. At birth, the length is normal; however, in childhood, the growth velocity follows a low

Table 16.5 Interpretation of the Estimated Height in Terms of Bone Age, Height Age, and Chronological Age

Familial SS	Height age (HA) < bone age (BA) = chronological age (CA) (Height age is less than the calculated bone age and bone age matches the chronological age)
Pathologic SS	BA < HA < CA Delay of 2 years or more in BA from CA is clearly abnormal
Constitutional SS	HA = BA < CA (Height age matches the bone age, which is less than the chronological age)

normal pattern. In addition to low growth velocity, there is a delay in attaining pubertal maturation. As a result, the height discrepancy as compared to peers is most apparent in pre-teenage years. At this time, the bone age is delayed and (as can be seen in Table 16.5) seems close to the height age. When such an individual enters puberty, catch-up growth occurs, and the ultimate height is in the normal adult range. The phenomenon of constitutional delay can be remembered by the phrase that such "individuals are late bloomers." Children are considered to be mature with no possible increase in height when bone age is 17 years in males and 15 years in females.

16.6 FURTHER WORKUP AND INVESTIGATIONS

The detailed workup of a short-statured child is beyond the scope of this book. The points to be remembered are to identify whether the child is pathologically short and to differentiate proportionate SS from disproportionate SS. Once the basic homework is done, the patient should be assessed by a pediatric endocrine specialist and geneticist for further workup and interpretation. Children with FSS need only reassurance, whereas children with CSS need close monitoring of growth.

REFERENCES

1. Khadilkar VV, Khadilkar AV. Revised Indian Academy of Pediatrics 2015 growth charts for height, weight and body mass index for 5 – 18-year-old Indian children. *Ind J Endocr Metab.* 2015;19:470–476.
2. Yadav S, Dabas A. Approach to short stature. *Ind J Pediatr.* 2015;82:462–470.
3. Turan S, Bereket A, Omar A, Berber M, Ozen A, Bekiroglu N. Upper segment/lower segment ratio and armspan–height difference in healthy Turkish children. *Acta Paediatrica.* 2005;94:407–413.
4. Engelbach W. Endocrinologic interpretation of normal weight, height and proportions. *Endokrinologie.* 1929;5:28–61.
5. Rose SR, Vogiatzi MG, Copeland KC. A general pediatric approach to evaluating a short child. *Pediatr Rev.* 2005;26:410–420.
6. Greulich WW, Pyle SI. *Radiographic atlas of skeletal development of the hand and wrist.* Stanford: Stanford University Press, 1950.
7. Tanner JM, Whitehouse RH, Cameron N, et al. *Assessment of skeletal maturity and prediction of adult height (TW2 Method).* London: Academic Press, 1983.
8. Tanner JM, Goldstein H, Whitehouse RH. Standards for children's height at ages 2–9 years allowing for heights of parents. *Arch Dis Child.* 1970;45:755–762.
9. Tanner JM. Normal growth and techniques of growth assessment. *Clin Endocrinol Metab.* 1986;15:411–451.

Evaluation of Pediatric Limb Deformities

SIDDHARTHA SHARMA

17.1 INTRODUCTION

This chapter will describe the examination of a child with lower limb deformity. In particular, it will focus on limb malalignment resulting from long-bone deformities. Assessment of upper limb, hip, knee, foot, and ankle deformities, etc. are discussed in Chapters 5, 6, 9–11.

The reader must remember that a lower limb deformity, or any deformity for that matter, can exist in the frontal (coronal), sagittal, or axial planes. Isolated deformities in the frontal, sagittal, or axial plane are termed as *uniplanar* deformities. It may so happen that the deformity may lie in a plane that is neither frontal nor sagittal but is at an angle in between the frontal and sagittal planes. This is known as an *oblique plane* deformity (Figure 17.1). Oblique plane deformities can be noted both from the front and from the side, giving the impression of the existence of two

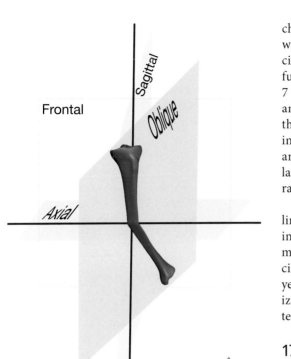

Frontal

Sagittal

Oblique

Axial

Figure 17.1 The concept of oblique plane deformity. The frontal, sagittal, and axial planes are depicted. The plane of this tibial deformity is neither frontal nor sagittal; it lies *obliquely* between the two. Hence, this is an *oblique plane* deformity.

deformities. However, the reader should bear in mind that oblique plane deformities are also uniplanar deformities.

The examination of a lower limb deformity should focus on addressing the following issues.

17.1.1 Differentiate Physiological Variants from True Deformity

The frontal plane alignment of the lower limb changes from physiological varus at birth to a neutral position by 18–24 months. Thereafter, the limb is in a valgus alignment, and peak values of 8–10° are attained by 3–4 years of age. Valgus alignment decreases thereafter, and adult values are attained around 7 years of age. Hence, it is important to know these changes in order to differentiate pathological deformities from physiological variation. Varus after 2 years of age, severe varus (>20°) in

children below 2 years of age, varus in children with short stature (<3rd percentile), and suspicion of a metabolic or genetic disorder necessitate further workup. Also, an increase in valgus after 7 years of age should be considered pathological and investigated accordingly. The reader must note that physiological varus results from smooth bowing that involves the entire proximal, midshaft, and distal parts of the femur and tibia. Focal angular deformity involving the proximal tibia should raise the suspicion of Blount's disease.

Similarly, the rotational alignment of the lower limb also undergoes a significant change during growth. Out-toeing is commonly observed in many infants and toddlers. In-toeing may be associated with physiological varus in infants below 2 years of age. Rotational variations usually normalize by 8 years of age, and any abnormality thereafter warrants careful evaluation.

17.1.2 Identify the Deformity Plane (Frontal/Sagittal/Oblique/Axial)

As discussed earlier in this chapter, the reader should ascertain the plane of the deformity. This is discussed further in Section 17.5 of this chapter.

17.1.3 Identify the Deformity Site (Epiphysis and Metaphysis versus Diaphysis)

Deformities near the joint, i.e., epiphyseal and metaphyseal deformities, tend to alter the joint range of motion and may become less apparent with the motion of the joint (Table 17.1). Furthermore, deformities occurring at the level of the physis also tend to result in marked limb-length discrepancy, depending on the contribution of the physis to the growth of the limb.

17.1.4 Quantify the Deformity

The magnitude of the deformity must be quantified. Methods for quantification are described in Section 17.5 of this chapter. When quantifying the deformity, it is essential to perform measurements in the standing position. This is because weight-bearing reveals the true magnitude of the deformity.

Table 17.1 Comparison of Clinical Features of Intra-Articular, Extra-Articular Metaphyseal, and Diaphyseal Deformities

Feature	Intra-Articular Deformity	Extra-Articular (Metaphyseal Deformity)	Diaphyseal Deformity
Progression	Usually progressive	May progress if the adjacent physis is also involved	Usually non-progressive
Limb-length discrepancy	Severe (depending on the physis involved)	Mild to moderate	Mild to moderate
Joint range of motion	May be painful and restricted	Arc of motion is changed; overall range remains same unless there are coexistent soft-tissue contractures	Generally normal, unless there are coexistent soft-tissue contractures
Effect of joint movement	May alter the appearance of deformity	May alter the appearance of deformity	Does not alter the appearance of deformity

17.1.5 Identify the Etiopathogenesis of the Deformity

History and examination should also focus on identification of the etiopathogenesis of the deformity. Are there any tell-tale signs of trauma or infection? Is the deformity a part of a generalized metabolic or genetic disorder? This is discussed in some more detail in Sections 17.2, 17.3, and 17.6 of this chapter.

17.1.6 Determine the Effects of the Deformity on Adjacent Joints and Gait

Finally, the examiner should make a note of the effect of the deformity on adjacent joints, as well as gait. This is discussed in Sections 17.4 and 17.5 of this chapter.

17.2 RELEVANT HISTORY

Although history-taking must be individualized, the following points need to be carefully ascertained:

- Was the deformity congenital or acquired? If acquired, how long has the deformity been present? In case of congenital deformities, a full antenatal history that includes maternal drug intake, substance abuse, infections, or other significant problems during pregnancy must be elicited.

- Was there a well-defined event that led to the deformity? History of trauma or infection may be elicited.
- Is the deformity static or progressive?
- Does the deformity result in limitation of function, activities of daily living, or abnormal gait?
- Developmental history should be elicited.

17.3 RELEVANT GENERAL EXAMINATION

General examination should focus on determining whether the deformity is part of a generalized skeletal disorder. As is the case with history-taking, the examination should be individualized, but the following points should be ascertained:

- Are there any features of skeletal dysplasias? Short stature, abnormal facies, disproportionate segmental measurements, etc. may be important pointers.
- Are there any features suggestive of metabolic disorders, for example, rickets? Chest wall abnormalities, hypotonia, problems with dentition, etc. may be noted.

17.4 ASSESSMENT OF GAIT

A careful assessment of gait is mandatory in all cases. It is beyond the scope of this chapter to discuss pathological gait, however, a few gait patterns relevant to lower limb deformities are mentioned below.

17.4.1 Varus Thrust Gait

Varus (or lateral) thrust gait is indicative of a dynamic deformity and refers to a visible and sudden worsening of a varus deformity in the stance phase of gait. A varus deformity leads to increased weight-bearing through the medial femoral and tibial condyles. In stance phase, this effect is exaggerated, and the lateral joint line of the knee opens up as a varus moment is created about the knee. This phenomenon is observed as a "thrust" on the lateral side of the knee. As the limb enters into swing phase, the varus moment and the varus deformity visibly decrease.

17.4.2 Valgus Thrust Gait

This phenomenon is similar to the varus thrust gait. A valgus deformity leads to increased weight-bearing on the lateral femoral and tibial condyles. In the stance phase of gait, the valgus moment increases, leading to the opening up of the medial joint line. This is visualized as a worsening of the valgus deformity and a thrust on the medial side. As the limb goes into swing phase, the valgus moment, as well the valgus deformity, visibly decreases.

17.4.3 Dynamic Knee Recurvatum

This refers to compensatory hyperextension of the knee during stance phase of the gait and is seen in patients with an equinus deformity. As the patient is unable to place the foot in a plantigrade position during stance phase, this is compensated by hyperextension of the knee, which allows the heel to be placed on the ground. Over a period of time, this dynamic knee hyperextension may become significant, and may be visualized as a *thrust*, similar to a varus or valgus thrust.

17.4.4 In-Toeing and Out-Toeing

In-toeing and out-toeing refer to inward and outward deviation of the foot in standing and walking. As mentioned earlier, this should be differentiated from physiological variants. Torsional deformities can result in pathological in-toeing and out-toeing. It is pertinent to mention here that varus deformities are invariably associated with in-toeing.

17.5 EXAMINATION OF LOWER LIMBS

Examination of the lower limbs should be done by the *look-feel-move* scheme, as is done for any region or joint. Some aspects of examination specific to a patient with lower limb deformity are described below.

17.5.1 Assessment of Frontal Plane Limb Alignment and Deformity

The reader must remember that assessment of lower limb alignment should always be done with the patient *standing*. The patient is asked to stand straight with both patellae pointing straight ahead (Figure 17.2). In this position, one of three scenarios may be observed:

- The medial femoral condyles touch each other, but the medial malleoli do not. This happens when the limb alignment is in *valgus*. The *intermalleolar distance* is used in these cases to quantify the amount of valgus (Figure 17.2). To measure this distance, the examiner ensures that both limbs are fully extended and that the medial femoral condyles are in contact with each other. The most prominent points on both medial malleoli are marked, and a ruler or tape is used to measure the distance, in centimeters, between the two malleoli. It must be remembered here that many obese children may have corpulent thighs, which may prevent the legs from touching each other during standing. This gives the appearance of a pseudovalgus alignment.
- The medial malleoli touch each other, but the medial femoral condyles do not. In this case, the limb alignment is in *varus*. The *intercondylar distance* is used in these cases to quantify the varus deformity (Figure 17.3). To measure this distance, the examiner ensures that both limbs are fully extended and that both medial malleoli are in contact with each other. Both medial femoral epicondyles are marked, and a ruler or a tape is used to measure the distance, in centimeters, between the two epicondyles.

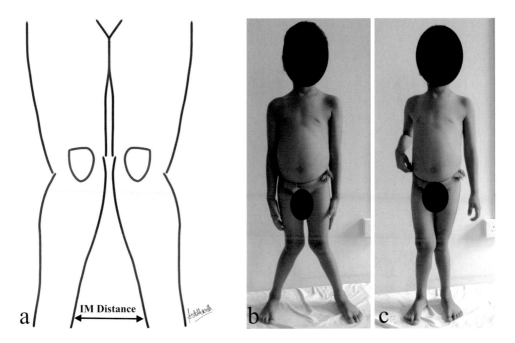

Figure 17.2 (a) Valgus alignment and intermalleolar (IM) distance. (b) Bilateral genu valgum – the child is standing with both patellae facing forwards. In this position, the true magnitude of the valgus deformity can be appreciated. (c) The same child standing with both feet forward, the patellae are facing outwards. The valgus deformity is masked.

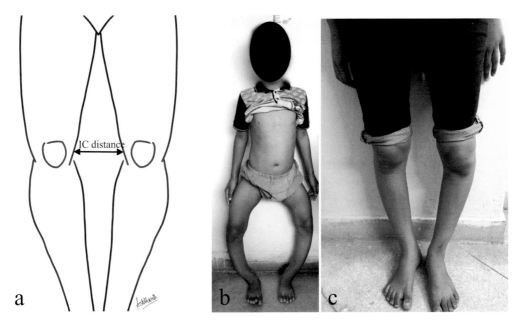

Figure 17.3 (a) Varus alignment and intercondylar distance. (b) A child with severe, bilateral symmetrical varus of the femur and tibia, also known as the "O" deformity. (c) Left-sided unilateral varus deformity of the tibia.

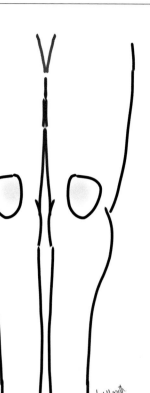

Figure 17.4 Rectus alignment.

- Both medial femoral epicondyles and medial malleoli may touch each other. In this scenario, the limb alignment is neutral or *rectus* (Figure 17.4).

Frontal plane limb alignment can also be quantified clinically by measuring the *tibiofemoral* angle. In terms of deformity correction, this is the angle formed between the *anatomic axes* of the femur and tibia. It must be remembered that under normal circumstances, the anatomic and mechanical axes of the tibia are similar. Before starting measurements, the examiner should ensure that the patient is standing straight with both limbs in full extension and both patellae facing forwards. The patella forwards (rather than the foot forwards) position is important to ensure that the limb is in neutral rotation before any measurements are made. The anatomic axis of the femur is marked by a line joining the anterior superior iliac spine to the center of the patella. The anatomic axis of the tibia is marked by a line joining the center of the patella to the center of the ankle joint. The angle between the two axes gives the tibiofemoral angle.

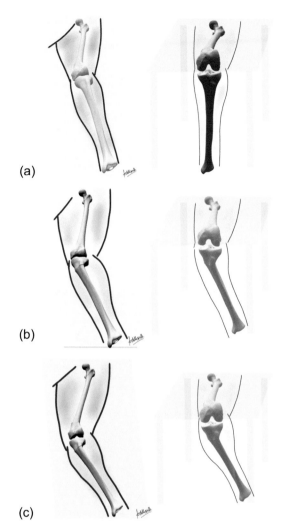

(a)

(b)

(c)

Figure 17.5 (a) Flexion test – femoral valgus deformity. The valgus disappears on knee flexion. (b) Flexion test – tibia valgus deformity. The valgus persists on knee flexion. (c) Flexion test – combined femoral and tibial valgus. The valgus decreases but does not disappear.

In case a frontal plane deformity is noted, the *"flexion test"* can be used to determine whether the deformity lies within the femur, tibia, or both bones. The anatomical basis of the test can be understood by appreciating the fact that in knee flexion, the tibial plateau articulates with the posterior part of the femoral condyles. Therefore, if the deformity lies within the femur, knee flexion brings the tibial plateau in contact with the normal posterior aspect of the femoral condyles, and the deformity disappears (Figure 17.5a). However, if the deformity lies within the tibia, the deformity will not decrease with flexion (Figure 17.5b). If there is a combined deformity of the femur and tibia, the magnitude of deformity will decrease with flexion but will not be completely obliterated (Figure 17.5c). This test needs two important prerequisites. First of all, there should be no deformity of the posterior femoral condyles, or the test may be wrongly interpreted. Secondly, rotation of the limb must be prevented during flexion, or the deformity may be erroneously masked. This may be done by firmly grasping the thigh during knee flexion or by asking the patient to sit on a couch with the knee and leg hanging free off the couch. In the sitting position, the thigh can be easily stabilized to prevent rotation, and this is the author's preferred method of performing the flexion test.

It must be remembered that standing full-length radiographs are a must for accurate assessment of limb alignment and must be performed in all cases where deformity needs to be assessed.

17.5.2 Assessment and Quantification of Sagittal Plane Deformity

Assessment of sagittal plane deformity is done by examining the patient from the side. This is done by measuring the angle subtended between the long axes of the femur and tibia. In normal limbs, this measurement is usually 0°. Flexion (procurvatum) or hyperextension (recurvatum) deformities may be picked up (Figure 17.6).

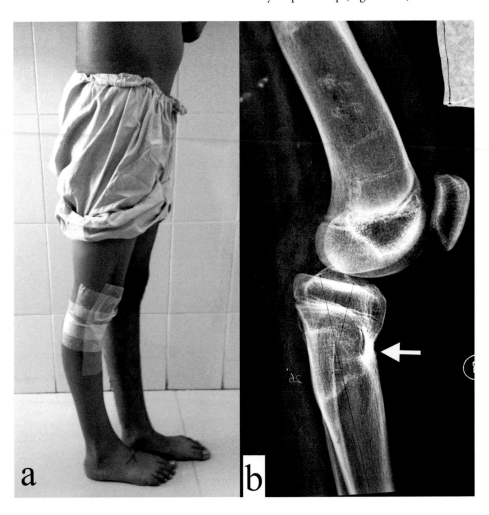

Figure 17.6 Recurvatum deformity of the tibia after tibial tubercle physeal arrest. (a) Recurvatum is appreciated by examining the patient from the side. (b) Lateral radiograph shows tibial recurvatum; a tibial tubercle physeal bar is noted (white arrow).

17.5.3 Assessment and Quantification of Axial Plane (Rotational) Deformity

Assessment of the rotational profile of the lower limb is mandatory in all cases and has been described in Chapter 9 on hip examination. Briefly, the examiner should assess the overall rotational alignment of the limb by measuring the *foot-progression angle* during walking. Torsional deformities of individual segments are assessed next. Femoral anteversion can be determined by *Craig's test*. Torsional deformity of the leg is assessed by means of the *thigh-foot angle*. Adduction (or abduction) of the foot can be quantified by the *heel-bisector* method.

17.5.4 Assessment of Limb-Length Discrepancy

Assessment of limb-length discrepancy is a must in all cases presenting with limb deformity. The Allis and Galeazzi tests may be used to quickly ascertain the presence and location of limb-length discrepancy. True and apparent lengths must be ascertained, taking into account any deformities around the hip, knee, and ankle. Segmental limb-length measurements should be performed to identify whether there is shortening in the femur, tibia, or both.

17.5.5 Assessment of Joint Range of Motion

As is the case with any orthopedic patient, joints adjacent (proximal and distal) to, or those involved with the deformity itself, must be carefully examined. Both active and passive range of motion needs to be ascertained.

17.6 OTHER RELEVANT EXAMINATION

The distal neurovascular status must be assessed in every case. Furthermore, depending on the type of deformity encountered, the examiner may need to examine other regions, including the spine, hip, knee, ankle, and foot. For example, valgus malalignment is invariably associated with pes planus and possibly with patellar instability.

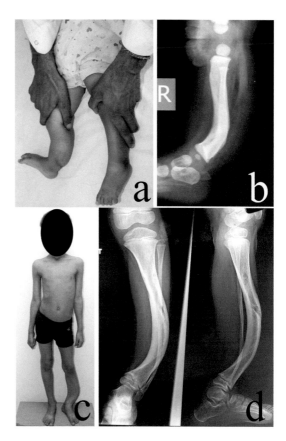

Figure 17.7 (a) Clinical image. (b) Lateral radiograph of a child with posteromedial bowing of the tibia. (c) Clinical image. (d) Anteroposterior (AP) and lateral radiographs of a child with anteromedial bowing due to congenital pseudarthrosis of the tibia.

Examination of these regions is discussed in detail in Chapters 10 and 11.

Of special note is bowing of the tibia in young children. In these cases, it is important to differentiate between anterolateral bowing (indicative of congenital pseudarthrosis of the tibia), anteromedial bowing (indicative of fibular hemimelia), and congenital posteromedial bowing (Figure 17.7). The three conditions are compared in Table 17.2.

17.7 SUMMARY

To conclude, the examination of a child with deformity warrants careful assessment of the type, site(s), magnitude, and etiopathogenesis of the deformity. Physiological variations should be kept in mind and differentiated from truly pathologic deformity. The examiner must not forget to evaluate the sagittal

Table 17.2 Comparison of Congenital Anterolateral, Anteromedial, and Posteromedial Bowing in Children

Feature	Anterolateral Bowing	Anteromedial Bowing	Posteromedial Bowing
Pathogenesis	Pathological (congenital pseudarthrosis of tibia)	Pathological (Fibular hemimelia)	Usually physiological
Site	Middle-distal third	Middle third	Middle-distal third
Genetic association	Neurofibromatosis Type 1 (in 55–60% of patients)	Sonic hedgehog gene	None
Associated deformities	Ankle instability	LLD, missing lateral toes, genu valgum, equinovalgus foot, tarsal coalition	Calcaneovalgus foot
Possible long-term sequelae (if untreated)	Pseudarthrosis, recurrent fractures, LLD of around 5 cm at skeletal maturity	Varying degrees of LLD depending on disease severity, ankle instability, knee instability	3–5 cm LLD at skeletal maturity

Abbreviation: LLD, limb-length instability.

plane and rotational deformities, in addition to frontal plane deformities. Additionally, evaluation of limb-length discrepancy and assessment of the proximal and distal joint function and distal neurovascular status is mandatory in all cases. Finally, radiographic examination by means of full-length standing radiographs with the patella forwards is a must in all cases to accurately assess all elements of the deformity.

BIBLIOGRAPHY

1. Paley D, Herzenberg JE, Tetsworth K, McKie J, Bhave A. Deformity planning for frontal and sagittal plane corrective osteotomies. *Orthop Clin North Am.* 1994;25(3):425–465.

2. Silva MS, Fernandes ARC, Cardoso FN, Longo CH, Aihara AY. Radiography, CT, and MRI of hip and lower limb disorders in children and adolescents [published correction appears in radiographics. 2019;39(4):1232. *Radiographics.* 2019;39(3):779–794.

3. Benard MA. Pediatric considerations. *Clin Podiatr Med Surg.* 2020;37(1):125–150.

4. Staheli LT, Corbett M, Wyss G, King H. Lower extremity rotational problems in children. Normal values to guide management. *J Bone Joint Surg Am.* 1985;67:39–47.

5. Gautam VK, Maini L, Gupta R, Sabharwal A, Arora S. Flexion test in the coronal plane deformities of knee. *J Clin Orthop Trauma.* 2013;4(3):115–118.

18

Miscellaneous Topics

PRATEEK BEHERA, KARTHICK RANGASAMY,
AND NIRMAL RAJ GOPINATHAN

18.1 RICKETS

Rickets is a common metabolic disorder resulting from the defective mineralization of immature bones (Figure 18.1).[1] Rickets can result from vitamin D deficiency, abnormal metabolism of vitamin D, or an abnormal metabolism and/or excretion of inorganic phosphate and/or calcium.

18.1.1 Presenting Complaints

Parents most often consult a pediatrician for complaints like bony deformities, failure of growth, delayed dentition, generalized weakness, and sometimes muscular spasms. The child is then referred to an orthopedic specialist for their opinion and timely diagnosis of the disorder.

18.1.2 History

Examination should start with an appropriate history. The child's age, dietary habits, and the socioeconomic status of the parents provide background knowledge of the condition.[1] A history of frequent abdominal pain, convulsions, muscular spasms, oliguria, polyuria, hematuria, diarrhea, and constipation should be taken in addition to a history of intake of any medication like anticonvulsants and steroids.

231

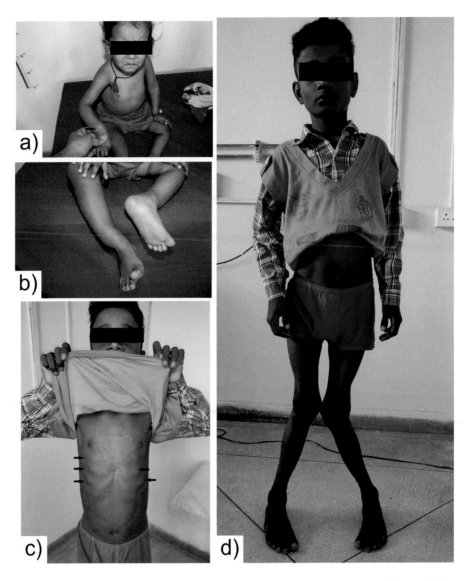

Figure 18.1 Rickets: (a) widened wrist, protuberant abdomen due to hypotonia, (b) distal tibia deformity, (c) rachitic rosary at costochondral junction, (d) genu valgum.

18.1.3 Examination

The examination should then start with the measurement of the child's biometric parameters. The gait can be examined when the child walks into the room. A child might not be able to walk properly from generalized hypotonia in severe cases. A genu varum or valgum is the most obvious abnormality noted in majority of the children.

The physical examination should start from the head, looking for frontal bossing, craniotabes, widened and open cranial sutures, and delayed and abnormal dentition (enamel and dentine defects). The examiner then should progress caudally. Pectus carinatum, uncommonly pectus excavatum, rachitic rosary (seen and palpated at the costochondral junctions), and Harrison's sulcus (groove along the lower rib cage and the diaphragmatic attachment) are the usual findings of the chest. These children can have a pot belly. Examine for spinal deformities like kyphosis, scoliosis, or a combination of both.[1] Limb deformities become prominent as and when the immature metaphyses are subjected to loading and pressure. Widening of the lower end of the radius is seen when a child starts to crawl and puts pressure on the wrists. Lower limb deformities become pronounced when the child starts to stand and walk. Genu varum and valgum are the common deformities around the knees. Genu varum occurs with the onset of disease at a young age (less than 2 years), and genu valgum occurs in an older child as the knee alignment progresses from varus to valgus normally. The ankles, too, undergo a widening, producing what is called a double malleoli sign marked by the presence of two distinct medial bony prominences. The proximal one is formed by the overgrowth of cartilage cells in the rachitic maturation zone, and it mimics the presence of a second medial malleolus on the true medial malleolus (formed by the epiphysis). In severe cases, both the femur and tibia are bowed anterolaterally, producing an "O" deformity. The examination should conclude with an evaluation of muscle tone and a neurological examination. Look for findings suggestive of resistant rickets like alopecia in vitamin D dependent rickets type II and defective dentition due to repeated dental abscesses in hypophosphatemic rickets, etc.

18.2 MUSCULAR DYSTROPHIES AND MYOPATHIES

Muscular dystrophies are rare genetic disorders seen in children.[2] Myopathies can be of genetic origin, or they can be secondary to inflammatory, endocrinological, nutritional, and drug-induced causes. The muscular dystrophies that are encountered in clinical practice are Duchenne muscular dystrophy (DMD), Becker muscular dystrophy (BMD), and congenital muscular dystrophy (CMD). Of these, DMD and BMD are seen in males (X-linked inheritance). DMD is the most common hereditary neuromuscular disease affecting all races and ethnic groups.[2] From the perspective of clinical presentation, DMD and BMD appear in preschool children. While a child with DMD tends to become bedridden by 10–12 years, those with BMD tend to be ambulatory even into their adulthood. Parents consult a physician with complaints regarding their child's weakness, inability to walk in a previously walking child, frequent falls, difficulty in climbing stairs, and abnormal swelling of the calf musculature.

18.2.1 History and Findings

The history in children suspected of muscular dystrophy should focus on perinatal history, developmental milestones, family history, and history of any drug intake. While poor head control in infancy may be the first sign of weakness, most children achieve their milestones with no or mild delay only. Children with muscular dystrophies often have a waddling gait. They tend to have an exaggerated lumbar lordosis, and many children walk on their toes. It is not uncommon to find intellectual impairment in children with DMD. Their voice may be of nasal quality. Persistent tachycardia is a common feature.[2] Children with DMD show Gower's sign, usually by 5–6 years of age. After being confined to a wheelchair and bed, they tend to develop scoliosis. Contractures are seen around the knees, ankles, hips, and elbows. Children with BMD have similar complaints, but the severity of symptoms and the extent of disability is less than that of DMD.

Children with myopathies also present with complaints of muscular weakness. They tend to have more systemic features than those of muscular dystrophy. These features are dependent on the underlying pathology of the myopathy. These patients primarily have involvement of the proximal muscles of a limb, and it is a major differentiating factor from neuropathies.

18.3 ARTHROGRYPOSIS

The term "arthrogryposis multiplex congenita" (AMC) refers to a heterogeneous group of muscular, neurological, and connective tissue anomalies that present with two or more joint contractures at birth as well as muscle weakness (Figure 18.2).[3] Arthrogryposis is not a diagnosis per se but rather is a descriptive term with many etiologies and clinical presentations. Of all the etiologies, neurological factors account for 70–80% of cases. Based on the clinical presentation, signs, and etiology, AMC is divided into subgroups. Amyoplasia and distal arthrogryposis are the two most common subgroups.[3] Children with amyoplasia are often bedridden. They tend to have a midfacial hemangioma. They primarily affect the limbs. Table 18.1 summarizes the clinical features of these two subgroups.

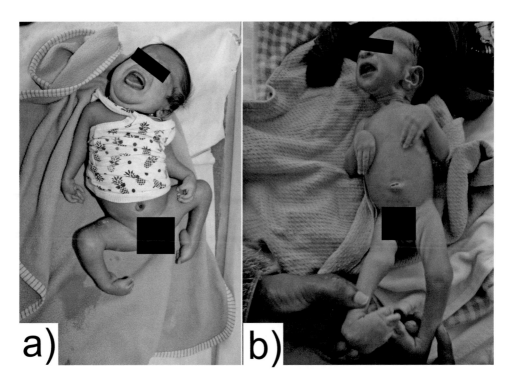

Figure 18.2 Arthrogryposis multiplex congenita with multiple joint contractures.

Children with arthrogryposis have difficulty in ambulation. Most patients with amyoplasia are unable to walk. Those with distal arthrogryposis can ambulate but have a lower activity level and walk slowly with small steps.

The history should focus on maternal illness, trauma, drug use, decreased fetal movements in the prenatal phase, and complications of the antenatal period. The examination should focus on the child as a whole and then proceed onto the expected orthopedic features. Features of various syndromes that can be associated with arthrogryposis must be actively searched for in the child.

18.4 INFECTIVE CONDITIONS (OSTEOMYELITIS/SEPTIC ARTHRITIS)

Infective conditions affecting the musculoskeletal system are not uncommon. Osteomyelitis, septic arthritis, pyomyositis, and a combination of all three are often the reason for a specialist consult. While the details of the organisms and the pathophysiology of the infections are beyond the scope of this book, the reader is advised to be aware of these important aspects.

18.4.1 Findings

Osteomyelitis is more common in boys than girls, and this results primarily from a greater number of traumas experienced by them.[4] Clinical presentation of acute osteomyelitis varies with the age of the child. Neonates and young children often present with a refusal to move their affected limb (pseudoparalysis) or incessant cry (due to pain) on attempted movements. They may not have the typical symptom of fever, toxic look, or pain. Local erythema, edema, and warmth might be absent too. These classical features are, however, the common presentation in older children. Refusal to bear weight should also raise suspicion. Tenderness on the affected bone is invariably found in these children.

Acute septic arthritis has a similar presentation as osteomyelitis in young children as the transphyseal spread of infection is common.[5] Older children present with fever and pain. Localizing signs such as swelling, erythema, and warmth of the affected joint can be elicited. Refusal to bear weight is an associated feature. In superficial joints like the knee, ankle, wrists, and elbows, septic arthritis can lead to swelling of the synovium and the joint can be diffusely swollen.

Table 18.1 Features of Amyoplasia and Distal Arthrogryposis

| Subgroup | Upper Limb | | | | Lower Limb | | |
	Shoulder	Elbow	Wrist	Fingers	Hip	Knee	Foot
Amyoplasia	Internal rotation and adduction	Extension with the forearms in pronation	Flexed and in many cases ulnar deviation	Flexed	Frequently dislocated	Extended, valgus or varus deformities are possible	Severe equinovarus feet
Distal arthrogryposis			Flexed wrists	Medially overlapping fingers, clenched fists, ulnar deviation of fingers, camptodactyly, thumb in palm deformity			Calcaneovalgus/ equinovarus/ vertical talus/ metatarsus adductus

Children with chronic osteomyelitis have a waxing and waning course of infection. They often present with a history of incision and drainage or inadequate surgical debridement of their osteomyelitis. Discharging sinuses are commonly seen. While seropurulent discharge is almost always noticed, some patients can have small bony spicules coming out. The local skin is involved, and it is not uncommon to find localized edema. Some children can present with pathological fractures. Tenderness, raised temperature, irregular surface of the bone, fixed sinus, and scars of previous surgeries are the common palpatory findings. Stiffness of the adjacent joints can be seen. Localized lymphadenopathy is an adjunct finding. Draining lymph nodes provides valuable diagnostic access (fine needle aspiration cytology) in tubercular infections and are to be examined without fail (Figure 18.3).

Children with Pott's spine can present with back pain and can also have neurological involvement. Some children present with an inability to extend their hip. This limitation of hip extensions in the absence of any hip pathology is termed as pseudoflexion deformity of the hip and often results from Pott's spine with a psoas abscess. This can be differentiated from a hip pathology by evaluating the range of motion of the hip, especially the internal and external rotations, which are unaffected by a psoas abscess. A mass can often be palpated along the iliac fossa. Further confirmation can be obtained with an ultrasound examination or an MRI.

18.5 CHILD ABUSE

Child abuse can be in the form of an act of commission or an act of omission (when the harm could have been prevented but was not).[6] Child abuse can be physical, sexual, or psychological. From an orthopedic viewpoint, awareness of physical abuse is essential. A pediatric orthopedic surgeon might have to provide treatment to a victim of child abuse, and he/she might be called on for expert advice on the injuries sustained by a child.

18.5.1 History and Findings

A detailed history must be obtained from the caregiver of a child, and the injuries that have been sustained are to be corroborated with the history. The lack of a plausible history other than inflicted trauma is the key element in making a diagnosis of child abuse.[6] Sentinel injuries may be noted in approximately 25% of abused infants and may precede the diagnosis by weeks or even months from the sentinel event.[6] Bruises are the most common form of injury sustained by victims of abuse. Atypical age and atypical location of the bruises are often indicative of the possibility of child abuse. Bruises are often multiple in number and location and are of different ages. Additionally, their shapes might be different too. Bites, burns, and fractures are the other injuries that, if present, should alert the orthopedic surgeon. Fractures that can be suggestive of abuse include classic metaphyseal lesions, posterior rib fractures, and fractures of the scapula, sternum, and spinous processes, especially in young children. Fractures of these regions need forces much greater than that sustained by the child due to a fall at home. The differential diagnosis includes osteopenia of prematurity and osteogenesis imperfecta, metabolic and nutritional disorders (e.g., scurvy, copper deficiency, rickets), renal osteodystrophy, and congenital insensitivity to pain, etc. Appropriate radiographic evaluation is also necessary.

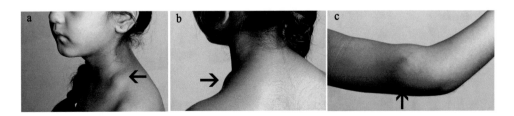

Figure 18.3 Tubercular osteomyelitis of the distal humerus with abscess formation and significant supraclavicular lymphadenopathy. The lymph node was subjected to aspiration cytology analysis, which helped in diagnosis.

18.6 SURFACE-MARKING OF PERIPHERAL NERVES

18.6.1 Median Nerve

18.6.1.1 IN THE ARM

Firstly, mark the brachial artery by connecting the following points. Mark the first point on the lower edge of the lateral axillary wall. Mark the second point medial to the biceps brachii tendon at the radial neck level. The artery begins on the medial aspect of the arm in the upper half and runs downwards and slightly lateral in the lower half to end on the elbow front.[7]

The median nerve can then be marked on the lateral side of the brachial artery in the upper half of the arm and on the medial side of the artery in the lower part of the arm. At the mid-part of the arm, the median nerve crosses the brachial artery anteriorly.

18.6.1.2 IN THE FOREARM

The median nerve can be marked by connecting the two points mentioned below.

- At the bend of the elbow, mark a point on the medial side of the brachial artery.
- In the anterior aspect of the wrist, mark a point over the palmaris longus tendon or at 1 cm medial to the flexor carpi radialis tendon.

18.6.1.3 IN THE HAND

The median nerve passes deep to the flexor retinaculum to enter the palm and then it divides immediately into the medial and lateral branches. The lateral branch innervates the thenar eminence muscles and divides into three branches to supply the thumb and lateral aspect of the index finger. The medial branch provides branches to the adjoining sides of the index finger, middle, and ring finger. The nail beds on the lateral three and a half fingers are also supplied by the median nerve.

18.6.2 Radial Nerve

18.6.2.1 IN THE ARM

The radial nerve can be traced by connecting the following three points:

- Mark the first point at the lower limit of the lateral wall of the axilla.

- Draw a line connecting the lateral epicondyle to the deltoid insertion. Mark the junction of the upper one-third and lower two-thirds of the above line as the second point.
- Mark the third point on the front of the elbow below the lateral epicondyle level at 1 cm lateral to the biceps brachii tendon.

The first and second points are then joined through the back of the arm marking the oblique course of the radial nerve in the spiral (radial) groove of the posterior compartment. Join the second and third points on the front side of the arm to label the vertical course of the radial nerve in the anterior compartment.[7]

18.6.2.2 IN THE FOREARM

A superficial branch of the radial nerve can be traced by connecting the following points:

- Mark the first point at 1 cm on the lateral side of the biceps brachii tendon slightly below the lateral epicondyle.
- Mark the second point on the lateral border of the forearm at the junction of the superior two-thirds and inferior one-third, just slightly on the lateral side of the radial artery.
- Mark the third point on the anatomical snuff box.

The nerve follows a vertical course from the first to the second point, and from the second point, it goes backward and reaches the anatomical snuff box.

18.6.3 Posterior Interosseous Nerve or Deep Branch of Radial Nerve

This nerve can be marked by connecting the following points:

- Mark the first point at 1 cm on the lateral side of the biceps brachii tendon slightly below the lateral epicondyle.
- Mark the second point at the juncture of the upper third and lower two-thirds of the line connecting the center point of the radial head on the posterior aspect and Lister's or dorsal tubercle on the lower end of the radius.

- Mark the third point on the posterior aspect of the wrist at 1 cm medially from the dorsal tubercle.

It supplies the muscles on the posterior compartment of the forearm.[7]

18.6.4 Ulnar Nerve

18.6.4.1 IN THE ARM

The ulnar nerve is labeled by connecting the following points:

- The first point is at the inferior border of the teres major on the lateral wall of the axilla.
- The second point is at the center of the medial border of the arm.
- The third point is at the back of the base of the medial humeral epicondyle.[7]

18.6.4.2 IN THE FOREARM

The ulnar nerve is marked by connecting the following two points:

- The first point is behind the base of the medial humeral epicondyle.
- The second point is marked laterally to the pisiform bone.

Along the lower two-thirds of the forearm, the ulnar nerve lies in medial relation to the ulnar artery.

18.6.4.3 IN THE HAND

The ulnar nerve passes superficially on the medial side of the flexor retinaculum in medial relation to the ulnar vessels and divides into superficial and deep branches. The superficial branch supplies the palmaris brevis muscle and gives branches to the medial one-and-a-half fingers along with the nail bed. A deep branch courses behind and in between the pisiform bone and hook of the hamate bone and lies in the concavity of the deep palmar arch.

18.6.5 Sciatic Nerve

The sciatic nerve is labeled by connecting the following three points:

- A point 2.5 cm laterally from the midpoint of the line joining the posterior superior iliac spine and ischial tuberosity.

- The second point is marked just medially to the midpoint of the line connecting the ischial tuberosity and the greater or outer trochanter.
- The third point is marked on the back of the thigh in the midline at the upper two-thirds and lower one-third junction (apex of popliteal fossa).[8]

18.6.6 Common Peroneal Nerve

Marking of the common peroneal nerve is done by connecting the following points:

- The first point is at the summit of the popliteal fossa.
- The second point is at the back of the fibula neck.[8]

18.6.7 Deep Peroneal Nerve

The deep peroneal nerve is marked by connecting the following points:

- The first point is on the lateral side of the fibula neck.
- The second point is on the anterior aspect of the ankle in the midpoint between the two malleoli.
- The third point is at the first interosseous space.

The nerve lies in lateral relation to the anterior tibial artery in the upper one-third and lower one-third, whereas in the middle one-third, it lies anterior to the artery.[8]

18.6.8 Superficial Peroneal Nerve

Marking of the superficial peroneal nerve is done by connecting the following points:

- The first point is on the lateral side of the fibula neck.
- The second point is at the juncture of the upper two-thirds and lower one-third of the leg over the anterior margin of the peroneus longus muscle.

At its lower end, it is divided into medial and lateral branches.[8]

18.6.9 Medial Plantar Nerve

The medial plantar nerve is marked by connecting the following points:

- The first point is at the midpoint between the medial malleolus and heel prominence.
- The second point is midway between the heel and base of the big toe over the navicular bone.

The medial plantar nerve is lateral to the medial plantar artery.[8]

18.6.10 Lateral Plantar Nerve

The lateral plantar nerve is labeled by connecting the following points:

- The first point is at the midpoint between the medial malleolus and heel prominence.
- The second point is 2.5 cm medially from the tuberosity of the fifth metatarsal bone.

The lateral plantar nerve lies medial to the lateral plantar artery.[8]

REFERENCES

1. Laxamanaswamy A. *Clinical pediatrics – history taking and case discussion*, 3rd ed. Gurgaon: Walters Kluwer Health, 2010.
2. Sarnat HB. Muscular dystrophy. In: Kliegman RM, Stanton BF, Schor NF, st Gene III JW, Behrman RE, editors. *Nelson textbook of pediatrics*, 20th ed. Philadelphia: Elsevier; 2016. pp. 2975–3986.
3. Horstmann HM, Conroy CM, Davidson RS. Arthrogryposis. In: Kliegman RM, Stanton BF, Schor NF, st Gene III JW, Behrman RE, editors. *Nelson textbook of pediatrics*, 20th ed. Philadelphia: Elsevier; 2016. pp. 3310–3314.
4. Kaplan SL. Osteomyelitis. In: Kliegman RM, Stanton BF, Schor NF, st Gene III JW, Behrman RE, editors. *Nelson textbook of pediatrics*, 20th ed. Philadelphia: Elsevier; 2016. pp. 3322–3326.
5. Kaplan SL. Septic arthritis. In: Kliegman RM, Stanton BF, Schor NF, st Gene III JW, Behrman RE, editors. *Nelson textbook of pediatrics*, 20th ed. Philadelphia: Elsevier; 2016. pp. 3327–3329.
6. Dubowitz H, Lane WG. Abused and neglected children. In: Kliegman RM, Stanton BF, Schor NF, st Gene III JW, Behrman RE, editors. *Nelson textbook of pediatrics*, 20th ed. Philadelphia: Elsevier; 2016. pp. 236–248.
7. Chaurasia BD. *Human anatomy. Upper limb and thorax*, 6th ed. New York: CBS Publishers and Distributors, 2013. Chapter 11, Surface marking and radiological anatomy. pp. 162–166.
8. Chaurasia BD. *Human anatomy. Lower limb, abdomen and pelvis*, 6th ed. New York: CBS Publishers and Distributors, 2013. Chapter 14, Surface and radiological anatomy. pp. 168–169.

Index